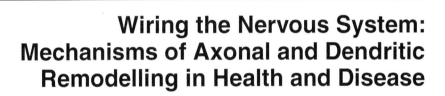

Wiring the Nervous System: Mechanisms of Axonal and Dendritic Remodelling in Health and Disease

RIVER PUBLISHERS SERIES IN BIOTECHNOLOGY AND MEDICAL RESEARCH

Series Editors

PAOLO DI NARDO
University of Rome Tor Vergata,
Italy

PRANELA RAMESHWAR
Rutgers University,
USA

ALAIN VERTES
London Business School,
UK and NxR Biotechnologies,
Switzerland

Aiming primarily at providing detailed snapshots of critical issues in biotechnology and medicine that are reaching a tipping point in financial investment or industrial deployment, the scope of the series encompasses various specialty areas including pharmaceutical sciences and healthcare, industrial biotechnology, and biomaterials. Areas of primary interest comprise immunology, virology, microbiology, molecular biology, stem cells, hematopoiesis, oncology, regenerative medicine, biologics, polymer science, formulation and drug delivery, renewable chemicals, manufacturing, and biorefineries.

Each volume presents comprehensive review and opinion articles covering all fundamental aspect of the focus topic. The editors/authors of each volume are experts in their respective fields and publications are peer-reviewed.

For a list of other books in this series, visit www.riverpublishers.com

Wiring the Nervous System: Mechanisms of Axonal and Dendritic Remodelling in Health and Disease

Editors

Tracy S. Tran

Rutgers University, NJ, USA

Avraham Yaron

Weizmann Institute of Science, Rehovot, Israel

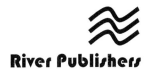

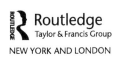

NEW YORK AND LONDON

Published 2025 by River Publishers

River Publishers

Broagervej 10, 9260 Gistrup, Denmark

www.riverpublishers.com

Distributed exclusively by Routledge

605 Third Avenue, New York, NY 10017, USA

4 Park Square, Milton Park, Abingdon, Oxon OX14 4RN

Wiring the Nervous System: Mechanisms of Axonal and Dendritic Remodelling in Health and Disease / Tracy S. Tran and Avraham Yaron.

Routledge is an imprint of the Taylor & Francis Group, an informa business

ISBN 978-87-7022-852-7 (hardback)
ISBN 978-87-7004-053-2 (paperback)
ISBN 978-10-0381-220-3 (online)
ISBN 978-1-032-63269-8 (ebook master)

While every effort is made to provide dependable information, the publisher, authors, and editors cannot be held responsible for any errors or omissions.

The use of general descriptive names, registered names, trademarks, service marks, etc. in this publication does not imply, even in the absence of a specific statement, that such names are exempt from the relevant protective laws and regulations and therefore free for general use.

The publisher, the authors and the editors are safe to assume that the advice and information in this book are believed to be true and accurate at the date of publication. Neither the publisher nor the authors or the editors give a warranty, express or implied, with respect to the material contained herein or for any errors or omissions that may have been made.

This work was supported by funding from the U.S. National Science Foundation (NSF), The Division of Integrative Organismal Systems (BIO/IOS, grant # 2034864), the New Jersey Commission on Spinal Cord Research (grant # CSCR16IIRG013), and the NJ Governor's Council for Medical Research and Treatment of Autism (grant # CAUT17BSP022) to Tracy S. Tran (T.S.T.). In addition, this work was supported by funding from the Israel Science Foundation (grant # 2495/2) and NSF and the U.S.-Israel Binational Science Foundation (BSF, grant # 2020633) to Avraham Yaron (A.Y.) who is also an incumbent of the Jack & Simon Djanogly Professorial Chair in Biochemistry at the Weizmann Institute.

Contents

List of Contributors

Calhan, O. Yipkin, *Department of Biology, University of Virginia, USA; Program in Fundamental Neuroscience, University of Virginia, USA*

Cao, Ying, *IDG/McGovern Institute for Brain Research, Center for Life Sciences, School of Life Sciences, Peking University, China*

Coz, Madeleine Le, *Molecular Neuroscience Unit, Okinawa Institute of Science and Technology Graduate University, Japan*

Curran, Bridget M., *Department of Neuroscience, Jefferson Center for Synaptic Biology, Vickie and Jack Farber Institute for Neuroscience, Sydney Kimmel Medical College, Thomas Jefferson University, USA*

Deppmann, Christopher D., *Department of Biology, University of Virginia, USA; Program in Fundamental Neuroscience, University of Virginia, USA*

Gamage, Kanchana, *Department of Biology, University of Virginia, USA*

Han, Chun, *Weill Institute for Cell and Molecular Biology and Department of Molecular Biology and Genetics, Cornell University, USA*

Hertzler, James I., *The Huck Institutes of the Life Sciences and Biochemistry and Molecular Biology, The Pennsylvania State University, USA*

Hunter-Chang, Sarah, *Department of Biology, University of Virginia, USA; Program in Fundamental Neuroscience, University of Virginia, USA*

Ji, Hui, *Weill Institute for Cell and Molecular Biology and Department of Molecular Biology and Genetics, Cornell University, USA*

Kucenas, Sarah, *Department of Biology, University of Virginia, USA; Program in Fundamental Neuroscience, University of Virginia, USA*

Kumar, Sushanth, *Department of Biology, University of Virginia, USA; Program in Fundamental Neuroscience, University of Virginia, USA*

Ma, Le, *Department of Neuroscience, Jefferson Center for Synaptic Biology, Vickie and Jack Farber Institute for Neuroscience, Sydney Kimmel Medical College, Thomas Jefferson University, USA*

Rolls, Melissa M., *The Huck Institutes of the Life Sciences and Biochemistry and Molecular Biology, The Pennsylvania State University, USA*

Moese, Elizabeth R., *Department of Neuroscience, Jefferson Center for Synaptic Biology, Vickie and Jack Farber Institute for Neuroscience, Sydney Kimmel Medical College, Thomas Jefferson University, USA*

Rosenthal, Justin, *Dendrite Morphogenesis and Plasticity Unit, National Institute of Neurological Disorders and Stroke, USA*

Stepanova, Ekaterina, *Department of Biology, University of Virginia, USA; Program in Fundamental Neuroscience, University of Virginia, USA*

Terenzio, Marco, *Molecular Neuroscience Unit, Okinawa Institute of Science and Technology Graduate University, Japan*

Yang, Jing, *IDG/McGovern Institute for Brain Research, Center for Life Sciences, School of Life Sciences, Peking University, China*

Yong, Yu, *Department of Biology, University of Virginia, USA*

Yuan, Quan, *Dendrite Morphogenesis and Plasticity Unit, National Institute of Neurological Disorders and Stroke, USA*

Zakhia, Sarah, *Molecular Neuroscience Unit, Okinawa Institute of Science and Technology Graduate University, Japan*

List of Figures

List of Tables

Introduction: An overview and with acknowledgements to seminal, historical discoveries in the field

Tracy S. Tran[1] and Avraham Yaron[2]

[1]Department of Biological Sciences, Rutgers University, Newark, NJ, USA.
[2]Department of Biomolecular Sciences, Department of Molecular Neuroscience, Weizmann Institute of Science, Rehovot, Israel
Email: tstran@rutgers.edu; avraham.yaron@weizmann.ac.il

From a historical perspective the metaphor of the nervous system being like electrical wires have been used for the past two centuries since the time of the invention of the telegraph or telephone in the 1800s to the more recent abstract term of a wiring diagram from connectome work in the 21st century. Starting from the mid-1800s, several doctors and scientists made comparisons of the nerves in the human body to electrical wires carrying external sensory information to the brain (Smee, 1850; Thomson and Smith, 1853; Helmholtz, 1875). Fast-forward to the 20th century, the first cell-level wiring diagram that mapped the connections of the *C. elegans* nervous system was published in 1986 from Sydney Brenner's group (White et al 1986). Then more than 20 years later, the Human Connectome Project was launched in 2009 (Bardin 2012). However, in the vast landscape of scientific inquiry and since Ramón y Cajal's time over a century ago, there are few fundamental questions such as the mechanisms of neuronal wiring that remain intriguing to the scientific community. Indeed, from the unique branching patterns of dendritic arbors to the precise guidance of axons to their synaptic targets, this extraordinary neuronal connectivity that forms functional circuits is the foundation for complex networks that shape our behavior. From simple sensory-motor reflexes to complex skills of learning and memory and higher cognitive functions that dictates our thoughts, this functional connectivity of the nervous system results from an orderly series of events. It begins with neuronal stem cells or neuronal precursors proliferation, differentiation, migration, axon guidance and dendrite growth during embryonic development, then continues with synaptogenesis, axon and dendrite pruning, and synaptic plasticity during postnatal stages. These events are orchestrated by myriad of molecular and cellular mechanisms, which were discovered over the past century from groundbreaking research that collectively establish our current understanding of the dynamic process of neuronal wiring.

In this book, we will review the current understanding of key aspects in neuronal wiring with a focus on the emerging mechanisms underlying the major progressive processes in neuronal morphogenesis (Part I). However, it would be remiss of us if we did not first mention the numerous significant contributions Ramón y Cajal has made to the field of neuroscience, especially from his groundbreaking work on the basic principles of the organization of the nervous system, which for the large part is documented in the monumental (two-volumes) work of *Histology of the Nervous System of Man and Vertebrates* (1995, N. Swanson and L.W. Swanson Trans. from French, Oxford University Press). This definitive body of work on the cellular morphology and organization of the vertebrate nervous system not only holds-up over time by its accuracy but few other biological publications could match its scope. One of Ramón y Cajal's greatest discovery, the growth cone, which he described as a *"living battering ram...which advances, pushing aside... the obstacles which it finds in its way,"* remains a fascination to numerous developmental neuroscientists attempting to further unravel its mysteries. The notions of the axon as an outgrowth of the cell soma, the functions of the growth cone, the existence and probable role of molecular cues (or chemical factors as better known in Ramón y Cajal's time) that guide axons to their targets, and the exuberant early production of neuronal processes and their later refinement by a process he called *"process resorption"*, which now called pruning. The revolutionary foundation and some of the most important ideas that currently inform the field of neural development. Thus, the first chapter (1) in this book provides a summary of the recent findings and highlights up-to-date views on some of the major molecular and cellular mechanisms regulating axon morphogenesis. Next in chapter 2, the reader is introduced to the complex process of dendritic development, which involves neuronal activity and cell surface receptor to nuclear signaling, working together to modify the dendritic arbor from branching patterns, arbor size, spine density and maturity. In the last chapter (3) of Part I, the authors provided a concise but thorough historical perspective regeneration in the nervous system and then discuss the mechanisms of dendritic degeneration and regeneration following injury and disease. Concluding with the fundamental questions of do dendrites have an active degeneration program, and are the molecular pathways governing dendritic regeneration distinct from axon regeneration?

In the second half (Part II) of this book we will focus on some of the latest concepts on the major regressive processes in neuronal remodelling. However, the questions related to neuronal injury, axon degeneration, remodelling and regeneration are not new to the field of neuroscience. Again, Ramón y Cajal has a say on these topics from *Degeneration and Regeneration of the Nervous System* translated from his original work (1991, J. DeFelipe and E.G. Jones Ed., Oxford University Press). Although less well-unknown than *Histology of the Nervous System* and often overlooked by those working in the field of neuronal plasticity. Some of the most important conceptional issues facing neuroscientists today were foreshadowed when Ramón y Cajal proposed the "dynamic polarity" of the neuron, by which he meant the unidirectional flow of information from the dendrites through the cell body to the axon and finally its terminal branches, a concept that lead to the anticipated discovery of axonal transport and the prescient prediction that neurons and their processes are not static but dynamic structures. Thus, new neuronal connections could form throughout life, and axons are capable of regeneration after injury. However, immediately following neuronal injury, the damaged neurons and their processes must first be cleared from the injury site, often by phagocytes in the nervous system, in order for the repair and regeneration to begin. Or in the case seen in neural development, exuberant neuron processes and synapses are eliminated by engulfment performed by phagocytes. Therefore, it is fitting that Part II of this book begins with a chapter (4) to review the current experimental systems used to study phagocytosis during neuronal remodelling in both invertebrates and vertebrates and the emerging molecular pathways underlying phagocytosis during neural development. Next in Chapter 5, the authors explored the mechanisms of how overabundance of neurons, axons and synapses is selectively pruned and refined to establish functional circuits. The notion of chemotrophic factors in the nervous system and the concepts of axons competing for trophic cues for survival to more recent discovery of distinct axonal death signaling pathways are reviewed. While program cell death and axonal pruning is required for the proper development of functional neural circuits, the process of pathological axonal degeneration is a sinister hallmark of neurodegenerative diseases. In the following chapter (6), the authors discussed the distinct mechanisms of pathological axonal degeneration which is often linked to neuronal metabolism. The hope is that recent findings will lay the groundwork for future investigations to delay, or even prevent, pathological axonal damage, which could be a potential treatment for neurodegenerative diseases. Finally, we end the book with a chapter (7) on the complex roles and implications of local mRNA translation in axons during neuronal development, injury, and in neurodegeneration.

It is worth noting that it is unintentional but rather unavoidable that the editors opened this introduction by highlighting Ramón y Cajal's work. His observations were so careful and his interpretation of the histological images so astute that no one seriously interested in how the nervous system is organized and wired can afford to ignore. While Ramón y Cajal's research laid the groundwork for modern neuroscience and continues to inspire and influence the field to this day, we also acknowledge how much the field has grown in the number of seminal discoveries since his time. This is, by far, not an exhaustive list but just to mention a few of the notable contributions: Roger Sperry's chemoaffinity theory (Sperry 1963) which led to the birth of the axon guidance field, and the discovery and successful isolation of the first neurotrophic factors, Nerve Growth Factor (NGF) by Rita Levi-Montalcini and Stanley Cohen (Cohen 1960, Cohen & Levi-Montalcini 1956, Levi-Montalcini & Cohen 1956) demonstrating that neurons require target derived chemotrophic factors for survival, but even earlier Donald Hebb published his theory of Hebbian plasticity (Hebb 1949), which provided the bases for learning and memory. It is with regret that we are unable to discuss each one of these seminal discoveries in detail as each topic deserves its own book or books, which others have already reviewed elsewhere. Indeed, there are also numerous works that are ongoing, within the past few decades, such as synaptic pruning, stem cell biology and transplantation following neuronal injury for regeneration, and the discovery that new neurons continue to be generated in specific brain regions throughout adulthood. While on their own these topics can stand alone, but when looking at the big picture each one of these discoveries either contributed to the overall molecular and cellular mechanisms or are associated with the process of neuronal wiring. We might start with Ramón y Cajal's work, especially his beautiful histological drawings illustrating the diversity of neuronal morphologies that provided the initial inspiration for the modern field of neuroscience. However, we also want to acknowledge all the molecular and cellular mechanistic work, including those briefly mentioned above, that followed. Thus, the goal of this book is to merge these fundamental aspects of neuronal morphogenesis and remodellng of axons and dendrites, and the required underlying molecular mechanisms coordinating these processes during development and injury or disease, which are crucial for the proper wiring of the nervous system.

References

Bardin J. 2012. Neuroscience: Making connections. *Nature* **483**: 394–396

Cohen S. 1960. Purification of a Nerve-Growth Promoting Protein from the Mouse Salivary Gland and Its Neuro-Cytotoxic Antiserum. *Proc Natl Acad Sci U S A* **46**: 302–311

Cohen S, Levi-Montalcini R. 1956. A Nerve Growth-Stimulating Factor Isolated from Snake Venom. *Proc Natl Acad Sci U S A* **42**: 571–574

Hebb DO. 1949. *The organization of behavior; a neuropsychological theory.* New York,: Wiley. xix, **335** p. pp.

Helmholtz, H. (1875). On the Sensations of Tone as a Physiological Basis for the Theory of Music. London: Longmans, Green. doi: 10.1037/10838-000

Levi-Montalcini R, Cohen S. 1956. In Vitro and in Vivo Effects of a Nerve Growth-Stimulating Agent Isolated from Snake Venom. *Proc Natl Acad Sci U S A* **42**: 695–699

Ramón y Cajal, Santiago and others (eds), *Cajal's Degeneration and Regeneration of the Nervous System*, History of Neuroscience (New York, 1991; online edn, Oxford Academic, 22 Mar. 2012), https://doi.org/10.1093/acprof:oso/9780195065169.001.0001

Ramón y Cajal, Santiago (1995). Histology of the Nervous System of Man and Vertebrates Volume I and II, History of Neuroscience No. 6 and 7 (N. Swanson and L.W. Swanson, Trans. from French). Oxford University Press. (Original work published in Spanish from 1899-1904).

Smee, A. (1850). Instinct and Reason Deduced from Electro-Biology. London: Reeve, Benham and Reeve. doi: 10.1037/12035-000

Sperry RW. 1963. Chemoaffinity in the Orderly Growth of Nerve Fiber Patterns and Connections. *Proc Natl Acad Sci U S A* **50**: 703–710

Thomson, S., and Smith, H. (1853). A Dictionary of Domestic Medicine and Household Surgery. Philadelphia: Lippincott.

White JG, Southgate E, Thomson JN, Brenner S. 1986. The structure of the nervous system of the nematode Caenorhabditis elegans. *Philos Trans R Soc Lond B Biol Sci* **314**: 1–340

PART I

1

Molecular and Cellular Mechanisms of Axon Morphogenesis

Bridget M. Curran*, Elizabeth R. Moese*, and Le Ma

Department of Neuroscience, Jefferson Center for Synaptic Biology, Vickie and Jack Farber Institute for Neuroscience, Sydney Kimmel Medical College, Thomas Jefferson University, Philadelphia, USA
Email: le.ma@jefferson.edu
*Bridget M. Curran and Elizabeth R. Moese contributed equally to this work.

Abstract

Axons allow neurons to transmit electrical information to target cells with synaptic connections. Axons often have stereotypic morphologies accompanied by various branched structures that connect with multiple synaptic targets. Developing these branched morphologies is critical to building complex neural circuits. In this chapter, we discuss our general understanding of axon morphogenesis, with a focus on three steps, growth, guidance, and branching, which are often repeated to generate the diverse morphologies in the nervous system. We summarize some recent findings with the goal of providing a broad, but up-to-date, view of general molecular and cellular mechanisms of this important developmental process.

1.1 Introduction

Neurons are the fundamental functional unit of the nervous system. Each neuron has only one axon to relay the information collected at various synaptic sites on the dendrites and soma. The information is integrated and then propagated along the axons by action potentials generated at the axonal hillock, the specialized region connecting the axon with the soma, and then passed on to target cells via synaptic connections at axonal terminals. Often, axons have various types of branches, such as terminal branches that allow synaptic connections with similar targets and collateral branches that connect with different targets. Throughout the nervous system, axons display different morphologies that are defined by the axon length and trajectory as well as branch shape, size, and pattern (Gibson and Ma, 2011; Kalil and Dent, 2014). These diverse morphologies are tailored to the functional needs of neural circuits underlying complex animal behaviors. For example, in the olfactory system, each olfactory sensory neuron has one simple axon that synapses with mitral cell dendrites in a specific glomerulus of the olfactory bulb, while mitral cells send long axons to different regions of the cortex via multiple collateral branches. Another example is found in the reflex arc of the spinal cord. There, sensory neurons in the dorsal root ganglion (DRG) collect somatic sensory information from branched nerve endings of their peripheral projections in the body's periphery. The information is relayed through their central collateral branches that connect directly or indirectly with motor neurons inside the spinal cord. Motor neurons then extend long axons from the spinal cord and reach the muscle targets where they form highly arborized terminal branches.

The diverse axonal morphologies have captivated the attention of neurobiologists studying different regions of the nervous system in the past century. A fundamental question that has been constantly asked is how to generate the stereotypic axonal morphologies for various neural circuits. Past studies have provided a general framework for addressing this seemingly simple question. Studies using live cell imaging in culture or in tissues have demonstrated that axon morphogenesis starts with axonogenesis, the formation of an axon from the soma (Polleux and Snider, 2010), a step that is characterized by neuronal polarization, neurite outgrowth, and axon specification (Figure 1.1A). Several excellent reviews summarized the recent understanding of this critical step (Alfadil and Bradke, 2023; Arikkath, 2020; Funahashi et al., 2020; Schelski and Bradke, 2017; Takano et al., 2019). Following axonogenesis, axons continue to develop through axon growth, guidance, and branching, three steps that are repeated multiple times to generate the eventual axon morphology that is intimately associated with synaptic function (Figures 1.1B and 1.1C) (Gibson and Ma, 2011; Kalil and Dent, 2014). Early cell biological studies have revealed that these steps are highly controlled by the two cytoskeleton components, namely actin and microtubule, which are protein polymers made of subunits that can dynamically assemble and disassemble (Figure 1.1D) (Atkins et al., 2023; Dent et al., 2011; McCormick and Gupton, 2020; Menon and Gupton, 2016). In addition, trafficking of various membrane organelles inside the axon is critical for where to make branches, how to grow or increase branch length, and how to guide them (Bodakuntla et al., 2021; Winkle et al., 2016). Moreover, biochemical and genetic studies in the past three decades

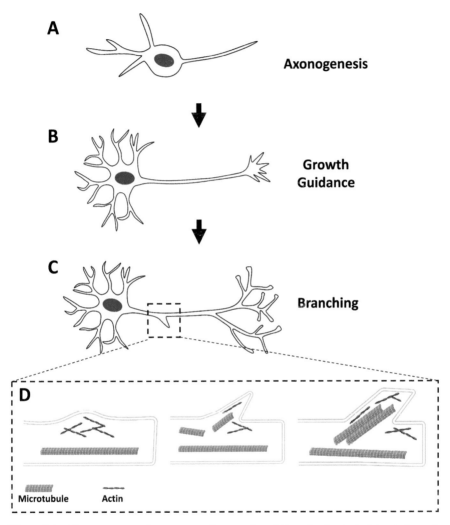

Figure 1.1 Commons steps in axon morphogenesis and the role of cytoskeleton in branch formation. (A–C) Schematic drawings depicting different steps leading to the generation of complex axon morphologies. **(D)** Schematic drawings depicting the stages of axon branch formation governed by the cytoskeleton. Actin patches accumulate where a new branch is to be initiated. Actin filaments are then assembled into filopodia-like structures. Microtubules undergo remodeling and invade the newly formed branch.

have identified various molecular cues in the embryonic environment that regulate both cytoskeletal and membrane dynamics via cell surface receptors (Bashaw and Klein, 2010; Chedotal and Richards, 2010; Kolodkin and Tessier-Lavigne, 2011). Many extracellular cues are common in regulating these steps, but the intracellular mechanisms are often unique to each step.

In this chapter, we discuss the general concept related to these steps, with a focus on recent investigations that have spawned new ideas and made disease connections. We hope to provide readers with a broad but more current view of the molecular and cellular mechanisms of axon morphogenesis.

1.2 Regulation of the Cytoskeleton

1.2.1 Actin

The actin cytoskeleton is essential for axon growth, guidance, and branching. It is best studied in the growth cone, the motile tip that explores the environment and leads to the growth and guidance of a growing axon or branch (Lowery and Van Vactor, 2009). Growth cone motility is largely mediated by dynamic assembly and disassembly of actin filaments in two membrane protruding structures: filopodia, a needle-like membrane protrusion that is composed of filamentous actin bundles, and lamellipodia, the veil-like structure composed of filamentous actin networks (Figure 1.2A) (Gomez and Letourneau, 2014). Actin assembly in these structures allows the growth cone to spread out and move forward (Lowery and Van Vactor, 2009). Any asymmetrical protrusion and rearrangement of actin assembly allows the growth cone to turn to a different direction. Actin also plays a role in initiating new branches from the main axonal shaft, where actin polymerization in a structure called "actin patch" precedes branch formation (Gallo, 2011) (Figure 1.1D).

Much of our understanding of actin dynamics has been derived from neurons cultured on flat substrates (Lowery and Van Vactor, 2009). Two recent studies (Clarke et al., 2020a; Clarke et al., 2020b) used live cell imaging to examine actin assembly in the growth cone of TSM1 pioneer axons from the developing *Drosophila* wing. They revealed that in the *in vivo* three dimensional (3D) environment, the TSM1 axonal growth cone is mainly composed of filopodia-like structures. Here, in the growth cone, actin was highly dynamic with the accumulation of actin filaments at distal portions of the axon, leading to a biased prediction of net outgrowth and protrusion. This actin distribution and distal accumulation were regulated by Abl kinase signaling (Clarke et al., 2020b). Abl is a signaling molecule downstream of some of the most conserved axon guidance molecules including Robo (Bashaw et al., 2000; Yu et al., 2002) and Netrin/Frazzled (Forsthoefel et al., 2005). Blocking Abl signaling altered the growth cone morphology and actin assembly. Using a multitude of parameters, such as number of protrusions, branches, and actin peaks, the study found two distinct correlative clusters that represent the morphological differences with and without Abl signaling

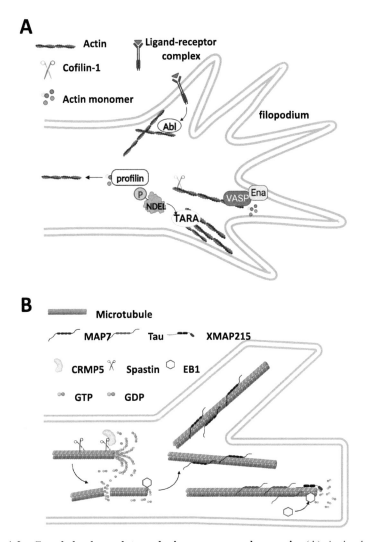

Figure 1.2 Cytoskeletal regulators during axon morphogenesis. (A) Actin dynamics contribute to axon morphogenesis through regulation of filopodia and growth cone motility. These processes can be regulated directly by actin binding proteins such as Ena/VASP to promote polymerization or indirectly through various signaling cascades such as NDEL signaling. Abl mediates ligand receptor signaling that regulates actin dynamics ultimately effecting growth cone morphology. **(B)** The dynamics and stability of microtubules contribute to axon branching and morphogenesis. MAP7 binds microtubules to promote axon branching through stabilizing newly formed branches. Other MAPs such as tau stabilizes microtubule polymerizing ends to allow for EB1 and XMAP215 to promote polymerization and axon elongation. CRMP5 and spastin physically interact to control microtubule length and polymerization.

(Clarke et al., 2020a). These studies thus demonstrate the coordinated actin regulation in directing growth cone motility *in vivo* (Figure 1.2A).

Actin assembly is regulated by a number of actin binding proteins (Figure 1.2A). They include: 1) the Arp2/3 complex and formin, which nucleate actin to generate new filaments to form actin networks or bundles respectively; 2) profilin, a protein that binds to actin monomers and aids actin filament polymerization; 3) Ena/VASP, a family of proteins that cooperate with profilin to promote polymerization; and 4) cofilin-1, which destabilizes actin filaments and regulates actin length (Svitkina, 2018). These actin regulators participate in many steps of axon morphogenesis. For example, the Arp2/3 complex is activated by the wave complex, which is recruited by the guidance receptor Robo in midline repulsion (Chaudhari et al., 2021); profilin, Ena/VASP, and formin work in different combinations to control axon regrowth and sprouting in *Drosophila* neurons (Yaniv et al., 2020); and cofilin controls the growth rate of developing motor axons (Frendo et al., 2019).

How these actin regulators are controlled is a key question in uncovering the molecular mechanisms of axon morphogenesis (Figure 1.2A). Recent studies of nuclear distribution element-like 1 (NDEL1) suggest the complexity of such regulation. NDEL1 and its homolog NDEL play many roles in early neural development including neuronal differentiation, migration, and maturation, as well as cytoskeletal reorganization (Sasaki et al., 2005; Hayashi et al., 2010; Ye et al., 2017). NDEL1 expression is first observed in the nervous system during embryonic development and this expression persists throughout adulthood (Pei et al., 2014). Its function is thought to regulate dynein activity and the localization of katanin, both of which are microtubule regulatory proteins (see discussion below) (Shu et al., 2004; Toyo-Oka et al., 2005). However, there is evidence for the interaction of NDEL1 with the actin cytoskeleton (Hong et al., 2016) which is mediated by trio-associated repeat on actin (TARA), an actin bundling protein that directly binds to and stabilizes actin filaments (Hong et al., 2016). A recent study using rat and mouse hippocampal and cortical neurons showed that phosphorylation of NDEL1 at S336 and S332 by DYRK2 and GSK3β kinases is critical for increasing neurite outgrowth. Using biochemical fractionation to distinguish actin filaments vs. monomers, the study demonstrated that phosphorylated NDEL1 was associated with high filamentous actin levels in the growth cone, and when phosphorylation was suppressed, actin filaments were decreased (Woo et al., 2019). As NDEL1 phosphorylation depends on TARA and the recruitment of DYRK2/GSKβ kinases to actin, it is interesting to investigate how NDEL1 regulates actin dynamics via the cordination of actin binding proteins during neurite outgrowth. These studies illustrate the importance of regulating actin assembly by various signaling molecules as well as the potential connection with the microtubule cytoskeleton. Although it was studied for axon growth, tsuch actin regulation likely plays critical roles in axon guidance and branching during axon morphogenesis.

1.2.2 Microtubule

In addition to actin, microtubules are highly regulated in axon morphogenesis. Made up of α- and β-tubulin heterodimers that assemble into 25-nm hollow cylinders, microtubules provide structural support for mechanical strength and tracks for motor-based transport. Microtubules are not static structures, but rather dynamically polymerize and depolymerize at each end. This inherent property, termed dynamic instability, allows cycles of growth and shrinkage of microtubules, and thereby provides a mechanism to rapidly remodel microtubules during axon growth, guidance, and branching. In the growth cone, most microtubules are concentrated in the center, but some can assemble and extend into the peripheral domain that has active actin remodeling (Figure 1.2B) (Lowery and Van Vactor, 2009). There, dynamic microtubule assembly/disassembly is not only important for the forward advancement of axons but also for controlling their growth direction (Lowery and Van Vactor, 2009). When microtubules polymerize in the center but depolymerize from the edge, the growth cone moves forward; when microtubules polymerize on one side but depolymerize from the other side, the growth cone can reorient and change axon growth direction. When new growth cones are generated from axonal shafts through actin patches (Gallo, 2011), microtubules are critical to generating and stabilizing nascent branches via polymerization or transport as short fragments.

Many molecular players have been identified to control microtubule dynamics and stability at different assembly/disassembly steps (Armijo-Weingart and Gallo, 2017; Kevenaar and Hoogenraad, 2015), and they can regulate axon morphology (Figure 1.2B). Microtubule associated proteins (MAPs), such as tau, MAP1B, and MAP2, bind to the microtubule lattice and stabilize microtubules, and all were shown to function to promote axon morphogenesis (Dehmelt and Halpain, 2005; Kapitein and Hoogenraad, 2015). Severing proteins, including spastin and katanin, differentially participate in axon branch formation by severing microtubules and creating ends to allow for new polymerization to occur (Ghosh et al., 2012; Yu et al., 2008). Also, motor proteins that move cargos along microtubules contribute to axon morphogenesis through anterograde and retrograde transport of proteins, RNAs, vesicles, and organelles (Guillaud et al., 2020). However, how these molecules coordinate to regulate microtubule structure and function during different stages of axonal morphogenesis remains a major question. Here, we describe several recent studies that illustrate the complexity of such regulation.

Spastin is an AAA-ATPase severing protein that regulates microtubule dynamics by producing small microtubule segments and thus promotes neuronal branching possibly via increased fragment transport and new microtubule assembly (Kuo et al., 2019; Yu et al., 2008). However, the underlying mechanism for this role has remained elusive. One study suggests spastin accumulates at the ends of microtubules, severs the shrinking ends, and then increases the total mass and number of microtubules through an ATP-independent regrowth mechanism (Kuo et al., 2019). How does severing allow for the regrowth of microtubules? A recent study has identified a connection between spastin and CRMP5, a member of the collapsin-response mediator protein (CRMP) family proteins that are known to promote microtubule assembly and neuronal development (reviewed in (Hotta et al., 2005; Nakamura et al., 2020; Yamashita et al., 2011)). The group found a direct physical interaction, through immunoprecipitation, between the N-terminal of spastin and the C-terminal of CRMP5. This interaction is important for increasing microtubules in HeLa cells in which co-transfection of CRMP5 and spastin reduced the loss of total tubulin levels caused by spastin alone. Based on rescue and overexpression analysis in hippocampal neurons, the study showed that this interaction is important for axon growth and branching (Ji et al., 2018). This new study supports the notion that spastin-induced severing could then be closely followed by another microtubule polymerization stimulating factor to promote overall microtubule assembly needed for axon growth and branching.

The notion that different microtubule regulators work in a coordinated manner to mediate axon morphogenesis is supported by another recent study of the interplay between three microtubule regulators, XMAP215, tau, and EB1 (Hahn et al., 2021). XMAP215 is a microtubule polymerase that promotes microtubule growth and elongation *in vitro* by catalyzing the addition of tubulin dimers at the plus end (Brouhard et al., 2008). XMAP215 was shown to play a critical role in growth cone morphology and axon guidance by regulating microtubule dynamics downstream of guidance cues (Slater et al., 2019). Tau is most widely known for stabilizing microtubules in neurons. However, recent evidence suggests that tau is not required for microtubule stabilization but enables microtubules to have long lived labile domains for growth and polymerization (Kadavath et al., 2015; Qiang et al., 2018). Additional work in hamster neurons has shown that tau is enriched in growth cones and associated with dynamic and stable microtubules as well as actin filaments to promote neurite outgrowth and growth cone turning (Biswas and

Kalil, 2018). EB1 (also known as end binding protein 1) is a microtubule plus end tracking protein associated with microtubule extension, and it localizes at the distal axons and growth cones to track the growing microtubule plus end (Akhmanova and Hoogenraad, 2005). The current study screened individual microtubule regulator in cultured *Drosophila* neurons (Hahn et al., 2021) and found that genetic ablation of any one of these genes resulted in reduced polymerization, curling of the microtubules into the formation of bundles, and defects in axon growth. Trans-heterozygous and epistatic analysis further showed a role of their genetic interaction in promoting microtubule bundle formation and polymerization based on shared mutant phenotypes, i.e., reduced axon growth, EB1 comet sizes, numbers, and velocities (Hahn et al., 2021). Using several truncation mutants in rescue experiments, the study suggested a model in which tau outcompetes EB1 for space on GDP tubulin, therefore allowing EB1 to bind and stabilize the GTP tubulin cap that is needed for XMAP215 mediated polymerization. The study also linked these three proteins to spectraplakin-dependent guidance of microtubule bundle formation needed for axon growth and maintenance.

While the above study illustrates the importance of local regulation of microtubule assembly via multiple regulators during axon growth, local regulation is also important for microtubule stability and transport function during axonal branch development. This is illustrated by recent studies of MAP7, a MAP that upregulates its expression during the development of collateral branches of sensory neurons from the DRG (Tymanskyj and Ma, 2019; Tymanskyj et al., 2017; Tymanskyj et al., 2018). Knockout of MAP7 in cultured DRG neurons reduces branch formation, whereas overexpression of MAP7 increases branches (Tymanskyj and Ma, 2019; Tymanskyj et al., 2017). Interestingly, endogenous MAP7 localizes at mature branch junctions, but in nascent branches, MAP7 follows the newly arrived microtubules (Tymanskyj et al., 2017; Tymanskyj et al., 2018). This delay is attributed to its ability to bind to acetylated microtubules and avoid tyrosinated microtubules at the dynamic plus ends. This unique binding feature is mediated by two microtubule binding domains, thus allowing MAP7 to stabilize microtubules and prevent nascent branch retraction. Furthermore, MAP7 is shown to interact with the motor protein kinesin-1 via its carboxyl domain and affect kinesin recruitment to microtubules (Monroy et al., 2018; Tymanskyj et al., 2018). This unique ability allows MAP7 to change intracellular transport via a potential track switching mechanism to promote branch growth (Tymanskyj et al., 2018). In fact, analyses of MAP7 domains that interact with microtubules or kinesins in DRG neurons are consistent with its role in regulating branch formation and growth, two steps that are essential to axon morphogenesis. MAP7 has two additional gene homologs expressed in mammalian neurons. MAP7D1 localizes in the proximal region of cortical neurons and enhances outgrowth of callosal neurons through phosphorylation by DCLK1 *in vivo* (Koizumi et al., 2017). MAP7D2 was recently shown to localize at the proximal region of cortical neurons and recruit kinesin-1 to enhance transport and cortical branching (Pan et al., 2019). Since other MAPs, such as tau, not only localize to certain parts of microtubules but also interacting with kinesin motors (Dixit et al., 2008), these studies raise the importance of localized control of transport by various MAPs in supporting axon morphogenesis.

1.3 Regulation of Intracellular Membrane Organelles

1.3.1 Energy metabolism and mitochondria

The creation of various axon morphologies is an energetically demanding process. Led by motile growth cones, axons can travel great distances and navigate through many different tissues in order to find their correct targets. Depending on local cues, branches can be formed and retracted along this developmental journey. As mentioned earlier in this chapter, axon growth, guidance, and branching invovle cytoskeletal rearrangement and motor-based organelle transport, both require energy. Where is the energy produced to support these processes and how does the neuron use energy to create the diverse array of neuronal subtypes and specific compartments such as axons and dendrites?

ATP is the main energy source for many cellular processes such as signaling cascades, actin and microtubule re-reorganization, and motor-based long distance transport (Figure 1.3) (reviewed in (Gallo, 2020)). Cellular ATP is primarily generated through oxidative phosphorylation in mitochondria, which relies on the movement of electrons through the electron transport chain to produce large amounts of ATP with the consumption of oxygen. Mitochondria are transported through the cell by kinesin-based transport to sites of high energy demand. This role of mitochondria at developing branch junctions has been shown by live imaging of cultured DRG neurons where mitochondria stall prior to sites of branch formation (Spillane et al., 2013). Disruption of mitochondria transport and localization is implicated in numerous development and degenerative diseases such as Parkinson's disease (Liu et al., 2012). Therefore, transport and localization of mitochondria to areas of high energy demand is particularly important for neuronal morphogenesis.

Previous studies have shown that Lkb1, a tumor-suppressor protein, regulates mitochondrial motility and axon morphogenesis of the central

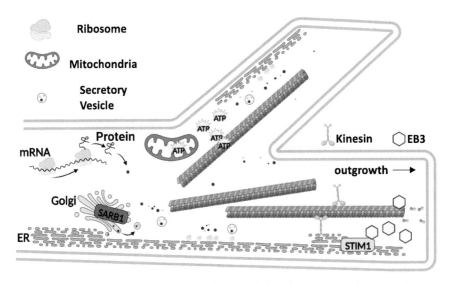

Figure 1.3 Intracellular organelles enriched within a branch junction contribute to axon morphogenesis. Schematic drawings depicting the energy and local translation machineries that are enriched within a branch junction. Endoplasmic reticulum (ER), Golgi apparatus, mRNA transcripts, ribosomes, and mitochondria are present to support protein synthesis and secretory vesicle formation during branch formation and extension. Interplay between microtubules, kinesins, and ER could shape neuronal morphology as ER interacting proteins, such as STIM1, promote the recruitment of EB3 to plus ends of microtubules allowing for outgrowth.

nervous system (CNS) neurons *in vivo* (Courchet et al., 2013; Spillane et al., 2013). A recent study of the transcriptome of Lkb1 knockout neurons has identified Efhd1, a calcium-binding protein in the inner mitochondrial membrane to be the downstream effector of Lkb1. Utilizing both *in vitro* DRG explants and *in vivo* limb analysis in knockout mice, the authors showed that loss of Efdh1 led to decreased ATP production, shortened mitochondria, and aberrant axon morphology such as reduced axon elongation and reduction in axon branching (Ulisse et al., 2020). Interestingly, however, these defects are not related to mitochondrial motility, but rather caused by increased stress responses mediated by two kinases (AMPK and Ulk) (Ulisse et al., 2020). Since mitochondria are known to be involved in many metabolic functions and critical for energy production, this new study demonstrates additional roles that mitochondria play in axon morphogenesis (Figure 1.3).

ATP can be also produced by glycolysis, which enzymatically adds phosphate to ADP with the conversion of glucose into pyruvate. Glycolysis is oxygen independent and is faster but less efficient than oxidative phosphorylation. Recent studies demonstrate the requirement of the glycolytic pathway for high energetic needs of morphogenesis in a faster and local manner.

Axons and growth cones of sensory DRG axons in culture were shown to have glycolysis enzymes. With the necessary materials present, the authors showed that growth cone dynamics and axon extension depend on glycolysis (Ketschek et al., 2021). Considering its additional role in synaptic development (Jang et al., 2016), the non-mitochondrial sources of ATP could provide another way to regulate axon morphogenesis, specifically in the creation of new branches.

1.3.2 Local translation, endoplasmic reticulum, and the Golgi apparatus

In addition to energy demands, the highly asymmetric structures of neurons contain different compositions of proteins and organelles in their axons. How is a neuron able to produce the needed proteins to maintain its function across vast distances? The emerging idea of local protein synthesis (LPS) suggests that specialized neuronal branches and distal regions of axons locally produce necessary proteins instead of relying on transport-based protein delivery. The presence of the protein synthesis machinery at distal regions and distinct branch sites provides evidence of local translation away from the soma (reviewed in (Holt et al., 2019)). Supported by proteomic analysis, fluorescent-based live cell imaging, and *in vivo* knockdown of ribosomal proteins (Holt et al., 2019; Wong et al., 2017), specific regulation of local protein synthesis is recognized as an important characteristic of highly polarized and morphologically complex neurons (Figure 1.3).

New techniques such as *in situ* cryo-electron tomography (CryoET) have allowed for a finer look at the axon branch to understand the complexity of the morphological distinction of subcellular components. CryoET examines protein 3D structures at high resolution in their intact, cryo preserved, native environment by repeated exposure of electrons to the sample at rotating angles. Recently, CryoET was utilized for the identification of organelles and molecular machinery present in two morphologically distinct stages of axonal branches (Nedozralova et al., 2022). It revealed that immature branches contained mainly actin patches, while mature branches contained microtubules and more structured actin. Small mitochondria were often localized at branch sites. Complex association of microtubules, mitochondria, and endoplasmic reticulum (ER) was found at mature branches, suggesting their important roles. Interestingly, clusters of ribosomes were also found in dense patches at branches, supporting the idea of locally synthesized proteins and providing evidence that branches are hubs of axon development and outgrowth (Nedozralova et al., 2022). Identification of these ribosomal clusters further supports the concept that instead of being transported to long distances, proteins are able to be made locally. The co-presence of these LPS machineries in the axon branch junction reinforces the necessity of cytoskeleton and membrane remodeling needed for branch morphogenesis.

The interplay between microtubules and ER in determining neuronal polarity and axon specification is further supported by additional studies. The ER has two main subtypes: tubules and cisternae. In unpolarized cells, the ER is organized in perinuclear cisternae that are connected with tubular structures in the cell periphery. These two ER subtypes were found to localize in developing neurons based on marker staining, with ER tubules in the axons and ER cisterna in the soma and dendrites. This differential distribution depends on the interaction of ER with microtubules via the kinesin motor KIF5A (Figure 1.3). Conversely, ER tubules also regulate microtubule organizations by facilitating the stabilization of microtubules and correct localization of proteins required for the development of the axon initial segment. Importantly, recruitment of ER tubules into one nascent neurite is required for axon specification and it involves an ER shaping protein P180, which regulates microtubule stabilization (Farías et al., 2019). The result suggests a greater role of the concerted effort of ER and microtubules in axon morphogenesis. Indeed, remodeling of the growth cone also requires a concerted effort of reorganization of microtubules and ER. The ER-calcium sensor stromal interacting molecule 1 (STIM1) was shown to regulate the recruitment of polymerizing microtubules through EB3 movement into filopodia of sensory DRG neurons *in vitro* and *in vivo* (Pavez et al., 2019). Neurons with STIM1 knockdown were unable to recruit microtubules to the steering edge of the growth cone. This study provides a potential mechanism not only linking ER and microtubules but also connecting calcium signaling to growth cone dynamics, which ultimately can regulate branching and outgrowth, leading to the formation of the diverse morphologies of neurons (Pavez et al., 2019).

Trafficking from the ER to the Golgi apparatus is part of normal cellular function, pivotal in secreting proteins throughout the neurons to specified destinations. Recent studies investigating disruption of this process suggest a role of the Golgi apparatus in early stages of neuronal development such as axon polarization and axonogenesis (Figure 1.3). This is demonstrated by the study of SAR1B, a member of the Arf GTPase family involved in the fusion and budding of vesicles in the secretory pathway from the ER to the Golgi (Li et al., 2020). SAR1B was shown to express in the developing cortex. SAR1B knockdown in the developing mouse cortex led to defects in radial migration and axon morphogenesis of cortical neurons, as neurons were unable to orient in the proper layers of the cortex and had altered processes with more unpolarized morphologies, and disrupted Golgi localization

(Li et al., 2020). Another example is from the study of Efa6, an Arf activa-tor (Qu et al., 2019). Interestingly, Efa6 is a membrane-associated protein that inhibits microtubule outgrowth by binding to tubulin directly through its microtubule elimination domain. This ability allows Efa6 to exclude micro-tubules from filoppdial protrusions and inhibit microtubule polymerization, thus controlling the location of branching (Qu et al., 2019).

Since the Golgi apparatus plays a role in cellular trafficking of pro-teins, axonal specification and outgrowth have been linked to Golgi dynam-ics (Rosso et al., 2004). One example of this regulation is demonstrated by SCY1-like pseudokinase 1 (SCYL1), a catalytically inactive protein kinase that interacts with the COP protein and controls Golgi morphology. SCYL1 is expressed in the brain and its variants cause brain developmental delay (Schmidt et al., 2007b). A recent study further demonstrated that SCYL1 knockdown altered Golgi morphology and inhibited axon outgrowth in Rat1-cells. Interestingly, it was identified that arginine methylation of SCYL1 is pivotal in normal Golgi morphology and subsequent outgrowth of hippocam-pal neurons (Amano et al., 2020). Biochemical analysis showed that SCYL1 was methylated in brain tissues, and pharmacological inhibition of protein arginine methyltransferase 1 (PRMT1) led to the similar Golgi and axon out-growth defects. Finally, wild-type SCYL1, but not the arginine methylation deficient SCYL1 mutant, rescued the SCYL1 knockdown defects. Although the mechanism mediating this methylation regulation remains to be resolved, the organization of membrane structures within the developing axon will continue to show their critical albeit complex roles in axon morphogenesis.

1.4 Cell Surface Signaling

Axon morphogenesis involves the integration of information in the surround-ing environment with temporal–spatial specificity. Neighboring cells and extracellular matrix often provide molecular cues. Neurons can detect these cues through ligand-receptor mediated signaling cascades. During develop-ment, these signaling cascades control axon growth, guidance, and branching, ultimately giving rise to the diverse shapes tailored for specialized neuronal functions (reviewed in (Bashaw and Klein, 2010; Gibson and Ma, 2011; Kalil and Dent, 2014)).

The classical signaling cascade involves transmembrane receptors bound by specific extracellular ligands activating downstream proteins to alter growth cone responses, typically through cytoskeletal rearrangement (Figure 1.4) (Bashaw and Klein, 2010). Many of these receptors are type I transmembrane proteins that, once bound to ligands, dimerize and engage

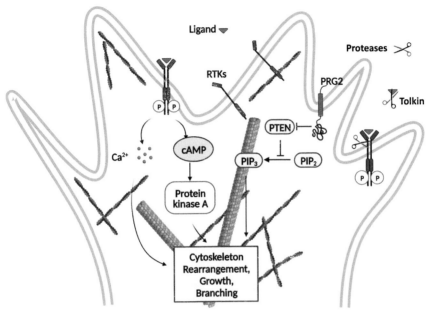

Figure 1.4 Signaling from cell surface receptors in axon morphogenesis. Schematic drawing of extracellular ligands binding to receptor tyrosine kinases (RTKs), which leads to receptor autophosphorylation and downstream signaling via second messengers, such as calcium (Ca^{2+}), cAMP and lipids (PIP_2 and $PIPI_3$). This signaling leads to rearrangement of cytoskeletal components and ultimately axon growth, guidance, and branching. Interacting proteins, such as PRG2/PTEN, balance positive and negative regulators to reorganize the cytoskeleton. Cell surface receptors can be regulated by other factors, including proteases, such as Tolkin, that can cleave both ligands and receptors.

downstream signaling molecules either through phosphorylation or direct binding. Four main families of ligands and receptors were initially identified for guiding axons: netrins and their DCC, Unc5, and neogenin receptors (Kennedy, 2000); Slits and their Robo receptors (Brose and Tessier-Lavigne, 2000); semaphorins and their plexins and neuropilins receptors ((Pasterkamp and Kolodkin, 2003); and ephrins and their Eph receptors (Kullander and Klein, 2002). Since the initial identification of these families, additional factors like the morphogens (BMP, sonic hedgehog, and Wnt) as well as growth factors (such as neurotrophins and neuregulin) have been shown to mediate axon guidance and morphology (Augsburger et al., 1999; Charron et al., 2003; Lyuksyutova et al., 2003; Markus et al., 2002). Although additional factors may be found, there is a finite number of genes encoding these factors in the genome. What are the mechanisms that increase the versatility of molecular pathways to generate complex axon morphologies in the developing nervous system?

One mechanism is to regulate receptor function. This can be illustrated by Slit/Robo signaling involved in midline crossing during commissural axon development in the spinal cord. Commissural axons project across the floorplate at the midline making connections on the contralateral side. Prior to crossing, secreted Slit ligands at the ventral midline are unable to influence the axons. This is partly due to the inhibition of the surface expression and the activity of the Slit receptors, Robo1/2, by other proteins such as Robo3. Post crossing, Robo3 expression is downregulated and Slits are able to interact with Robo1/2 receptors and repel the growth cone from the floorplate to prevent recrossing (Chedotal, 2019).

Additionally, proteolytic regulation of ligands and receptors could provide a mechanism for specificity (Figure 1.4). This can be again illustrated by Slit/Robo signaling in axon guidance. A previous biochemical purification study has suggested that Slit is cleaved into N and C fragments (Wang et al., 1999). While the N fragment functions similar to the full length (FL) Slit to mediate repulsive guidance of commissural axons in the midline, the C fragment is shown to bind to PlexinA1 to regulate postcrossing commissural axons (Delloye-Bourgeois et al., 2015). In *Drosophila*, commissural axons expressing a cleavage-blocking Slit mutant caused a longitudinal guidance defect but not midline repulsion. Further biochemical and genetic analyses of the two Slit receptors, Robo and Dscam, suggest a model in which FL-Slit binds Robo complex to cause repulsion while the cleaved N fragment binds Dscam and Robo complex to promote axonal outgrowth after midline crossing (Alavi et al., 2016). Recently, the protease responsible for the cleavage was identified to be Tolkin (Tok) based on both *in vitro* and *in vivo* analyses (Kellermeyer et al., 2020). Utilizing *Drosophila* S2 cells, the study identified that only co-transfected cells with Slit-FL and Tok had processed Slit. *In vivo*, genetic manipulation of Tok through knock-out and rescue demonstrated that Slit-FL processing into Slit-N and Slit-C is critical for spinal cord midline guidance. While Tok may be a Slit-specific protease, understanding how extracellular ligands undergo cleavage to alter the guidance response can shed light on how morphology can be shaped as circuits develop.

Another proteolytically regulated family of cell surface proteins is neuregulins (Nrgs), which are implicated in having a neural developmental role since mutations of Nrgs pose as a high-risk factor and are associated with greater incidences of psychiatric disorders (reviewed in (Mei and Nave, 2014)). Nrgs are transmembrane proteins that exist in two topologies and undergo proteolytic cleavage by extracellular proteases including BACE1.

In type I topology, proteolysis causes membrane tethered Nrgs to release a diffusible epidermal growth factor (EGF)-like containing polypeptide that interacts with ErbB receptors to elicit a conical signaling cascade. In type II topology, BACE1 cleavage generates a transmembrane form that contains the EGFL domain to interact with ErbB to elicit transmembrane-dependent signaling. A recent study showed that in cortical GABA positive interneuron cultures, the soluble form of three Nrg homologs (Nrg1–3) was able to increase neurite outgrowth of interneurons by increasing branch number, complexity, and length (Rahman-Enyart et al., 2020). Another study aimed at understanding the sites of transmembrane forms of Nrgs using an optogenetic cleavage reporter, LA[143]-NRG3 (Ahmad et al., 2022). It was found that mature membrane Nrg3 emerges on the somatodendritic plasma membrane where it is re-endocytosed and transported into axons via transcytosis. Mature Nrg3 also accumulates on the presynaptic membrane through a "transsynaptic retention model". Thus, the mechanism mediating the processing of cell surface signaling molecules could diversify the regulation of their normal function in axon outgrowth and the ability to make proper connections.

While the regulation of ligands and their cell surface receptors is important for the diversity of responses from axons, dissecting the downstream signal transduction pathways provides a more complete understanding of how the axon can navigate its environment, giving rise to the necessary morphologies. Second messengers, including cAMP, cGMP, Ca^{2+}, and lipid-based messengers such as phosphoinositides, are important components of the pathways to propagate signals more broadly across the navigating axon (Figure 1.4). For example, most receptor tyrosine kinases, when they dimerize after ligand binding, undergo a conformational change allowing them to autophosphorylate to provide binding sites as well as to activate downstream targets through phosphorylation. The targets include membrane voltage gated $Ca2^{+}$ channels, Ryanodine receptors that release calcium from intracellular stores, cyclic nucleotides, phosphoinositides such as phosphatidylinositol 3,4,5-trisphosphate (PIP3) at the plasma membrane, and other second messengers (Newton et al., 2016). These second messengers allow for the membrane localized signaling to propagate away from the cell surface to more precise mediators like cytoskeletal regulators needed for creating the diverse neuronal morphologies (Figure 1.4).

Another way to generate diverse axonal morphologies in developing axons is the regulation of competing signaling pathways leading to both positive and negative outcomes. The lipid signaling involving PIP3 provides a good example to illustrate this mechanism. PIP3 is generated by phosphoinositide 3-kinase at the plasma membrane and promotes axon elongation and axon branching by reorganizing the actin cytoskeleton. Interestingly, this positive signaling can be attenuated by PTEN, a phosphatase that dephosphorylates PIP3 and reverses axon growth and branching. As PTEN is expressed at high levels in neurons, how does PIP3 overcome this antagonizing molecule? A recent study (Brosig et al., 2019) found a PTEN interacting protein that can resolve this conflict. It involves plasticity-related gene 2 (PRG2), a transmembrane protein that inhibits the phosphatase activity of PTEN and thus supports localized PIP3 production needed for actin remodeling. Overexpressing PRG2 in embryonic stem cell-derived neurons induced filopodia and branches along axons, whereas PRG2 knockout in hippocampal neurons reduced filopodia and branch formation. Importantly, the branching defect in the PRG2 knockout neurons can be rescued by the knockdown of PTEN or expressing FL-PRG2 but not the deletion mutant that does not bind PTEN. Although it remains to be determined how PRG2 is controlled, the inhibitory release model demonstrates the balancing act to control positive and negative signaling pathways in developing axons. Here, a mechanism to attenuate the PTEN block allows PIP3 signaling to facilitate the cytoskeletal rearrangement that is required for axon growth, guidance, and branch formation.

1.5 Posttranslational Modifications

Axon morphogenesis is a complex and dynamic process that requires tight regulation of a variety of protein functions. Posttranslational modifications (PTMs) increase the diversity of a protein through the covalent modification of their structures after protein synthesis. Here, we focus on PTMs that add functional groups, such as phosphates, small molecules, amino acids, peptides, or lipids. These types of PTMs affect protein structure, function, localization, stability, and proteolytic cleavage (Ramazi and Zahiri, 2021). Each of these PTM processes can modify the neuronal cytoskeleton such as microtubules, as well as signaling molecules that play a role in different steps of axon morphogenesis. The following section will discuss several recent studies and provide examples of four PTMs that play important roles in axon morphogenesis.

1.5.1 Phosphorylation

Phosphorylation is the addition of a phosphate group onto a protein by a protein kinase; this results in the protein being more negatively charged. Phosphorylation is a common method of protein regulation in the nervous system and can occur on a variety of proteins, structures, and other molecules. This PTM functions to reversibly mediate a wide variety of protein functions during axon development and morphogenesis such as: microtubule stability, energy and mitochondrial metabolism, and neuronal polarization (Barbier et al., 2019; Igarashi et al., 2020; Ulisse et al., 2020). Each of these events is required for axon development and morphogenesis as previously mentioned in this chapter. For example, as discussed above, phosphorylation of AMPK and Ulk in the mitochondrial inner membrane decreases energy production and metabolism in *Efhd1* knockout neurons and results in decreased branching, demonstrating that phosphorylation plays a role in axon morphogenesis (Ulisse et al., 2020) (Figure 1.5A).

1.5.2 Acetylation of tubulin

Acetylation is the transfer of an acetyl group onto the lysine residue of a protein by the lysine acetyltransferase, resulting in the change of protein functionality and localization. Acetylation is widely known to occur in many cell types and cellular processes, but how it contributes to axon morphogenesis depends on the modified site in the target protein. Here, we use microtubule acetylation as an example to illustrate this point. Microtubules can undergo a variety of modifications such as acetylation, tyrosination, phosphorylation, and ubiquitination (Wloga et al., 2017). Acetylation of tubulin is known to be associated with microtubule behaviors in cells. Among multiple acetylation sites, lysine 40 (K40) on α-tubulin has been well characterized. This site is inside the lumen of microtubules, and its acetylation is correlated with stable and long-lived microtubules. Interestingly, recent studies have identified >12 other sites, and one of them, lysine 394 (K394), is highly conserved and located at the α–β tubulin interface (Figure 1.5B). Using the *Drosophila melanogaster* neuromuscular junction (NMJ) as a model system, a recent study (Saunders et al., 2022) examined the role of K394 in neuronal morphogenesis. They found that genetically blocking acetylation in a K394 mutant reduced microtubule stability and increased the number of synaptic boutons associated with the growth of axonal terminals. This mutant has decreased MAP1B-induced microtubule loops in axon terminals as well as an increased sensitivity to nocodazole, suggesting a role of microtubule stability supported by K394 acetylation. Consistent with the idea, increasing microtubule stability by various methods, including taxol treatment and overexpression of MAP1B (Futsch) or a tubulin chaperon, rescued the mutant phenotype similar to the wild-type level. They were also able to show that HDAC6, a deacetylase, is likely the key enzyme that controls the level of

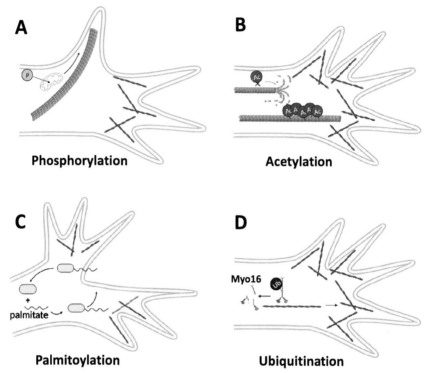

Figure 1.5   Posttranslational modifications in axon morphogenesis. (A) Phosphorylation of the mitochondrial inner membrane regulates energy production and plays a role in axon branching. **(B)** Acetylation (Ac) of tubulin is an important PTM regulating microtubule dynamics. Tubulin acetylation stabilizes microtubules allowing for axons and branches to be maintained. **(C)** Palmitoylation signals for proteins to be associated with the membrane. Palmitoylation functions in growth cone splitting allowing for the formation of two daughter branches. **(D)** Some proteins can be tagged for ubiquitination and subsequent degradation during axon development. A family of TRIM E3 ligases interact with unconventional Myo16 to promote axon growth.

K394 acetylation and consequently microtubule stability in the boutons. The study demonstrates the importance of microtubule acetylation in neuronal morphogenesis. Additional work determining other acetylation targets such as molecular motors, synaptic proteins, and receptors, as well as specific sites in these proteins could help provide a more detailed insight into how acetylation plays a role in axon morphogenesis.

1.5.3 Palmitoylation

Palmitoylation is the addition of a lipid group, such as palmitic acid, to a protein that results in membrane association and trafficking of the protein through intracellular membrane compartments. A recent study (Dumoulin et al., 2018) suggests that palmitoylation contributes to neuronal morphogenesis through growth cone shaping and subsequent axon bifurcation (Figure 1.5C). The study used embryonic DRG neurons that exhibited a stereotyped axon bifurcation in the dorsal spinal cord (Gibson and Ma, 2011). This process is controlled by cGMP-dependent signaling, which involves a secreted peptide hormone CNP, its receptor Npr2, a membrane guanylyl cyclase that produces cGMP, and the cGMP-dependent protein kinase 1 (cGKI) (Schmidt et al., 2009; Schmidt et al., 2007a; Zhao and Ma, 2009; Zhao et al., 2009). In culture, CNP induced DRG growth cone enlargement, a potential step leading to bifurcation, through activation of cGKI (Dumoulin et al., 2018). Interestingly, cGKI is localized to vesicular structures that are associated with palmitoylated proteins, and cGKI activation leads to increased levels of protein palmitoylation. Using pharmacological reagents, the study showed that blocking S-palmitoylation, a reversible modification via thioester linkages, attenuated growth cone enlargement stimulated by CNP, whereas blocking de-palmitoylation increased growth cone size and axon elongation. These results suggest that S-palmitoylation could function downstream of cGKI to mediate CNP-mediated growth cone remodeling and subsequent axon bifurcation.

While this study is the first to explore the role of S-palmitoylation in growth cone remodeling, it is important to note that palmitoylation can also occur via amide-linkages (N-palmitoylation) to generate irreversible attachment of palmitate to the N-terminus of a protein. N-palmitoylation has previously been shown to regulate sonic hedgehog (Shh), a morphogen involved in cell proliferation and differentiation (Ji et al., 2016; Pepinsky et al., 1998). Therefore, many proteins involved in axonal development, such as guidance cues and receptors, could be regulated this way, and identifying the palmitoylation target proteins will provide useful clues to this type of regulation during axon morphogenesis.

1.5.4 Ubiquitination

Ubiquitination is an enzymatic reaction that adds a small protein ubiquitin to a cellular protein that is typically destined for degradation. The target protein is recognized by a substrate-specific E3 ligase, which in conjunction with the E2 ubiquitin-conjugating enzyme catalyzes the addition of single or multiple ubiquitins (Stack et al., 2000). Ubiquitination is known to play a role throughout the life of a neuron, from neurite outgrowth to presynaptic formation as well as degeneration (Pinto et al., 2021). Interestingly, ubiquitination can also enhance neurite outgrowth by tagging and degrading proteins that inhibit axon growth (Konishi et al., 2004; Yang et al., 2010). A recent study showed that a family of E3 ubiquitin ligases contributes to axon guidance and morphology through destabilizing actin in response to extracellular cues (Figure 1.5D) (Pinto et al., 2021).

The TRIpartitite Motif (TRIM) proteins are a family of ubiquitin E3 ligases found to have critical roles in morphogenesis of cortical and hippo-campal neurons. Two members, TRIM9 and TRIM67, interact with DCC, the netrin-1 receptor, to promote axon guidance and exhibit contrasting aberrant phenotypes when deleted (Boyer et al., 2018; Winkle et al., 2014). Deletion of TRIM9 in the cortex results in the thickening of the corpus callosum, which could be due to aberrant branching (Boyer et al., 2018). However, cortical deletion of TRIM67 results in the opposite phenotype, leading to thinning of the corpus callosum. Additional studies have demonstrated that TRIM9 and TRIM67 regulate cytoskeletal dynamics by modulating the ubiq-uitination of VASP, an actin polymerase (Menon et al., 2015). Interestingly, TRIM9 and TRIM67 have opposite roles in branching. *Trim9*$^{-/-}$ neurons have increased basal level branching and no change in Netrin-1-induced branch-ing, whereas *Trim67*$^{-/-}$ neurons have no change in basal level branching but affect Netrin-1 branching, suggesting additional substrates for these ligases that could mediate such differences. Using a BioID-based proteomics approach, a recent study (Menon et al., 2021) identified a host of new candi-dates that TRIM9 and TRIM67 interact with based on their proximities. One candidate is an unconventional myosin, Myo16, which is localized along the axon as well as the tip of growth cone filopodia. Myo16 was found to inter-act with TRIM9 and TRIM67 at specific sites, and knockdown analysis sug-gests that Myo16 regulates netrin-dependent axon branching. Interestingly, Myo16 knockdown blocked netrin-induced branching seen in *Trim67*$^{-/-}$ neu-rons as well as basal branching seen in *Trim9*$^{-/-}$ neurons. These data suggest a possible regulatory mechanism in which TRIM9 and TRIM67 recognize Myo16 for ubiquitination for subsequent basal-level and netrin-dependent branching (Menon et al., 2021). Because the study has also revealed critical interactions with several other cytoskeletal components such as MAPs and tubulin isoforms, it is not surprising that additional regulation of cytoskeletal components by ubiquitination is present to fine-tune the cytoskeletal organi-zation during neuronal morphogenesis (Menon et al., 2021).

1.6 Transcriptional Control

The complexity and diversity of neuronal subtypes is a hallmark of the mam-malian nervous system. Historically, the classification of neurons has been determined by morphology or functional roles. The morphologically specific features are associated with neuronal differentiation that is often accompanied by transcriptional regulation. Recent technological advances including single-cell isolation and next-generation sequencing allow for transcriptomic analysis of individual cells. Identification of the precise transcriptional signature of each neuron helps to understand the diversity of neurons and their morphologies (reviewed in (Armand et al., 2021)). An emerging idea is that defined neuronal cell types are determined not only by their distinct morphological features but also by their transcriptional profiles (Winnubst et al., 2020; Yuste et al., 2020). Additionally, studying distinct compartments (axon vs. soma) can link transcriptional profiles of axons or synapses to neurological diseases (reviewed in (Di Paolo et al., 2021)).

Alternative splicing is another mechanism that can expand the diversity of proteins produced for building axon morphologies. Pre-mRNA constructs can be spliced into a multitude of mRNAs that encode protein isoforms that shape neuronal subtypes. The *Drosophila* down syndrome cell adhesion molecule (Dscam) uses splicing to generate >19,000 isoforms with variable extracellular domains. These isoforms provide a unique self-surface recognition or tagging mechanism that is critical to self-avoidance, a patterning mechanism to generate non-overlapping branches (Grueber and Sagasti, 2010). A recent study examined not just the isoform expression, but their localization through lipid trafficking between dendritic and axonal compartments. When DSCAM trafficking and localization were disrupted through perturbed sphingolipid biosynthesis, *Drosophila* mushroom body axons lost the ability to segregate axon branches at distal axonal regions (Goyal et al., 2019). Alternative splicing and distinct localization of those isoforms thus can give neurons the diverse protein-building blocks to form the complex array of patterning of neuronal circuits.

Recent advances in transcriptomics allow for identification of alternative splicing in neuronal subtypes for a specific gene. Using cultured cortical neurons pre- and post-axon specification, a recent study found a strong association of axon specification and neuron-specific alternative splicing (Zhang et al., 2019). PTBP2, an RNA binding protein that is enriched in neurons at the time of axonogenesis, is required for proper axon formation both *in vitro* and *in vivo*. The importance of splicing is further demonstrated by one of the PTBP2 targets, Shtn1, which is involved in neuronal polarization. Normally, Shtn1 switches from a long isoform (Shtn1L) to a short one during axonogenesis. This switching depends on PTBP2 and is critical to axon formation because each isoform has different activities in actin polymerization (Zhang et al., 2019).

The complexity of vertebrae neuronal cells has also been expanded by the study of non-coding genomic regions (Closser et al., 2022). Enhancers, the gene regulatory sequences that alter gene transcription, were shown to have varying promoter interaction profiles between neuronal and non-neuronal cell types. Additionally, the use of mouse embryonic stem cells and *in vivo* mouse embryonic spinal cord allowed a closer examination of motor neurons at different developmental stages. During these stages with distinct connectivity and morphological shapes, motor neurons have unique gene regions that are accessible for transcriptional factors. In addition, the authors showed the evolutionary differences in the complexity of regulatory elements, providing a possible explanation to how the nervous system increases its complexity with a relatively small difference in the total number of genes (Closser et al., 2022). The diverse array of neuronal cell types requires some intrinsic mechanisms to dictate them and, as the understanding of genetic regulation expands, these mechanisms can add additional control of distinct axonal morphologies and hence diverse cell types.

1.7 Axon Morphogenesis in Neurodegeneration and Nerve Regeneration

Neurodegeneration can lead to drastic changes in neuronal morphology, due to activation of abnormal cell death pathways and cell death (Jellinger, 2001). There are a wide variety of neurodegenerative diseases, including, but not limited to, amyotrophic lateral sclerosis (ALS), Alzheimer's disease (AD), and Parkinson's disease (PD). While it is known that the key contributors to each of these disease result in neuronal death, less is known about their role, if any, in neural development and maintenance. Not surprisingly, though, the recent identification of an evolutionary conserved Wnk kinase demonstrates the cross-function of a developmental gene in neurodegeneration (Izadifar et al., 2021). Identified through reverse genetic screening in *Drosophila* and corroborated in mouse cortical neurons *in vivo*, Wnk was found to be required for branch extensions and stabilization, as well as maintenance of adult neurons with a role in programed degeneration. Interestingly, downstream factors of Wnk include Nmnat, Axed, and Sarm1, proteins known to have opposite functions in axonal maintenance and destruction, suggesting that axonal development and maintenance share intrinsic mechanisms. Thus, in this section, we discuss some recent investigations of key neurodegeneration players in axonal growth and morphology. Understanding their roles in axon morphogenesis may provide insights and potential therapeutic targets for neurodegenerative diseases. In addition, we will expand the discussion to nerve regeneration, the opposite of degeneration, when axon morphogenesis is crucial to functional recovery after nerve injury.

1.7.1 Amyotrophic lateral sclerosis

TDP-43 is a transcriptional repressor well-known for its involvement in ALS and the related disorder, frontotempoal dementia (FTD). Mutations in TDP-43 produce cytosolic aggregates in post-mortem tissue, a hallmark of ALS and FTD (Suk and Rousseaux, 2020). The aberrant expression and mislocalization of TDP-43 are associated with neurite abnormalities and subsequent degeneration of motor neurons (Brettschneider et al., 2014; Vickers et al., 2009; Zhou et al., 1998). Although TDP-43 is predominantly localized to the nucleus, it is involved in transporting messenger ribonucleoprotein particles along axons. A recent study (Atkinson et al., 2021) links TDP-43 expression to neuronal morphology and cytoskeleton regulation during development. It shows that changes in TDP-43 expression levels might affect the neuronal cytoskeleton by upregulating actin cytoskeletal proteins. Using primary cortical mouse neurons that expressed either one or two copies of human wild-type TDP-43, the group used a proteomic approach to show that two copies of TDP-43 significantly upregulated actin-binding proteins, which are required for axon guidance, receptor trafficking, and synaptic plasticity. Interestingly the group found that expressing one copy of human TDP-43 increased the number of branches in DIV3 cortical neurons compared to wild-type neurons; however, no change in the overall length or density of neurites was observed. Additional data established that neurons expressing two copies of TDP-43 did not show any morphological changes compared to the wild-type neurons potentially due to an increase in cytoplasmic TDP-43. This suggests that changes in TDP-43 expression can result in changes in neuronal branch complexity but do not result in changes in overall neuron growth. Together with the proteomics data, TDP-43 expression could contribute to changes in branch complexity through the interaction with the cytoskeleton (Atkinson et al., 2021). Other molecules such as FUS and SOD1 have been previously described to have similar branching phenotypes (Garone et al., 2021; Osking et al., 2019). As many actin proteins are involved in growth cone dynamics and outgrowth, further studies are required to parse out the relationship and the mechanisms governing the regulation of the actin cytoskeleton by these ALS-linked genes.

1.7.2 Alzheimer's disease

Amyloid precursor protein (APP) is most widely known for its association with AD. APP typically undergoes cleavage by β and γ secretase. Aberrant cleavages caused by genetic mutations result in the accumulation of APP and subsequent AD symptoms. Under normal conditions, APP is a transmembrane protein that contributes to a wide variety of cellular events including axonal outgrowth, synaptic development, and plasticity as well as receptor-like signaling (reviewed by (Muller et al., 2017)). APP is highly expressed during early development and is also found in stem cells in the adult brain, suggesting that it might be critical for neurogenesis (Wang et al., 2014). While the pathological role of APP is widely studied, its role in axon growth was only investigated recently. Using cultured hippocampal neurons, a recent study (Southam et al., 2019) provides the evidence for the role of APP in axonal morphogenesis, as APP knockout neurons displayed a decrease in the distal axonal and dendritic outgrowth compared to wild-type neurons. However, immunohistochemistry and Western blots showed no alteration in synaptic markers. Interestingly, APP mutant neurons adhered more strongly to poly-L-lysine substrates in culture, raising the question about the role of APP as a cell adhesion molecule. This potential role could be important for axon growth and development since axons need to be attached to a substrate prior to growth (Southam et al., 2019).

While this study lays a solid framework for the role of APP in axon and dendrite morphogenesis, further studies are required to parse out the relationship between synaptic loss and axonal or dendritic loss. Furthermore, as studies have begun to characterize a myriad of biological and physiological roles of APP, loss of APP expression in hippocampal neurons could result in impaired intracellular signaling that could impact axon growth and branching.

1.7.3 Parkinson's disease

Alpha-synuclein (α-synuclein) is well-known for its role in PD. The pathogenic form of α-synuclein accumulates to form aggregates called Lewy bodies that are typically the precursor to neuronal degeneration. Many studies have shown under normal physiological conditions that α-synuclein localizes in the presynaptic terminals and alterations in localization result in changes of neurotransmission (reviewed in (Stefanis, 2012)). Additional studies have shown that α-synuclein associates with cellular membranes, but its functions in axonal morphogenesis are not well understood. A recent study (Schechter et al., 2020) showed that α-synuclein plays a significant role in axon growth and elongation. In cultured α-synuclein null mouse cortical neurons, overexpressing either wild-type (WT) α-synuclein or the A53T α-synuclein mutation that is associated with familial early-onset PD, led to longer axons and more collateral branches compared to control neurons. Interestingly,

A53T α-synuclein branch length was also significantly longer than WT collaterals. The authors further established a relationship between α-synuclein and PI4,5P$_2$, a phosphoinositide found at neuronal membranes and known to function in axon growth. The study revealed that α-synuclein expression increased together with PI4,5P$_2$ levels, which corresponded with increased axon growth and collateral branching. They also observed increased density of striatal white matter tracts *in vivo* consistent with the phenotypes seen *in vitro* (Schechter et al., 2020). These results support a role for α-synuclein in axon growth and branching. Further studies are necessary to better understand the role of membrane-associated α-synuclein in axon growth and guidance and parse out the functional difference between the axonal and synaptic pools of α-synuclein.

1.7.4 Nerve regeneration

Understanding the cellular and molecular mechanisms of axon regeneration is important for treating devastating human conditions following traumatic injury. Most research attempts to parse out the mechanisms governing regrowth of injured nerves in the central and peripheral nervous system. Extracellular factors such as proteins associated with myelin have been found to inhibit axonal regeneration, whereas intrinsic mechanisms can be altered to overcome such inhibition and increase the growth capacity (Mukhopadhyay et al., 1994; Qiu et al., 2002). The details of those mechanisms specifically related to the central nervous system can be found in a comprehensive review by Frank Bradke (2022). Interestingly, however, another way to promote nerve regeneration is through axon branching from injured or spared nerves. This is often referred to as "nerve sprouting" in the regeneration field and has been shown to be a potentially effective way to achieve functional recovery (Tuszynski and Steward, 2012). Relatively little is known how sprouting can be achieved and whether it can be promoted by targeting developmental mechanisms. Regardless, recent analysis using single-cell RNA sequencing (scRNA-seq) in various injury models (Matson et al., 2022, Li et al, 2022, Jacobi et al, 2022) could provide new insights into this important problem.

1.8 Concluding Remarks

Recent studies have provided many new insights into axon morphogenesis. Building on the key framework, we have begun to appreciate the complexity of molecular and cellular regulation of axon growth, guidance, and branching. Aided by new technologies, such as super resolution imaging and single-cell sequencing, future studies will continue to explore the mechanisms that endow the morphological diversity that are essential for building complex neural circuits. Several key questions need to be addressed. How does transcriptional regulation specify axon morphology? What controls the expression of a specific set of genes that are critical to defining axon morphology? How do neurons respond to environmental cues? And how are the expression and localization of these cues controlled? A recent study of the transcriptional regulation of dendrite development provides a good example of how to address these questions (Xie et al., 2022).

The molecular and cellular mechanisms of axon morphogenesis would help understand human brain disorders. For example, many axon guidance molecules are associated with autism and schizophrenia, whereas animal models with mutations in these molecules have revealed neural deficits found in human disorders (Van Battum et al., 2015). As described above, many genes related to neurodegeneration have begun to be found to play roles in axon growth, guidance, and branching. Further investigation of their roles in axonal development may provide a better understanding of their contribution to various neurodegenerations in adult brain. Finally, the mechanism identified during development would help find ways to promote axon regeneration after injury and regain the normal morphology for functional recovery (Hoersting and Schmucker, 2021). The recent study of the Wnk kinases and its evolutionary conserved role in axon branch development, maintenance, and degeneration (Izadifar et al., 2021) provides an excellent example. Therefore, continuing investigation of axon morphogenesis using a combinatorial approach will not only provide a better answer of a basic science question but also shed lights on many clinically relevant problems.

References

Ahmad, T., Vullhorst, D., Chaudhuri, R., Guardia, C.M., Chaudhary, N., Karavanova, I., Bonifacino, J.S., and Buonanno, A. (2022). Transcytosis and trans-synaptic retention by postsynaptic ErbB4 underlie axonal accumulation of NRG3. Journal of Cell Biology **221**, e202110167.

Akhmanova, A., and Hoogenraad, C.C. (2005). Microtubule plus-end-tracking proteins: mechanisms and functions. Current opinion in cell biology **17**, 47–54. 10.1016/j.ceb.2004.11.001.

Alavi, M., Song, M., King, G.L.A., Gillis, T., Propst, R., Lamanuzzi, M., Bousum, A., Miller, A., Allen, R., and Kidd, T. (2016). Dscam1 forms a complex with Robo1 and the N-terminal fragment of slit to promote the growth of longitudinal axons. PLoS biology **14**, e1002560.

Alfadil, E., and Bradke, F. (2023). Moving through the crowd. Where are we at understanding physiological axon growth? Semin Cell Dev Biol **140**, 63–71. 10.1016/j.semcdb.2022.07.001.

Amano, G., Matsuzaki, S., Mori, Y., Miyoshi, K., Han, S., Shikada, S., Takamura, H., Yoshimura, T., and Katayama, T. (2020). SCYL1 arginine methylation by PRMT1 is essential for neurite outgrowth via Golgi morphogenesis. Mol Biol Cell **31**, 1963–1973. 10.1091/mbc.E20-02-0100.

Arikkath, J. (2020). Mechanisms of axon polarization in pyramidal neurons. Mol Cell Neurosci **107**, 103522. 10.1016/j.mcn.2020.103522.

Armand, E.J., Li, J., Xie, F., Luo, C., and Mukamel, E.A. (2021). Single-cell sequencing of brain cell transcriptomes and epigenomes. Neuron **109**, 11–26.

Armijo-Weingart, L., and Gallo, G. (2017). It takes a village to raise a branch: Cellular mechanisms of the initiation of axon collateral branches. Mol Cell Neurosci. 10.1016/j.mcn.2017.03.007.

Atkins, M., Nicol, X., and Fassier, C. (2023). Microtubule remodelling as a driving force of axon guidance and pruning. Semin Cell Dev Biol **140**, 35–53. 10.1016/j.semcdb.2022.05.030.

Atkinson, R.A.K., Fair, H.L., Wilson, R., Vickers, J.C., and King, A.E. (2021). Effects of TDP-43 overexpression on neuron proteome and morphology in vitro. Mol Cell Neurosci **114**, 103627. 10.1016/j.mcn.2021.103627.

Augsburger, A., Schuchardt, A., Hoskins, S., Dodd, J., and Butler, S. (1999). BMPs as mediators of roof plate repulsion of commissural neurons. Neuron **24**, 127–141.

Barbier, P., Zejneli, O., Martinho, M., Lasorsa, A., Belle, V., Smet-Nocca, C., Tsvetkov, P.O., Devred, F., and Landrieu, I. (2019). Role of tau as a microtubule-associated protein: structural and functional aspects. Frontiers in aging neuroscience **11**, 204.

Bashaw, G.J., Kidd, T., Murray, D., Pawson, T., and Goodman, C.S. (2000). Repulsive axon guidance: Abelson and Enabled play opposing roles downstream of the roundabout receptor. Cell **101**, 703–715.

Bashaw, G.J., and Klein, R. (2010). Signaling from Axon Guidance Receptors. Cold Spring Harbor perspectives in biology **2**, a001941-a001941. 10.1101/cshperspect.a001941.

Biswas, S., and Kalil, K. (2018). The Microtubule-Associated Protein Tau Mediates the Organization of Microtubules and Their Dynamic Exploration of Actin-Rich Lamellipodia and Filopodia of Cortical Growth Cones. J Neurosci **38**, 291–307. 10.1523/JNEUROSCI.2281-17.2017.

Bodakuntla, S., Nedozralova, H., Basnet, N., and Mizuno, N. (2021). Cytoskeleton and Membrane Organization at Axon Branches. Front Cell Dev Biol **9**, 707486. 10.3389/fcell.2021.707486.

Boyer, N.P., Monkiewicz, C., Menon, S., Moy, S.S., and Gupton, S.L. (2018). Mammalian TRIM67 Functions in Brain Development and Behavior. eNeuro **5**. 10.1523/ENEURO.0186-18.2018.

Bradke, F. (2022). Mechanisms of Axon Growth and Regeneration: Moving between Development and Disease. Journal of Neuroscience **42**, 8393–8405.

Brettschneider, J., Arai, K., Del Tredici, K., Toledo, J.B., Robinson, J.L., Lee, E.B., Kuwabara, S., Shibuya, K., Irwin, D.J., Fang, L., et al. (2014). TDP-43 pathology and neuronal loss in amyotrophic lateral sclerosis spinal cord. Acta Neuropathol **128**, 423–437. 10.1007/s00401-014-1299-6.

Brose, K., and Tessier-Lavigne, M. (2000). Slit proteins: key regulators of axon guidance, axonal branching, and cell migration. Current opinion in neurobiology **10**, 95–102.

Brosig, A., Fuchs, J., Ipek, F., Kroon, C., Schrotter, S., Vadhvani, M., Polyzou, A., Ledderose, J., van Diepen, M., Holzhutter, H.G., et al. (2019). The Axonal Membrane Protein PRG2 Inhibits PTEN and Directs Growth to Branches. Cell Rep **29**, 2028–2040 e2028. 10.1016/j.celrep.2019.10.039.

Brouhard, G.J., Stear, J.H., Noetzel, T.L., Al-Bassam, J., Kinoshita, K., Harrison, S.C., Howard, J., and Hyman, A.A. (2008). XMAP215 is a processive microtubule polymerase. Cell **132**, 79–88. 10.1016/j.cell.2007.11.043.

Charron, F., Stein, E., Jeong, J., McMahon, A.P., and Tessier-Lavigne, M. (2003). The morphogen sonic hedgehog is an axonal chemoattractant that collaborates with netrin-1 in midline axon guidance. Cell **113**, 11–23.

Chaudhari, K., Gorla, M., Chang, C., Kania, A., and Bashaw, G.J. (2021). Robo recruitment of the Wave regulatory complex plays an essential and conserved role in midline repulsion. Elife **10**. 10.7554/eLife.64474.

Chedotal, A. (2019). Roles of axon guidance molecules in neuronal wiring in the developing spinal cord. Nat Rev Neurosci **20**, 380–396. 10.1038/s41583-019-0168-7.

Chedotal, A., and Richards, L.J. (2010). Wiring the brain: the biology of neuronal guidance. Cold Spring Harb Perspect Biol **2**, a001917. cshperspect.a001917 [pii] 10.1101/cshperspect.a001917.

Clarke, A., McQueen, P.G., Fang, H.Y., Kannan, R., Wang, V., McCreedy, E., Buckley, T., Johannessen, E., Wincovitch, S., and Giniger, E. (2020a). Dynamic morphogenesis of a pioneer axon in Drosophila and its regulation by Abl tyrosine kinase. Mol Biol Cell **31**, 452–465. 10.1091/mbc.E19-10-0563.

Clarke, A., McQueen, P.G., Fang, H.Y., Kannan, R., Wang, V., McCreedy, E., Wincovitch, S., and Giniger, E. (2020b). Abl signaling directs growth of a pioneer axon in Drosophila by shaping the intrinsic fluctuations of actin. Molecular biology of the cell **31**, 466–477.

Closser, M., Guo, Y., Wang, P., Patel, T., Jang, S., Hammelman, J., De Nooij, J.C., Kopunova, R., Mazzoni, E.O., Ruan, Y., et al. (2022). An expansion of the non-coding genome and its regulatory potential underlies vertebrate neuronal diversity. Neuron **110**, 70–85 e76. 10.1016/j.neuron.2021.10.014.

Courchet, J., Lewis, J., Tommy L, Lee, S., Courchet, V., Liou, D.-Y., Aizawa, S., and Polleux, F. (2013). Terminal Axon Branching Is Regulated by the LKB1-NUAK1 Kinase Pathway via Presynaptic Mitochondrial Capture. Cell **153**, 1510–1525. 10.1016/j.cell.2013.05.021.

Dehmelt, L., and Halpain, S. (2005). The MAP2/Tau family of microtubule-associated proteins. Genome Biol **6**, 204. 10.1186/gb-2004-6-1-204.

Delloye-Bourgeois, C., Jacquier, A., Charoy, C., Reynaud, F., Nawabi, H., Thoinet, K., Kindbeiter, K., Yoshida, Y., Zagar, Y., Kong, Y., et al. (2015). PlexinA1 is a new Slit receptor and mediates axon guidance function of Slit C-terminal fragments. Nat Neurosci **18**, 36–45. 10.1038/nn.3893.

Dent, E.W., Gupton, S.L., and Gertler, F.B. (2011). The growth cone cytoskeleton in axon outgrowth and guidance. Cold Spring Harbor perspectives in biology **3**. 10.1101/cshperspect.a001800.

Di Paolo, A., Garat, J., Eastman, G., Farias, J., Dajas-Bailador, F., Smircich, P., and Sotelo-Silveira, J.R. (2021). Functional Genomics of Axons and Synapses to Understand Neurodegenerative Diseases. Front Cell Neurosci **15**, 686722. 10.3389/fncel.2021.686722.

Dixit, R., Ross, J.L., Goldman, Y.E., and Holzbaur, E.L. (2008). Differential regulation of dynein and kinesin motor proteins by tau. Science **319**, 1086–1089. 10.1126/science.1152993.

Dumoulin, A., Dagane, A., Dittmar, G., and Rathjen, F.G. (2018). S-palmitoylation Is Required for the Control of Growth Cone Morphology of DRG Neurons by CNP-Induced cGMP Signaling. Front Mol Neurosci **11**, 345. 10.3389/fnmol.2018.00345.

Farías, G.G., Fréal, A., Tortosa, E., Stucchi, R., Pan, X., Portegies, S., Will, L., Altelaar, M., and Hoogenraad, C.C. (2019). Feedback-driven mechanisms between microtubules and the endoplasmic reticulum instruct neuronal polarity. Neuron **102**, 184–201. e188.

Forsthoefel, D.J., Liebl, E.C., Kolodziej, P.A., and Seeger, M.A. (2005). The Abelson tyrosine kinase, the Trio GEF and Enabled interact with the

Netrin receptor Frazzled in Drosophila. Development **132**, 1983–1994. 10.1242/dev.01736.

Frendo, M.E., da Silva, A., Phan, K.D., Riche, S., and Butler, S.J. (2019). The Cofilin/Limk1 Pathway Controls the Growth Rate of Both Developing and Regenerating Motor Axons. J Neurosci **39**, 9316–9327. 10.1523/JNEUROSCI.0648-19.2019.

Funahashi, Y., Watanabe, T., and Kaibuchi, K. (2020). Advances in defining signaling networks for the establishment of neuronal polarity. Curr Opin Cell Biol **63**, 76–87. 10.1016/j.ceb.2019.12.009.

Gallo, G. (2011). The cytoskeletal and signaling mechanisms of axon collateral branching. Dev Neurobiol **71**, 201–220. 10.1002/dneu.20852.

Gallo, G. (2020). The bioenergetics of neuronal morphogenesis and regeneration: Frontiers beyond the mitochondrion. Developmental neurobiology **80**, 263–276.

Garone, M.G., Birsa, N., Rosito, M., Salaris, F., Mochi, M., de Turris, V., Nair, R.R., Cunningham, T.J., Fisher, E.M., and Morlando, M. (2021). ALS-related FUS mutations alter axon growth in motoneurons and affect HuD/ELAVL4 and FMRP activity. Communications Biology **4**, 1025.

Ghosh, D.K., Dasgupta, D., and Guha, A. (2012). Models, Regulations, and Functions of Microtubule Severing by Katanin. ISRN Molecular Biology **2012**, 1–14. 10.5402/2012/596289.

Gibson, D.A., and Ma, L. (2011). Developmental regulation of axon branching in the vertebrate nervous system. Development **138**, 183–195.

Gomez, T.M., and Letourneau, P.C. (2014). Actin dynamics in growth cone motility and navigation. J Neurochem **129**, 221–234. 10.1111/jnc.12506.

Goyal, G., Zheng, J., Adam, E., Steffes, G., Jain, M., Klavins, K., and Hummel, T. (2019). Sphingolipid-dependent Dscam sorting regulates axon segregation. Nature communications **10**, 1–17.

Grueber, W.B., and Sagasti, A. (2010). Self-avoidance and Tiling: Mechanisms of Dendrite and Axon Spacing. Cold Spring Harb Perspect Biol.

Guillaud, L., El-Agamy, S.E., Otsuki, M., and Terenzio, M. (2020). Anterograde Axonal Transport in Neuronal Homeostasis and Disease. Front Mol Neurosci **13**, 556175. 10.3389/fnmol.2020.556175.

Hahn, I., Voelzmann, A., Parkin, J., Fulle, J.B., Slater, P.G., Lowery, L.A., Sanchez-Soriano, N., and Prokop, A. (2021). Tau, XMAP215/Msps and Eb1 co-operate interdependently to regulate microtubule polymerisation and bundle formation in axons. PLoS Genet **17**, e1009647. 10.1371/journal.pgen.1009647.

Hoersting, A.K., and Schmucker, D. (2021). Axonal branch patterning and neuronal shape diversity: roles in developmental circuit assembly:

Axonal branch patterning and neuronal shape diversity in developmental circuit assembly. Curr Opin Neurobiol **66**, 158–165. 10.1016/j. conb.2020.10.019.

Holt, C.E., Martin, K.C., and Schuman, E.M. (2019). Local translation in neurons: visualization and function. Nature structural & molecular biology **26**, 557–566.

Hong, J.H., Kwak, Y., Woo, Y., Park, C., Lee, S.A., Lee, H., Park, S.J., Suh, Y., Suh, B.K., Goo, B.S., et al. (2016). Regulation of the actin cytoskeleton by the Ndel1-Tara complex is critical for cell migration. Sci Rep **6**, 31827. 10.1038/srep31827.

Hotta, A., Inatome, R., Yuasa-Kawada, J., Qin, Q., Yamamura, H., and Yanagi, S. (2005). Critical role of collapsin response mediator protein-associated molecule CRAM for filopodia and growth cone development in neurons. Mol Biol Cell **16**, 32–39. 10.1091/mbc. e04-08-0679.

Igarashi, M., Honda, A., Kawasaki, A., and Nozumi, M. (2020). Neuronal signaling involved in neuronal polarization and growth: lipid rafts and phosphorylation. Frontiers in Molecular Neuroscience **13**, 150.

Izadifar, A., Courchet, J., Virga, D.M., Verreet, T., Hamilton, S., Ayaz, D., Misbaer, A., Vandenbogaerde, S., Monteiro, L., Petrovic, M., et al. (2021). Axon morphogenesis and maintenance require an evolutionary conserved safeguard function of Wnk kinases antagonizing Sarm and Axed. Neuron **109**, 2864–2883 e2868. 10.1016/j.neuron.2021.07.006.

Jacobi, A., Tran, N.M., Yan, W., Benhar, I., Tian, F., Schaffer, R., He, Z., and Sanes, J.R. (2022). Overlapping transcriptional programs promote survival and axonal regeneration of injured retinal ganglion cells. Neuron **110**, 2625–2645. e2627.

Jang, S., Nelson, J.C., Bend, E.G., Rodriguez-Laureano, L., Tueros, F.G., Cartagenova, L., Underwood, K., Jorgensen, E.M., and Colon-Ramos, D.A. (2016). Glycolytic Enzymes Localize to Synapses under Energy Stress to Support Synaptic Function. Neuron **90**, 278–291. 10.1016/j. neuron.2016.03.011.

Jellinger, K.A. (2001). Cell death mechanisms in neurodegeneration. Journal of Cellular and Molecular Medicine **5**, 1–17. 10.1111/j.1582-4934. 2001.tb00134.x.

Ji, Y., Bachschmid, M.M., Costello, C.E., and Lin, C. (2016). S- to N-Palmitoyl Transfer During Proteomic Sample Preparation. J Am Soc Mass Spectrom **27**, 677–685. 10.1007/s13361-015-1319-3.

Ji, Z., Zhang, G., Chen, L., Li, J., Yang, Y., Cha, C., Zhang, J., Lin, H., and Guo, G. (2018). Spastin Interacts with CRMP5 to Promote Neurite

Outgrowth by Controlling the Microtubule Dynamics. Dev Neurobiol **78**, 1191–1205. 10.1002/dneu.22640.

Kadavath, H., Hofele, R.V., Biernat, J., Kumar, S., Tepper, K., Urlaub, H., Mandelkow, E., and Zweckstetter, M. (2015). Tau stabilizes microtubules by binding at the interface between tubulin heterodimers. Proc Natl Acad Sci U S A **112**, 7501–7506. 10.1073/pnas.1504081112.

Kalil, K., and Dent, E.W. (2014). Branch management: mechanisms of axon branching in the developing vertebrate CNS. Nat Rev Neurosci **15**, 7–18. 10.1038/nrn3650.

Kapitein, L.C., and Hoogenraad, C.C. (2015). Building the Neuronal Microtubule Cytoskeleton. Neuron **87**, 492–506. 10.1016/j.neuron.2015.05.046.

Kellermeyer, R., Heydman, L.M., Gillis, T., Mastick, G.S., Song, M., and Kidd, T. (2020). Proteolytic cleavage of Slit by the Tolkin protease converts an axon repulsion cue to an axon growth cue in vivo. Development **147**. 10.1242/dev.196055.

Kennedy, T.E. (2000). Cellular mechanisms of netrin function: long-range and short-range actions. Biochemistry and Cell Biology **78**, 569–575.

Ketschek, A., Sainath, R., Holland, S., and Gallo, G. (2021). The axonal glycolytic pathway contributes to sensory axon extension and growth cone dynamics. Journal of Neuroscience **41**, 6637–6651.

Kevenaar, J.T., and Hoogenraad, C.C. (2015). The axonal cytoskeleton: from organization to function. Front Mol Neurosci **8**, 44. 10.3389/fnmol.2015.00044.

Koizumi, H., Fujioka, H., Togashi, K., Thompson, J., Yates, J.R., 3rd, Gleeson, J.G., and Emoto, K. (2017). DCLK1 phosphorylates the microtubule-associated protein MAP7D1 to promote axon elongation in cortical neurons. Dev Neurobiol **77**, 493–510. 10.1002/dneu.22428.

Kolodkin, A.L., and Tessier-Lavigne, M. (2011). Mechanisms and Molecules of Neuronal Wiring: A Primer. Cold Spring Harbor perspectives in biology **3**, a001727-a001727. 10.1101/cshperspect.a001727.

Konishi, Y., Stegmuller, J., Matsuda, T., Bonni, S., and Bonni, A. (2004). Cdh1-APC controls axonal growth and patterning in the mammalian brain. Science **303**, 1026–1030.

Kullander, K., and Klein, R. (2002). Mechanisms and functions of Eph and ephrin signalling. Nature reviews Molecular cell biology **3**, 475–486.

Kuo, Y.W., Trottier, O., Mahamdeh, M., and Howard, J. (2019). Spastin is a dual-function enzyme that severs microtubules and promotes their regrowth to increase the number and mass of microtubules. Proc Natl Acad Sci U S A **116**, 5533–5541. 10.1073/pnas.1818824116.

Li, X., Yan, M., Guo, Z., Yan, L., Feng, R., Zhu, H., Tu, X., Yu, S., and Chen, J.G. (2020). Inhibition of Sar1b, the Gene Implicated in

Chylomicron Retention Disease, Impairs Migration and Morphogenesis of Developing Cortical Neurons. Neuroscience **449**, 228–240. 10.1016/j. neuroscience.2020.09.044.

Li, E., Yan, R., Yan, K., Zhang, R., Zhang, Q., Zou, P., Wang, H., Qiao, H., Li, S., Ma, Q., and Liao, B. (2022). Single-cell RNA sequencing reveals the role of immune-related autophagy in spinal cord injury in rats. Front Immunol **13**, 987344. 10.3389/fimmu.2022.987344

Liu, S., Sawada, T., Lee, S., Yu, W., Silverio, G., Alapatt, P., Millan, I., Shen, A., Saxton, W., and Kanao, T. (2012). Parkinson's disease–associated kinase PINK1 regulates Miro protein level and axonal transport of mitochondria. PLoS genetics **8**, e1002537.

Lowery, L.A., and Van Vactor, D. (2009). The trip of the tip: understanding the growth cone machinery. Nat Rev Mol Cell Biol **10**, 332–343.

Lyuksyutova, A.I., Lu, C.-C., Milanesio, N., King, L.A., Guo, N., Wang, Y., Nathans, J., Tessier-Lavigne, M., and Zou, Y. (2003). Anterior-posterior guidance of commissural axons by Wnt-frizzled signaling. Science **302**, 1984–1988.

Markus, A., Patel, T.D., and Snider, W.D. (2002). Neurotrophic factors and axonal growth. Current opinion in neurobiology **12**, 523–531.

Matson, K.J., Russ, D.E., Kathe, C., Hua, I., Maric, D., Ding, Y., Krynitsky, J., Pursley, R., Sathyamurthy, A., and Squair, J.W. (2022). Single cell atlas of spinal cord injury in mice reveals a pro-regenerative signature in spinocerebellar neurons. Nature communications **13**, 5628.

McCormick, L.E., and Gupton, S.L. (2020). Mechanistic advances in axon pathfinding. Curr Opin Cell Biol **63**, 11–19. 10.1016/j.ceb.2019.12.003.

Mei, L., and Nave, K.-A. (2014). Neuregulin-ERBB signaling in the nervous system and neuropsychiatric diseases. Neuron **83**, 27–49.

Menon, S., Boyer, N.P., Winkle, C.C., McClain, L.M., Hanlin, C.C., Pandey, D., Rothenfusser, S., Taylor, A.M., and Gupton, S.L. (2015). The E3 Ubiquitin Ligase TRIM9 Is a Filopodia Off Switch Required for Netrin-Dependent Axon Guidance. Dev Cell **35**, 698–712. 10.1016/j. devcel.2015.11.022.

Menon, S., Goldfarb, D., Ho, C.T., Cloer, E.W., Boyer, N.P., Hardie, C., Bock, A.J., Johnson, E.C., Anil, J., Major, M.B., and Gupton, S.L. (2021). The TRIM9/TRIM67 neuronal interactome reveals novel activators of morphogenesis. Mol Biol Cell **32**, 314–330. 10.1091/mbc. E20-10-0622.

Menon, S., and Gupton, S.L. (2016). Building Blocks of Functioning Brain: Cytoskeletal Dynamics in Neuronal Development. Int Rev Cell Mol Biol **322**, 183–245. 10.1016/bs.ircmb.2015.10.002.

Monroy, B.Y., Sawyer, D.L., Ackermann, B.E., Borden, M.M., Tan, T.C., and Ori-McKenney, K.M. (2018). Competition between microtubule-associated proteins directs motor transport. Nat Commun **9**, 1487. 10.1038/s41467-018-03909-2.

Mukhopadhyay, G., Doherty, P., Walsh, F.S., Crocker, P.R., and Filbin, M.T. (1994). A novel role for myelin-associated glycoprotein as an inhibitor of axonal regeneration. Neuron **13**, 757–767.

Muller, U.C., Deller, T., and Korte, M. (2017). Not just amyloid: physiological functions of the amyloid precursor protein family. Nat Rev Neurosci **18**, 281–298. 10.1038/nrn.2017.29.

Nakamura, F., Ohshima, T., and Goshima, Y. (2020). Collapsin Response Mediator Proteins: Their Biological Functions and Pathophysiology in Neuronal Development and Regeneration. Front Cell Neurosci **14**, 188. 10.3389/fncel.2020.00188.

Nedozralova, H., Basnet, N., Ibiricu, I., Bodakuntla, S., Biertumpfel, C., and Mizuno, N. (2022). In situ cryo-electron tomography reveals local cellular machineries for axon branch development. J Cell Biol **221**. 10.1083/jcb.202106086.

Newton, A.C., Bootman, M.D., and Scott, J.D. (2016). Second messengers. Cold Spring Harbor perspectives in biology **8**, a005926.

Osking, Z., Ayers, J.I., Hildebrandt, R., Skruber, K., Brown, H., Ryu, D., Eukovich, A.R., Golde, T.E., Borchelt, D.R., and Read, T.-A. (2019). ALS-linked SOD1 mutants enhance neurite outgrowth and branching in adult motor neurons. Iscience **11**, 294–304.

Pan, X., Cao, Y., Stucchi, R., Hooikaas, P.J., Portegies, S., Will, L., Martin, M., Akhmanova, A., Harterink, M., and Hoogenraad, C.C. (2019). MAP7D2 Localizes to the Proximal Axon and Locally Promotes Kinesin-1-Mediated Cargo Transport into the Axon. Cell Reports **26**, 1988–1999.e1986. 10.1016/j.celrep.2019.01.084.

Pasterkamp, R.J., and Kolodkin, A.L. (2003). Semaphorin junction: making tracks toward neural connectivity. Current opinion in neurobiology **13**, 79–89.

Pavez, M., Thompson, A.C., Arnott, H.J., Mitchell, C.B., D'Atri, I., Don, E.K., Chilton, J.K., Scott, E.K., Lin, J.Y., Young, K.M., et al. (2019). STIM1 Is Required for Remodeling of the Endoplasmic Reticulum and Microtubule Cytoskeleton in Steering Growth Cones. J Neurosci **39**, 5095–5114. 10.1523/JNEUROSCI.2496-18.2019.

Pepinsky, R.B., Zeng, C., Wen, D., Rayhorn, P., Baker, D.P., Williams, K.P., Bixler, S.A., Ambrose, C.M., Garber, E.A., Miatkowski, K., et al. (1998). Identification of a palmitic acid-modified form of human Sonic hedgehog. J Biol Chem **273**, 14037–14045. 10.1074/jbc.273.22.14037.

Pinto, M.J., Tome, D., and Almeida, R.D. (2021). The Ubiquitinated Axon: Local Control of Axon Development and Function by Ubiquitin. J Neurosci **41**, 2796–2813. 10.1523/JNEUROSCI.2251-20.2021.

Polleux, F., and Snider, W. (2010). Initiating and Growing an Axon. Cold Spring Harbor perspectives in biology **2**, a001925-a001925. 10.1101/cshperspect.a001925.

Qiang, L., Sun, X., Austin, T.O., Muralidharan, H., Jean, D.C., Liu, M., Yu, W., and Baas, P.W. (2018). Tau Does Not Stabilize Axonal Microtubules but Rather Enables Them to Have Long Labile Domains. Curr Biol **28**, 2181–2189 e2184. 10.1016/j.cub.2018.05.045.

Qiu, J., Cai, D., Dai, H., McAtee, M., Hoffman, P.N., Bregman, B.S., and Filbin, M.T. (2002). Spinal axon regeneration induced by elevation of cyclic AMP. Neuron **34**, 895–903.

Qu, Y., Hahn, I., Lees, M., Parkin, J., Voelzmann, A., Dorey, K., Rathbone, A., Friel, C.T., Allan, V.J., Okenve-Ramos, P., et al. (2019). Efa6 protects axons and regulates their growth and branching by inhibiting microtubule polymerisation at the cortex. Elife **8**. 10.7554/eLife.50319.

Rahman-Enyart, A., Lai, C., and Prieto, A.L. (2020). Neuregulins 1, 2, and 3 Promote Early Neurite Outgrowth in ErbB4-Expressing Cortical GABAergic Interneurons. Mol Neurobiol **57**, 3568–3588. 10.1007/s12035-020-01966-7.

Ramazi, S., and Zahiri, J. (2021). Posttranslational modifications in proteins: resources, tools and prediction methods. Database (Oxford) **2021**. 10.1093/database/baab012.

Rosso, S., Bollati, F., Bisbal, M., Peretti, D., Sumi, T., Nakamura, T., Quiroga, S., Ferreira, A., and Caceres, A. (2004). LIMK1 regulates Golgi dynamics, traffic of Golgi-derived vesicles, and process extension in primary cultured neurons. Mol Biol Cell **15**, 3433–3449. 10.1091/mbc.e03-05-0328.

Saunders, H.A.J., Johnson-Schlitz, D.M., Jenkins, B.V., Volkert, P.J., Yang, S.Z., and Wildonger, J. (2022). Acetylated alpha-tubulin K394 regulates microtubule stability to shape the growth of axon terminals. Curr Biol **32**, 614–630 e615. 10.1016/j.cub.2021.12.012.

Schechter, M., Grigoletto, J., Abd-Elhadi, S., Glickstein, H., Friedman, A., Serrano, G.E., Beach, T.G., and Sharon, R. (2020). A role for alpha-Synuclein in axon growth and its implications in corticostriatal glutamatergic plasticity in Parkinson's disease. Mol Neurodegener **15**, 24. 10.1186/s13024-020-00370-y.

Schelski, M., and Bradke, F. (2017). Neuronal polarization: From spatiotemporal signaling to cytoskeletal dynamics. Mol Cell Neurosci **84**, 11–28. 10.1016/j.mcn.2017.03.008.

Schmidt, H., Stonkute, A., Juttner, R., Koesling, D., Friebe, A., and Rathjen, F.G. (2009). C-type natriuretic peptide (CNP) is a bifurcation factor for sensory neurons. Proc Natl Acad Sci U S A **106**, 16847–16852.

Schmidt, H., Stonkute, A., Juttner, R., Schaffer, S., Buttgereit, J., Feil, R., Hofmann, F., and Rathjen, F.G. (2007a). The receptor guanylyl cyclase Npr2 is essential for sensory axon bifurcation within the spinal cord. J Cell Biol **179**, 331–340.

Schmidt, W.M., Kraus, C., Hoger, H., Hochmeister, S., Oberndorfer, F., Branka, M., Bingemann, S., Lassmann, H., Muller, M., Macedo-Souza, L.I., et al. (2007b). Mutation in the Scyl1 gene encoding amino-terminal kinase-like protein causes a recessive form of spinocerebellar neurodegeneration. EMBO Rep **8**, 691–697. 10.1038/sj.embor.7401001.

Slater, P.G., Cammarata, G.M., Samuelson, A.G., Magee, A., Hu, Y., and Lowery, L.A. (2019). XMAP215 promotes microtubule-F-actin interactions to regulate growth cone microtubules during axon guidance in Xenopus laevis. J Cell Sci **132**. 10.1242/jcs.224311.

Southam, K.A., Stennard, F., Pavez, C., and Small, D.H. (2019). Knockout of Amyloid beta Protein Precursor (APP) Expression Alters Synaptogenesis, Neurite Branching and Axonal Morphology of Hippocampal Neurons. Neurochem Res **44**, 1346–1355. 10.1007/s11064-018-2512-0.

Spillane, M., Ketschek, A., Merianda, T.T., Twiss, J.L., and Gallo, G. (2013). Mitochondria coordinate sites of axon branching through localized intra-axonal protein synthesis. Cell reports **5**, 1564–1575.

Stack, J.H., Whitney, M., Rodems, S.M., and Pollok, B.A. (2000). A ubiquitin-based tagging system for controlled modulation of protein stability. Nature Biotechnology **18**, 1298–1302. 10.1038/82422.

Stefanis, L. (2012). -Synuclein in Parkinson's Disease. Cold Spring Harbor Perspectives in Medicine **2**, a009399-a009399. 10.1101/cshperspect.a009399.

Suk, T.R., and Rousseaux, M.W.C. (2020). The role of TDP-43 mislocalization in amyotrophic lateral sclerosis. Molecular Neurodegeneration **15**. 10.1186/s13024-020-00397-1.

Svitkina, T. (2018). The Actin Cytoskeleton and Actin-Based Motility. Cold Spring Harb Perspect Biol **10**. 10.1101/cshperspect.a018267.

Takano, T., Funahashi, Y., and Kaibuchi, K. (2019). Neuronal Polarity: Positive and Negative Feedback Signals. Front Cell Dev Biol **7**, 69. 10.3389/fcell.2019.00069.

Tuszynski, M.H., and Steward, O. (2012). Concepts and methods for the study of axonal regeneration in the CNS. Neuron **74**, 777–791. 10.1016/j. neuron.2012.05.006.

Tymanskyj, S.R., and Ma, L. (2019). MAP7 Prevents Axonal Branch Retraction by Creating a Stable Microtubule Boundary to Rescue Polymerization. J Neurosci **39**, 7118–7131. 10.1523/JNEUROSCI.0775-19.2019.

Tymanskyj, S.R., Yang, B., Falnikar, A., Lepore, A.C., and Ma, L. (2017). MAP7 regulates axon collateral branch development in dorsal root ganglion neurons. J Neurosci **37**, 1648–1661. 10.1523/JNEUROSCI.3260-16.2017.

Tymanskyj, S.R., Yang, B.H., Verhey, K.J., and Ma, L. (2018). MAP7 regulates axon morphogenesis by recruiting kinesin-1 to microtubules and modulating organelle transport. Elife **7**. 10.7554/eLife.36374.

Ulisse, V., Dey, S., Rothbard, D.E., Zeevi, E., Gokhman, I., Dadosh, T., Minis, A., and Yaron, A. (2020). Regulation of axonal morphogenesis by the mitochondrial protein Efhd1. Life Sci Alliance **3**. 10.26508/lsa.202000753.

Van Battum, E.Y., Brignani, S., and Pasterkamp, R.J. (2015). Axon guidance proteins in neurological disorders. Lancet Neurol **14**, 532–546. 10.1016/s1474-4422(14)70257-1.

Vickers, J.C., King, A.E., Woodhouse, A., Kirkcaldie, M.T., Staal, J.A., Mccormack, G.H., Blizzard, C.A., Musgrove, R.E.J., Mitew, S., Liu, Y., et al. (2009). Axonopathy and cytoskeletal disruption in degenerative diseases of the central nervous system. Brain Research Bulletin **80**, 217–223. 10.1016/j.brainresbull.2009.08.004.

Wang, B., Wang, Z., Sun, L., Yang, L., Li, H., Cole, A.L., Rodriguez-Rivera, J., Lu, H.-C., and Zheng, H. (2014). The Amyloid Precursor Protein Controls Adult Hippocampal Neurogenesis through GABAergic Interneurons. Journal of Neuroscience **34**, 13314–13325. 10.1523/jneurosci.2848-14.2014.

Wang, K.H., Brose, K., Arnott, D., Kidd, T., Goodman, C.S., Henzel, W., and Tessier-Lavigne, M. (1999). Biochemical purification of a mammalian slit protein as a positive regulator of sensory axon elongation and branching. Cell **96**, 771–784.

Winkle, C.C., McClain, L.M., Valtschanoff, J.G., Park, C.S., Maglione, C., and Gupton, S.L. (2014). A novel Netrin-1-sensitive mechanism promotes local SNARE-mediated exocytosis during axon branching. J Cell Biol **205**, 217–232. 10.1083/jcb.201311003.

Winkle, C.C., Taylor, K.L., Dent, E.W., Gallo, G., Greif, K.F., and Gupton, S.L. (2016). Beyond the cytoskeleton: The emerging role of organelles and membrane remodeling in the regulation of axon collateral branches. Dev Neurobiol. 10.1002/dneu.22398.

Winnubst, J., Spruston, N., and Harris, J.A. (2020). Linking axon morphology to gene expression: a strategy for neuronal cell-type classification. Current Opinion in Neurobiology **65**, 70–76.

Wloga, D., Joachimiak, E., Louka, P., and Gaertig, J. (2017). Posttranslational Modifications of Tubulin and Cilia. Cold Spring Harb Perspect Biol **9**. 10.1101/cshperspect.a028159.

Wong, H.H.-W., Lin, J.Q., Ströhl, F., Roque, C.G., Cioni, J.-M., Cagnetta, R., Turner-Bridger, B., Laine, R.F., Harris, W.A., and Kaminski, C.F. (2017). RNA docking and local translation regulate site-specific axon remodeling in vivo. Neuron **95**, 852–868. e858.

Woo, Y., Kim, S.J., Suh, B.K., Kwak, Y., Jung, H.J., Nhung, T.T.M., Mun, D.J., Hong, J.H., Noh, S.J., Kim, S., et al. (2019). Sequential phosphorylation of NDEL1 by the DYRK2-GSK3beta complex is critical for neuronal morphogenesis. Elife **8**. 10.7554/eLife.50850.

Xie, Q., Li, J., Li, H., Udeshi, N.D., Svinkina, T., Orlin, D., Kohani, S., Guajardo, R., Mani, D.R., Xu, C., et al. (2022). Transcription factor Acj6 controls dendrite targeting via a combinatorial cell-surface code. Neuron. 10.1016/j.neuron.2022.04.026.

Yamashita, N., Mosinger, B., Roy, A., Miyazaki, M., Ugajin, K., Nakamura, F., Sasaki, Y., Yamaguchi, K., Kolattukudy, P., and Goshima, Y. (2011). CRMP5 (collapsin response mediator protein 5) regulates dendritic development and synaptic plasticity in the cerebellar Purkinje cells. J Neurosci **31**, 1773–1779. 10.1523/JNEUROSCI.5337-10.2011.

Yang, Y., Kim, A.H., and Bonni, A. (2010). The dynamic ubiquitin ligase duo: Cdh1-APC and Cdc20-APC regulate neuronal morphogenesis and connectivity. Curr Opin Neurobiol **20**, 92–99. 10.1016/j.conb.2009.12.004.

Yaniv, S.P., Meltzer, H., Alyagor, I., and Schuldiner, O. (2020). Developmental axon regrowth and primary neuron sprouting utilize distinct actin elongation factors. J Cell Biol **219**. 10.1083/jcb.201903181.

Yu, T.W., Hao, J.C., Lim, W., Tessier-Lavigne, M., and Bargmann, C.I. (2002). Shared receptors in axon guidance: SAX-3/Robo signals via UNC-34/Enabled and a Netrin-independent UNC-40/DCC function. Nat Neurosci **5**, 1147–1154.

Yu, W., Qiang, L., Solowska, J.M., Karabay, A., Korulu, S., and Baas, P.W. (2008). The Microtubule-severing Proteins Spastin and Katanin Participate Differently in the Formation of Axonal Branches. Molecular biology of the cell **19**, 1485–1498. 10.1091/mbc.E07-09-0878.

Yuste, R., Hawrylycz, M., Aalling, N., Aguilar-Valles, A., Arendt, D., Armañanzas, R., Ascoli, G.A., Bielza, C., Bokharaie, V., and Bergmann, T.B. (2020). A community-based transcriptomics classification and nomenclature of neocortical cell types. Nature neuroscience **23**, 1456–1468.

Zhang, M., Ergin, V., Lin, L., Stork, C., Chen, L., and Zheng, S. (2019). Axonogenesis Is Coordinated by Neuron-Specific Alternative Splicing Programming and Splicing Regulator PTBP2. Neuron **101**, 690–706 e610. 10.1016/j.neuron.2019.01.022.

Zhao, Z., and Ma, L. (2009). Regulation of axonal development by natriuretic peptide hormones. Proc Natl Acad Sci U S A **106**, 18016–18021.

Zhao, Z., Wang, Z., Gu, Y., Feil, R., Hofmann, F., and Ma, L. (2009). Regulate axon branching by the cyclic GMP pathway via inhibition of glycogen synthase kinase 3 in dorsal root ganglion sensory neurons. J Neurosci **29**, 1350–1360.

Zhou, L., Miller, B.L., Mcdaniel, C.H., Kelly, L., Kim, O.J., and Miller, C.A. (1998). Frontotemporal dementia: Neuropil spheroids and presynaptic terminal degeneration. Annals of Neurology **44**, 99–109. 10.1002/ana.410440116.

2

Experience-dependent Structural Plasticity in Dendrite Development: Emerging Common Themes Across Model Systems

Justin Rosenthal and Quan Yuan

Dendrite Morphogenesis and Plasticity Unit, National Institute of
Neurological Disorders and Stroke, National Institutes of Health, USA
Corresponding Email: quan.yuan@nih.gov

Abstract

From flies to humans, the nervous system of animals is remarkably adept at
modifying itself in response to altered neuronal activity. One crucial component underlying this robust plasticity is a complex array of cellular and
molecular changes occurring on the dendritic arbor of postsynaptic neurons.
Both local events at the synapse, as well as broader effects, such as cell surface receptor-to-nuclear signaling, work together to adjust various features
of neuronal dendrites, including branching patterns, arbor size, spine density
and maturity. How dendrites respond to experience and activity are also influenced by their cellular environment and neighboring cells, such as astrocytes
and microglia. With updated research methods and new technologies, these
phenomena remain subjects of intense investigations. Studying dendrite plasticity not only helps us understand fundamental principles guiding the construction and modifications of circuit connectivity, but also begin to uncover
root causes for a wide spectrum of neurodevelopmental disorders and neuropsychiatric diseases.

Introduction

One of the essential features of our nervous system is its ability to adapt
to changes in both internal and external environments. How this flexibility

45

is regulated during development and in adulthood, and how it is altered in disease or injury, are fundamental questions that have long captivated neurobiologists' attention. Classic works performed a half century ago in the mammalian visual and somatosensory cortex demonstrated the profound influence of sensory experience on cortical development, and established activity-dependent modifications of neuronal structure and connectivity as critical components of circuit development and remodeling (LeVay, Wiesel et al. 1980, Katz and Shatz 1996) . During the past few decades, through extensive studies using a variety of experimental paradigms and model systems, we have learned that the way a neuron or a circuit responds to sensory experience or neural activity is largely determined by its genetic and cellular contexts, and directly linked to its functional properties. With recent technical innovations and the addition of invertebrate models, the repertoire of phenotypes and underlying molecular pathways associated with experience-dependent plasticity have been further enriched. At the same time, these advances also offer opportunities for comparative studies and help us extract common themes shared across systems.

In this chapter, we will focus on experience-dependent plasticity in dendrite and spine development. Amongst many dynamic cellular events occurring throughout circuit construction and remodeling, dendritic growth and patterning are particularly prone to the influences of experience (Wong and Ghosh 2002). In addition, altered spine dynamics and morphology are considered the cellular substrates for memory storage and are linked to cognitive decline observed in human neurological disorders (Nithianantharajah and Hannan 2006, Forrest, Parnell et al. 2018). There is a large body of literature accumulated on this topic, which we won't be able to cover adequately within the scope of this chapter. Instead, we will first briefly introduce some of the classic studies while referring the readers to broader and more detailed descriptions in excellent review articles (Whitford, Dijkhuizen et al. 2002, Smith, Heynen et al. 2009). We will then discuss the expression and regulation of structural plasticity in developing dendrites and compare studies performed in vertebrate and invertebrate model systems. Next, we will summarize the key molecular events induced by neuronal activity and sensory experience. Lastly, we will review exciting new discoveries exploring the role of non-autonomous contributions, such as neuron-glia interactions, in regulating dendritic plasticity, as well as shared molecular underpinnings between altered dendrite and spine morphology and human neurodevelopmental disorders. Despite the overwhelming degree of complexity and diversity associated with dendritic plasticity, and the many remaining questions, the molecular insights we have gained and the ever-growing new discoveries enabled by updated technologies have begun to reveal general principles and common pathways governing the dendrite morphogenesis and plasticity in central nervous systems across the animal kingdom.

2.1 Diverse Outcomes Associated with Experience-dependent Dendritic Plasticity

To study experience-dependent dendrite plasticity, numerous model systems have been adopted and each has its unique advantages. Collaboratively, they built the foundation of our knowledge on how developing nervous systems adapt to changes. Early studies have shown that monocular deprivation alters dendrite distribution in the lateral geniculate nucleus and visual cortex (Wiesel and Hubel 1963, Lendvai, Stern et al. 2000, Alvarez and Sabatini 2007), while the enriched environment for motor learning increases dendritic growth and branching in cortical neurons (Volkmar and Greenough 1972, Withers and Greenough 1989). More recently, *in vivo* time lapse imaging of *Xenopus* retinotectal neurons have provided compelling demonstrations of the close relationship between sensory input and dendritic development, where visual stimuli promote dendrite growth (Sin, Haas et al. 2002). Besides regulating growth, experience and synaptic activity also regulate dendritic branching patterns through dendritic remodeling, during which diffusely distributed dendrites retract and only correctly projected dendrites remain, ensuring the proper establishment of specified connectivity patterns during circuit maturation. Both mitral cells in the olfactory system and retinal ganglion cells are classic examples of activity-dependent dendrite remodeling (Malun and Brunjes 1996, Wang, Liets et al. 2001). With the development of two photon imaging techniques and genetically encoded synapse markers, the broad influence of sensory deprivation on both developing and established cortical circuits has been directly demonstrated *in vivo*, including reduced spine elimination in somatosensory cortex (Zuo, Yang et al. 2005), elevated rate of spine formation in visual cortex (Hofer, Mrsic-Flogel et al. 2009) and the abnormal pruning of dendrites in retinal ganglion cells (Tian and Copenhagen 2003). Thus, sensory influences on dendritic structure appear to be ubiquitous and exhibit a great deal of complexity and diversity.

Apart from making the obvious distinctions based on cell types and animal species, two additional factors must be taken into consideration to evaluate dendrite plasticity induced by sensory experience or activity: the cellular substrates being studied and quantified, such as dendrite length, volume, or branch dynamics; and the time window when the experiments are performed and the data are collected. The importance of these two factors is clearly demonstrated by studies summarized below.

2.1.1 Sensory experience impacts mammalian cortical development

Mammalian cortical development is broadly influenced by sensory experience. Cortical regions corresponding to visual and somatosensory systems are the two most heavily investigated areas and offer unique insights into how sensory deprivation affects circuit development and function in general. Descriptions of findings in other systems, such as auditory, motor, and navigation circuits, can be found in additional reviews (Fu and Zuo 2011).

Somatosensory cortex: In rodent primary somatosensory cortex (S1), the barrel cortex processes whisker-related information. The topographic pattern, or the distinct "barrels", can be disrupted by the ablation of vibrissae follicles. Almost 50 years ago, Van Der Loos and Woolsey first discovered that ablating a whisker follicle at birth disrupts the development of corresponding cortical representation of that whisker, while ablating the vibrissae follicles on the contralateral mystacial pad leads to a reorganization of the barrel patterning (Van der Loos and Woolsey 1973). These large-scale effects on barrel organization are most prominent during a developmental critical period and diminish in mature animals (Weller and Johnson 1975, Woolsey, Dierker et al. 1975).

In the following decades, researchers developed many techniques to produce sensory deprivation in the whisker-to-barrel system, including electrocauterization of whisker follicles, infraorbital nerve (ION) lesions, and whisker trimming in different patterns. Whisker follicle ablation at birth produces long lasting behavioral consequences, leading to reduced sensitivity even after whisker regrowth (Carvell and Simons 1996). In contrast, whisker trimming, a mild form of manipulation, leads to expansion of receptive fields and increased excitability of the barrel cells corresponding to the spared whiskers (Keller and Carlson 1999, Knott, Quairiaux et al. 2002). These manipulations also impose diverse impacts on the dendrite morphology in neurons occupying multiple cortical layers. Among many cell types in the neocortex, pyramidal and spiny stellate cells are the main excitatory glutamatergic types, while the basket, chandelier, double bouquet, and Martinotti cells are inhibitory GABAergic neurons. Consistent with their different functional roles, excitatory and inhibitory neurons show distinct responses to alterations in sensory experience. For instance, bilateral whisker trimming through the first postnatal month leads to dendrite expansion in layer 6 non-pyramidal neurons. The nearby pyramidal cells, however, showed increases in soma size and basilar dendritic arborization but a reduction in the apical dendrites (Chen, Steger et al. 2009, Chen, Tam et al. 2012). A similar redistribution of dendritic arbors was observed in layer 5 pyramidal neurons following one week of whisker trimming. On the other hand, GABAergic neurons in layer 5 only exhibit subtle changes in their dendritic processes (Zhang, Gao et al. 2013).

Given the variety of experimental techniques and the heterogeneity of cortical neurons, it is not surprising to observe a large range of sensory deprivation-induced phenotypes in the developing barrel cortex (Reviewed by (Chen and Brumberg 2021)). Importantly, the extent of the impact is significantly influenced by the timing and duration of experimental manipulation. In general, early onset of sensory deprivation, before postnatal day 4 (PND4), when the barrel pattern emerges, can cause changes in dendrite growth and patterning. By contrast, sensory deprivation applied in late juvenile developmental stages or adulthood does not lead to measurable changes in dendrite morphology. Instead, the main phenotypes are changes in the number, density, and dynamics of spines (Tian and Copenhagen 2003).

Although structural plasticity in dendritic spines has long been observed, fluorescent labeling techniques and multi-photon microscopy developed in recent years allow researchers to perform *in vivo* time-lapse imaging in living animals. These longitudinal studies helped reveal the dynamic features of spines and demonstrate how sensory experience and various learning paradigms impact circuit connectivity through changes in spine morphology and density. Similar to the case in dendrites, structural plasticity in spines also varies a great deal depending on the cell type, the timing and technique of the experimental manipulations and the specific parameters being evaluated. In general, sensory manipulation by whisker trimming affects spine motility and turnover during the early postnatal developmental period. In rats, trimming all whiskers unilaterally decreases both spine and filopodium motility in the contralateral barrel cortex during P11–13, without affecting spine size or density (Lendvai, Stern et al. 2000). In adolescent mice (1–3 months), sensory deprivation induced by plucking all whiskers on one side reduces spine elimination and delays spine pruning in the contralateral barrel cortex (Zuo, Yang et al. 2005). This diminishes as animals mature but persists into adulthood. Restoring sensory experience after the adolescent period accelerates spine elimination (Zuo, Yang et al. 2005). Interestingly, sensory stimulation induced by either an enriched environment or unilateral chessboard plucking increases spine turnover in this same brain region. In adult mice (>4 months), sensory manipulation continues to modify spine dynamics, but to a milder degree (Zuo, Yang et al. 2005). Together, studies of spine dynamics in the somatosensory cortex suggest that experience plays an important role in the net loss of synapses over an animal's lifetime, particularly during adolescence (Trachtenberg, Chen et al. 2002, Holtmaat, Wilbrecht et al. 2006, Yang, Pan et al. 2009).

Visual cortex: The mammalian visual cortex is another system highly amenable for investigating the role of sensory experience in regulating circuit development and plasticity. The visual activity can be manipulated relatively easily by raising animals in the dark, or by depriving visual input from one (monocular deprivation, MD) or both (binocular deprivation, BD) eyes. In addition, neurons in primary visual cortex (V1) and somatosensory cortex (S1) share common features in their dendritic organization (Staiger, Flagmeyer et al. 2004). Many of the principles regulating dendrite and spine plasticity in the somatosensory cortex also apply to the visual cortex (Fox and Wong 2005).

Because most mammals are born with their eyes closed, the initial activity-dependent wiring events are driven by spontaneous retinal activity (Del Rio and Feller 2006). Previous studies have shown that eye-specific segregation in the lateral geniculate nucleus (LGN) is regulated by spontaneous retinal waves, which are bursts of action potentials that spread across the retinal ganglion cell (RGC) layer before eye opening (Penn, Riquelme et al. 1998, Huberman, Stellwagen et al. 2002, Stellwagen and Shatz 2002, Feller 2009). After eye opening, however, patterned visual input is thought to be the main driver of maturation of the visual cortical circuit (Smith and Trachtenberg 2007). One example is the experience-dependent dendrite remodeling observed in the RGCs. RGCs reorganize their structure during development to restrict dendritic branching to either light-ON or light-OFF only lamina. This pruning event does not occur in dark-reared animals (Tian and Copenhagen 2003). In addition, dark rearing in mice or rats leads to a reduced number of spines in pyramidal cells of the V1 and a shifted distribution of dendritic branching of layer 4 stellate cells, potentially due to the loss of input within specific layers (Borges and Berry 1978, Majewska and Sur 2003, Tropea, Majewska et al. 2010).

In the 1960s, Hubel and Wiesel performed a series of experiments to demonstrate the strong impact of monocular deprivation on the establishment of ocular dominance columns (Hubel and Wiesel 1963, Wiesel and Hubel 1963). Monocular lid suture in visually inexperienced binocular mammals led to redistribution of afferents from the LGN in layer 4 and changed dendritic branching in spiny stellate cells (Kossel, Lowel et al. 1995). Physiologically, unbalanced input from the two eyes leads to bi-directional changes in visual cortex circuity (Smith, Heynen et al. 2009), rapid weakening of responses evoked through the deprived eye, followed by delayed strengthening of responses through the open eye. These seminal studies established ocular dominance plasticity (ODP) as a classic model for understanding how experience shapes circuit architecture and function during development (Wong and Ghosh 2002, Tropea, Van Wart et al. 2009, Sun, Espinosa et al. 2019).

Importantly, a series of experiments studying ODP have contributed to a molecular understanding of the mechanism controlling the opening and closing of the critical period. While cortical circuits have a distinct window of sensitivity towards activity manipulations, the sensitivity to MD is restricted to a critical period, which begins about 1 week after the eye opens (PND13) and peaks 1 month after birth in mice (Gordon and Stryker 1996). Studies by Tako Hensch and colleagues have shown that the onset of ODP can be delayed by preventing the maturation of GABA-mediated transmission through genetic deletion of Gad65, a gene encoding a GABA-synthetic enzyme, or by dark-rearing from birth (Hensch, Fagiolini et al. 1998, Morales, Choi et al. 2002, Maffei, Nelson et al. 2004). Conversely, the critical period can be advanced by enhancing GABA transmission using Benzodiazepines right after eye-opening, or by promoting interneuron maturation through Brain-Derived Neurotrophic Factor (BDNF) overexpression (Hanover, Huang et al. 1999, Huang, Kirkwood et al. 1999, Iwai, Fagiolini et al. 2003, Fagiolini, Fritschy et al. 2004).

Although V1 of rodents does not contain ocular dominance columns, a discrete binocular segment has been used extensively to characterize structural and functional rearrangement of cortical circuity in response to alteration in experience. One notable study was designed to capture synaptic restructuring following MD and tested whether the structural impact of the MD experience would outlast the functional changes. Using long-term live imaging studies, the dynamics of dendritic filopodia and spines were systematically evaluated in the binocular region (Hofer, Mrsic-Flogel et al. 2009). These results revealed that sensory experience leaves a long-lasting structural trace that facilitates the functional adaptations at a later time, suggesting a mechanism for storing prior experiences in cortical circuits.

2.1.2 Xenopus retinotectal system

Another classic system that offered many insights into the mechanisms of experience-dependent plasticity is the optic tectum of *Xenopus laevis* tadpoles, established by Hollis Cline and colleagues in the 1990s (Sin, Haas et al. 2002, Ruthazer, Akerman et al. 2003, Dong, Lee et al. 2009, Xu,

Khakhalin et al. 2011, Hiramoto and Cline 2014). This system allows genetically encoded morphology and synapse markers to be introduced into the specific region of developing tadpoles by electroporation, generating single-labeled tectal neurons that can be monitored throughout development by *in vivo* time-lapse imaging and electrophysiology. In a particularly informative study, Sin et al observed enhanced visual activity promotes dendritic arbor growth, which requires NMDA-mediated glutamatergic transmission (Sin, Haas et al. 2002).

A series of studies using this powerful system have further demonstrated how visual experience regulates dendritic arbor development through effects on both excitatory glutamatergic and inhibitory GABAergic synaptic transmission. Visual stimulation promotes maturation of the excitatory synapse by increasing the ratio of AMPA/NMDA type of glutamate receptors, which leads to the elaboration of dendritic arbors. Expressing the C-terminal peptides of GluA (GluA CTP) impairs AMPA Receptor (AMPAR) trafficking, reduces the number of excitatory synapses and decreases complexity of dendritic arbors (Haas, Li et al. 2006). Conversely, expressing the intracellular fragment of the GABA-Ag2 subunit reduces $GABA_A R$ presence at synapses, decreases inhibitory synaptic inputs, while also causing reduced complexity of dendritic arbors (Shen, Da Silva et al. 2009). These genetic manipulations prevent visual activity-dependent enhancement of dendrite arbor growth, supporting the critical function of synapse maturation in driving dendrite arbor development. Importantly, these observations are consistent with predications of the 'synaptotrophic hypothesis', originally proposed by Vaughn based on insight from electron microscopy studies, suggesting that synapse formation promotes the further elaboration of neuronal structures and ultimately circuit formation (Vaughn, Barber et al. 1988, Vaughn 1989).

Studies in *Xenopus* optic tectal neurons have placed synaptic integration of postsynaptic receptors, namely glutamatergic AMPA and NMDA receptors, as the major event regulating synapse maturation and dendrite elaboration. Several other factors involved in this process have since been identified through studies in the optic tectum, including neurexin-neuroligin cell adhesion complexes, glycosylphosphatidylinositol (GPI)-linked protein CPG15 and transcription factor MEF2 (Chen, Tari et al. 2010). Furthermore, experiments have shown that activity-dependent mechanisms can also restrict dendritic arbor growth. For example, elevated calcium and calmodulin-dependent kinase II (CaMKII) activity increases glutamatergic synaptic strength while stabilizing dendritic arbor structure by reducing rates of branch additions and retractions (Wu, Malinow et al. 1996, Wu and Cline 1998) . CaMKII is known to act downstream of synaptic activity-dependent increases in calcium to regulate synaptic strength and cytoskeletal dynamics, consistent with this observation (Lisman, Schulman et al. 2002, McVicker, Millette et al. 2015). More recently, Protein kinase Mζ (PKMz), an endogenous constitutively active kinase, was identified as a stabilizing factor for dendritic filopodia and restricts dendritic arbor growth (Liu, Tari et al. 2009).

While most of studies in *Xenopus* optic tectum have been performed on excitatory neurons, a recent study also evaluated experience-dependent morphological and physiological changes in inhibitory neurons. These results indicated that developing inhibitory neurons in the tectum, without applying distinguishable molecular markers, can be clustered into two groups that respond to visual stimulations in opposite ways (He, Shen et al. 2016). Half of them showed similar responses as excitatory neurons; upon visual stimulation, their dendritic arbor size and calcium response are both increased. The other half had reduced a dendrite size and calcium response. This study raised the interesting possibility that the inhibitory interneurons act as stabilizers in experience-induced circuit changes and contribute to maintaining Excitation/Inhibition balance during circuit development.

2.1.3 Developing motor and visual circuit in *Drosophila* exhibit homeostatic dendritic plasticity

Many of the initial molecular insights on neural plasticity have come from studies using simple invertebrate systems, such as *Aplysia* and *Drosophila*, which were excellent models for analyzing fundamental aspects of behavior and learning. The work by Eric Kandel and others have illustrated critical functions of members of the cAMP signaling pathway in activity-dependent synaptic potentiation, which were later demonstrated to be a conserved mechanism in many other animal models and were further linked to behavioral modifications such as learning and memory storage (Silva, Kogan et al. 1998). In recent years, powerful genetic systems have allowed *Drosophila* and *C. elegans* models to reveal important principles governing neural development and circuit organization (Dong, Shen et al. 2015). Notably, high-resolution *in vivo* imaging techniques, combined with large-scale forward genetic screens, have facilitated the identification of genetic mutants with defects in various aspects of dendrite development (Grueber and Jan 2004, Jan and Jan 2010, Hong, Park et al. 2014). Although coming on the scene relatively late, fly models have also been informative for questions related to dendrite plasticity and highlighted activity-dependent modifications as a common theme in neural development.

In the motor circuit of the *Drosophila* larval ventral nerve cord (VNC), dendrite morphology in the aCC and RP2 motoneurons are highly sensitive to synaptic activity. Here, homeostatic adjustments in dendrite fields are observed upon changes in presynaptic activity. The embryonic aCC motoneuron dendrite expands or shrinks following inhibited or enhanced neurotransmitter activity, respectively (Tripodi, Evers et al. 2008). Reducing intrinsic excitability during development, either through a temperature-sensitive mutant allele that reduces presynaptic acetylcholine release, or by overexpressing a transgene encoding the potassium channel Kir2.1 in the postsynaptic neurons, both led to an enlarged dendrite arbor size (Hartwig, Worrell et al. 2008). These studies were among the first to describe the activity-dependent homeostatic regulation of dendritic structures, which were later found in other *Drosophila* and mammalian systems (Yuan, Xiang et al. 2011, Kaneko and Stryker 2017), suggesting that structural homeostasis is a shared component in neural plasticity across animal species.

Taking advantage of the genetic tools available to the *Drosophila* system, a series of studies explored the cellular and molecular mechanisms governing homeostatic plasticity in the larval motor circuit. Specifically, genetic studies have identified reactive oxygen species (ROS) signaling pathway as a major regulator of activity-dependent plasticity. The Parkinson's disease-linked protein DJ-1β acts as a redox sensor in neurons, modulates the PTEN-PI3Kinase pathway and regulates structural development of dendrites (Oswald, Brooks et al. 2018). Furthermore, by evaluating the activity-induced changes in motor neuron dendrites, a recent study identified a critical period for the larval motor circuit, which is within 8 hours of larval hatching and strongly modulated by astrocyte-derived cell adhesion signaling and microtubule dynamics (Ackerman, Perez-Catalan et al. 2021) (also see discussion in Section 3).

The larval visual system of *Drosophila* has also been developed into a successful model for understanding the molecular underpinnings of experience-dependent dendrite plasticity. *Drosophila* larvae sense light through Bolwig's Organ (BO), a cluster of photoreceptors that send axonal projections into the brain and make cholinergic synaptic contacts with dendritic arbors of ventral lateral neurons (LNvs) (Malpel, Klarsfeld et al. 2002, Sprecher, Cardona et al. 2011). Importantly, synaptic activity induced by visual experience produces striking changes in the length of LNv dendrites: the amount of light exposure received by the animal is inversely correlated with the total dendritic length of LNvs (Yuan, Xiang et al. 2011). Through neuron specific manipulations, Yuan et al. demonstrated that compensatory structural changes in dendritic arbors could be driven by sensory experience, alterations in presynaptic neurotransmission or activity, or changes in the intrinsic excitability of postsynaptic neurons (Yuan, Xiang et al. 2011). This unique model allowed systematic *in vivo* analyses to identify molecules and pathways that regulate dendritic plasticity. The follow-up live imaging and genetic studies revealed dynamic dendritic filopodia as the cellular substrate targeted by activity in regulating synaptogenesis and subsequent dendrite expansion. Additionally, RNA sequencing (RNA-seq) guided genetic screens further identified neuron-glia lipid trafficking and nicotinic acetylcholine receptor (nAchR) signaling as two key pathways regulating activity-induced dendritic plasticity in the larval visual circuit (Yin, Gibbs et al. 2018, Rosenthal, Yin et al. 2021).

Beyond the motor and visual systems, which clearly show an experience-dependent structural plasticity during larval development, there are massive neural remodeling events associated with metamorphosis that affect many other cell types in the fly nervous system. In particular, the dendrite remodeling of *Drosophila* multi-dendritic peripheral nervous system (PNS) neurons have been used as a model to understand the molecular cascade responsible for controlling the dendrite degeneration and regrowth during the pupal stage (Singh, VijayRaghavan et al. 2010, Kanamori, Kanai et al. 2013).

In addition to *Drosophila*, neurons of the invertebrate model *C. elegans* also display experience-dependent structural plasticity. For example, calcium-dependent activity in dendrites of the chemosensory URX neurons, which respond to environmental oxygen levels, drives the expansion of dendrite tips during development (Cohn, Cebul et al. 2020). In the motor circuit, Tetrodotoxin-induced dampening of cholinergic synaptic activity in larval animals leads to a reduction of GABAergic neurotransmission at the NMJ and an increase in Postsynaptic Density (PSD) size on the muscle (Barbagallo, Philbrook et al. 2017). Another instance occurs during the peculiar dendrite-axon polarity reversal of the DD motoneuron, known as DD remodeling. Here, ACR-12-positive nAchR clusters emerge on what is originally the axonal neurite around the L1-to-L2 developmental transition. Although manipulation of synaptic activity does not physically impact the resulting dendrite, heightened or reduced circuit activity accelerates and delays, respectively, the timing of this remodeling (Jin and Qi 2018).

Outlook: Despite the complex phenotypes observed in these diverse model systems at different developmental stages, several common components integral for dendrite plasticity are shared across the systems, such as the determinant role of critical period, the intimate relationship with synaptogenesis, and the vital functions of neurotransmitter receptor signaling. Comparative studies combining the power of connectomics and transcriptomics, as well as bioinformatics analysis, will help us better understand this critical process and how it evolves within different animal species to better serve their physiological functions.

2.2 Molecular Regulation of Dendritic Structural Plasticity

In the past few decades, a large amount of research has been dedicated to searching for cellular and molecular substrates underlying experience-dependent changes in the brain, with the goal of finding the neural basis of human cognition. As a result, several well-conserved molecular pathways associated with activity-dependent structural plasticity in the postsynaptic compartment and dendrites have been identified (Koleske 2013, Nakahata and Yasuda 2018). Moreover, recent advances in two powerful technical approaches, transcriptome analysis and genetic lineage studies, have provided many candidate genes related to neurodevelopmental disorders and neuropsychiatric diseases. Intriguingly, a large proportion of the risk factors revealed by these studies are also key components of the pathways known to be involved in synapse development and plasticity (Forrest, Parnell et al. 2018). Detailed molecular studies using animal models will greatly facilitate our understanding of the network controlling the timing and extent of neurons or circuits responses to experience or activity. They will also be indispensable for identifying target molecules to be tested in therapeutic interventions.

While there are stereotypical transcriptional programs and signaling pathways associated with dendrite development and morphogenesis (Whitford, Dijkhuizen et al. 2002, Lefebvre, Sanes et al. 2015), sensory experience and activity often elicit cell- and context-specific responses, which are molecularly more complex and less understood. One exception is the established role of calcium-dependent signaling. Most of the activity-induced signaling cascades are triggered by changes in intracellular calcium concentration, either through calcium influx generated by calcium-permeable neurotransmitter receptors and voltage-gated calcium channels (VGCCs) at the postsynaptic cell surface, or the Ryanodine and IP_3 receptors on the endoplasmic reticulum membrane (Lohmann and Bonhoeffer 2008, Kanamori, Kanai et al. 2013, Lee, Soares et al. 2016).

Regardless of the source, $Ca2^+$ ions entering the cytoplasm can bind to the protein Calmodulin (CaM). The Ca^{2+}/CaM complex then activates the serine/threonine kinase CaMKII, a hub for multiple signaling events induced by neural activity (Lucic, Greif et al. 2008, Lee, Escobedo-Lozoya et al. 2009). Following the initial CaMKII activation, there is a second phase of inter-subunit autophosphorylation on T286/287 of a or b subunits that leads to persistent activation of CaMKII, which continues even after the dissociation of the Ca2+/CaM complex. This extended response is thought to prolong CaMKII's activity in order to exert its long-lasting effects on synaptic modifications, both functionally and structurally (Chang, Nakahata et al. 2019). This notion is supported by the observation that continuous NMDAR-dependent increases in intracellular calcium enhance CaMKII activity without leading to additional CaM binding to CaMKII. Moreover, despite peak CaMKIIa activation at 0.5 seconds, an extended decay period renders CaMKII partially active for up to 1 minute (Chang, Parra-Bueno et al. 2017). Besides the conformational change, activated CaMKII is translocated from the dendrite shaft to stimulated spines, a process that requires microtubules and actin networks, and is anchored to PSD components such as NMDAR subunits (Lemieux, Labrecque et al. 2012, Lu, MacGillavry et al. 2014, Rangamani, Levy et al. 2016). The terminal step in the CaMKII cycle is its eventual silencing by proteins phosphatases like PP1 (Rangamani, Levy et al. 2016). Additionally, another autophosphorylation event at an alternative site, T305/T306, reduces the enzyme's kinase activity (Lucic, Greif et al. 2008). Together, these distinct mechanisms collaboratively support the versatile and critical role of CaMKII in Ca^{2+} mediated synaptic plasticity.

2.2.1 Rho GTPases and their regulators

One of the most important regulatory mechanisms for dendrite and spine development involves a group of proteins called the Rho GTPases, which are members of the Ras GTPase superfamily of GTP-binding proteins (Govek, Newey et al. 2005, Stankiewicz and Linseman 2014). Through GTP binding and subsequent hydrolysis, Rho GTPases undergo transitions between an active and inactive form, and are key components involved in experience-dependent structural plasticity. They impose their influence through actin cytoskeleton modulation, which results in changes in dynamics and morphology of dendritic arbors and spines. Early investigations were performed in *Xenopus* optic tectal neurons, where increased activity of Rac and Cdc42, two well-studied Rho GTPases, is required for visual stimulation-induced dendrite branch dynamics and arbor growth (Sin, Haas et al. 2002). Conversely, RhoA activation was found to inhibit dendrite branch extension (Li, Van Aelst et al. 2000, Li, Aizenman et al. 2002, Sin, Haas et al. 2002)

Because RhoA and Cdc42 are activated by CaMKII, these small GTPases are capable of relaying transient CaMKII activation to synapse-specific, long-lasting signaling required for structural plasticity. This critical role is demonstrated by a set of sophisticated imaging experiments. The spatial activation pattern of RhoA and Cdc42 were probed in single dendritic spines using 2-photon fluorescence lifetime imaging microscopy (2pFLIM) and glutamate uncaging in cultured pyramidal neurons (Murakoshi, Wang et al. 2011). Both RhoA and Cdc42 were rapidly activated in the stimulated spine, followed by a dynamic and persistent phase of activity that lasted more than 30 min. Activated RhoA, which was necessary for initiating dendrite spine growth, diffuses and leaves the spine, whereas activated Cdc42 remains in the spine and maintains its morphology. In addition to these examples, there are many additional reports on Rho GTPases' contributions to dendrite plasticity, as well as those of the Rab protein family, which was found to facilitate activity-dependent AMPA receptor trafficking to the spine (Gerges, Backos et al. 2004, Hayashi-Takagi, Yagishita et al. 2015).

Rho GTPase activity itself is controlled by Rho Guanine nucleotide exchange factor (RhoGEFs) and Rho GTPase activating protein (RhoGAPs), molecules that toggle the GTPase between active and inactive states, respectively. One representative example is Kalirin, a RhoGEF involved in dendrite morphogenesis in early development. The *Kalirin* knockout mice display reduced hippocampal and cortical spine density and simplified dendritic arbors (Ma, Kiraly et al. 2008, Xie, Cahill et al. 2010). Similar to the Rho GTPases, Kalirin activation is induced by CaMKII-dependent phosphorylation following NMDA receptor activation. Activated Kalirin promotes enlargement of pre-existing dendrite spines and synaptic recruitment of AMPA receptors (Xie, Srivastava et al. 2007, Herring and Nicoll 2016). Counteracting the RhoGEFs are the RhoGAPs, such as OPHN1, which has been linked to metabotropic glutamate receptor (mGluR)-induced synaptic AMPA receptor removal observed during hippocampal Long-term Depression (LTD) (Nadif Kasri, Nakano-Kobayashi et al. 2011). However, OPHN1 is also implicated in synaptic strengthening through increased AMPA receptor density at NMDA receptor-stimulated dendrite spines (Nadif Kasri, Nakano-Kobayashi et al. 2009). These findings strongly suggest a context-dependent basis for RhoGAP and RhoGEF functionality.

Ultimately, the various Rho GTPases act on their own downstream targets, such as WASP and WAVE complex (Costa, Dines et al. 2020, Duman, Blanco et al. 2021). Rac1 and Cdc42 converge on these proteins, which in turn regulate the actin-branching protein complex Arp2/3 (Soderling, Guire et al. 2007, Watson, Owen et al. 2017). Additionally, Rac1 activation also induces a parallel kinase cascade that results in suppression of the depolymerizing factor Cofilin and thus stabilization of spines (Duman, Blanco et al. 2021).

2.2.2 Local translation

In contrast to general protein synthesis machinery localized in the cell body, a plethora of transcripts coding for synapse-related molecules are deliberately trafficked to synaptic sites so that their translation may be coupled to synaptic transmission (Ju, Morishita et al. 2004, Smith, Starck et al. 2005, Cajigas, Tushev et al. 2012). Other translational components, such as ribosomes and mRNA-binding proteins, have also been found in both dendritic and axonal compartments (Cajigas, Tushev et al. 2012, Younts, Monday et al. 2016, Scarnati, Kataria et al. 2018, Hafner, Donlin-Asp et al. 2019, Biever, Glock et al. 2020). These mRNAs and ribosomes support local translation near synapses and are required for long-lasting forms of synaptic plasticity that are elicited by glutamate binding to NMDA receptors or group I mGluRs. For instance, in the Ventral Tegmental Area (VTA) of juvenile mice, mGluR-induced LTD depends on rapid production of nascent NR2A subunit polypeptides, which shifts the iGluR composition on dopaminergic neuron dendrites in favor of lower ion conductance (Mameli, Balland et al. 2007). A similar finding was made in cultured hippocampal neurons, where locally transcribed mRNAs for CaMKII, β-actin and PSD-95 were examined. The study showed not only did both Long-term Potentiation (LTP) and mGluR-dependent LTD require local translation, but synaptic activity also induces the accumulation of mRNA for these transcripts near spines, indicating that activity-dependent RNA translocation is an additional contributing factor for regulating local translation (Miller, Yasuda et al. 2002, Donlin-Asp, Polisseni et al. 2021). Further investigations have also revealed how the translation instigated by synaptic activity is coordinated. In dentate gyrus cells of the hippocampus, for example, generation of LTP relies on the local translation of the NR2A subunit, which requires the function of poly(A) polymerase Gld2, the phosphorylation of RNA-binding protein CPEB, as well as the removal and downregulation of the deadenylase PARN and translation inhibitor Ngd (Udagawa, Swanger et al. 2012). Additionally, the RNA Induced Silencing Complex (RISC) has a significant contribution in regulating local translation. For example, in cultured hippocampal neurons, NMDA receptor stimulation induces the cooperative activity of phosphorylated Ago2 and miR-134, which represses translation of the cytoskeletal regulator LIMK1 and leads to a reduction in the size of dendritic spines (Rajgor, Sanderson et al. 2018).

Recent live imaging studies further demonstrate how activity-dependent local translation occurs in a stepwise fashion over an extended period. In cultured hippocampal neurons, postsynaptic stimulation through glutamate uncaging causes the recruitment, and long-lasting localization up to several hours, of β-actin mRNA from surrounding regions of the dendrite shaft to the base of acutely expanding dendrite spines (Yoon, Wu et al. 2016), followed by the translation of these mRNA molecules and the deposition of nascent β-actin polypeptides along the periphery of spine heads. Another advancement made possible by live imaging is single-molecule tracking of individual mRNA transcripts and newly translated peptides. Several studies have used fluorescently labeled RNA and proteins to investigate the differences between cytoplasmic vs. ER-localized translation, burst vs. sporadic translation, and monosome- vs. polysome-based translation (Tatavarty, Ifrim et al. 2012, Ifrim, Williams et al. 2015, Wu, Eliscovich et al. 2016). Notably, a recent study revealed that, basal levels of burst-type translation, for transcripts including PSD-95, ARC and FMRP, is enhanced in *Fmr1* knockout animals, a clinically important finding relevant to Fragile X Syndrome discussed in Section 4 (Richter and Klann 2009).

2.2.3 Activity-dependent transcriptional activation

Activity-dependent structural plasticity requires activation of transcriptional programs that translate synaptic activity to long-lasting morphological and physiological changes. Although this process can be studied in the context of individual cell types and isolated activity regulated genes (ARGs), in more recent years the blossoming of transcriptomic approaches have provided a route for a global understanding of how hundreds or thousands of genes are coordinately altered by neuronal activity in a cell-type specific fashion (West and Greenberg 2011, Yap and Greenberg 2018). From technologies like microarrays, tissue-specific RNAseq and single-cell RNAseq, we have learned that excitatory and inhibitory synapses share common upstream immediate early gene(s), such as a Fos and Egr1, but differ in the downstream factors, including members of the MAPK signaling pathway (Spiegel, Mardinly et al. 2014, Lacar, Linker et al. 2016). These type of analyses have also been applied to the classical visual deprivation model and revealed that ocular dominance relies on the regulation of temporally distinct transcriptional programs, which are perturbed in a dark-rearing condition (Majdan and Shatz 2006).

One of the most studied transcription factors is cAMP Response Element Binding protein (CREB), which is involved in various intracellular signaling events, coordinating changes in neurons and other cell types. Studies have identified a wide variety of extracellular stimuli that induce CREB phosphorylation and activation. In neurons, the part is often played by several CaMK members, which are potentiated upon cytoplasmic calcium influx generated by neuronal activity (Richter and Klann 2009). Besides CaMKII, which we discussed earlier, the expression of a constitutively-active form of CaMKIV in the developing rat brain elevates hippocampal dendrite spine density, accompanied by enhanced LTP and NMDA receptor-dependent synaptic current, as well as enhanced dendrite growth in cortical neurons (Redmond, Kashani et al. 2002, Marie, Morishita et al. 2005).

While CREB is a transcription factor, its function is partially controlled by its interactions with additional factors such as CREST, CBP and the neuronal-specific chromatin remodeling complex nBAF. Collectively, they modulate calcium-dependent dendrite growth (Aizawa, Hu et al. 2004, Wu, Lessard et al. 2007). Apart from this protein complex, CREB activity can also synergize with that of MKK1 to regulate neuronal morphology in rat Layer 3 visual cortex (Suzuki, Zhou et al. 2007). In addition to integrating diverse inputs, CREB-mediated transcription induces expression of a varied group of genes, including the secreted TrkB ligand BDNF and miRNAs, such as miRNA132 (Abdolahi, Zare-Chahoki et al. 2022). By negatively regulating its target p250GAP, miRNA132 promotes the formation of GluR1-containing spines (Shieh, Hu et al. 1998, Impey, Davare et al. 2010) Finally, although the CaMK-CREB signaling axis represents a major conduit for enacting activity-dependent transcription, many other pathways contribute to the process. For instance, MEF2, a transcription factor, has been shown to play a critical role in activity-dependent structural and functional plasticity in both rat and mouse models (Shalizi, Gaudilliere et al. 2006, Tu, Akhtar et al. 2017). Notably, genetic mutations in *mef2* gene have been linked to human neurological disorders in recent studies (Shalizi, Gaudilliere et al. 2006, Pfeiffer, Zang et al. 2010, Tsai, Wilkerson et al. 2017, Tu, Akhtar et al. 2017).

The second phase of long-term, activity-dependent modifications involves the transcriptional upregulation of immediate early genes (IEG). IEGs are rapidly transcribed upon neuronal stimulation, then act as transcription factors to control the expression of a group of effector molecules responsible for morphological adjustments on dendrites and postsynaptic sites (Lefebvre, Sanes et al. 2015). One example of a well-characterized IEG is Arc, or Arg3.1. Several studies suggest a homeostatic function for Arc in the rodent forebrain. Overexpression of Arc, simulating activity-induced Arc upregulation, leads to reduced AMPAR-dependent currents and decreases postsynaptic presence of the GluR2 and GluR3 subunits (Rial Verde, Lee-Osbourne et al. 2006). Reducing Arc level through RNA interference or a mutant form of Arc has the opposite effect (Rial Verde, Lee-Osbourne et al. 2006). The function of Arc is further supported by other mutant studies. In

Arc mutant mice, although vision is seemingly normal and baseline synaptic activity is intact, the visual system no longer exhibits experience-dependent synaptic depression (Gao, Sossa et al. 2010, McCurry, Shepherd et al. 2010). Other classical IEGs include c-Fos, whose potentiated expression has often been used as an indicator for neuronal activation, as well as Nr4a1, a critical transcriptional regulator for actin cytoskeletal rearrangements and spine formation (Murphy, Worley et al. 1991, Qiu and Ghosh 2008).

IEGs are also an important transducer of activity-dependent changes at inhibitory synapses. The transcription factor Npas4, is thought to be exclusively expressed in neurons, while c-fos and Nr4a members which also mediate signaling in the immune and muscular system. Nspas4 has been demonstrated to control GABAergic synapse number in both cell culture systems and mouse hippocampal neurons (Maxwell and Muscat 2006, Lin, Bloodgood et al. 2008). By regulating a unique set of inhibitory-specific, late-acting target genes, Npas4 adjusts the density of dendritic- vs somatic inhibitory synapses on CA1 pyramidal neurons (Lin, Bloodgood et al. 2008, Bloodgood, Sharma et al. 2013, Spiegel, Mardinly et al. 2014). In addition, one of the downstream targets of Npas4 is BDNF, which is a critical factor for specifying the number of synapses at specific locations (Lin, Bloodgood et al. 2008, Bloodgood, Sharma et al. 2013, Spiegel, Mardinly et al. 2014). Thus, circuit-wide activity will be used to adjust both excitatory and inhibitory connections, albeit through potentially distinct pathways.

2.2.4 Molecular events identified in invertebrate studies

As mentioned in Section 1, studies on activity-dependent dendrite plasticity in the invertebrate system are relatively new compared to vertebrate studies. However, there are well-established examples of activity-induced transcriptional programs that regulate structural plasticity in the invertebrate CNS. In the larval and pupal *Drosophila* ventral nerve cord, nAchR-mediated activation of MN5 motoneuron transiently induces the expression of AP-1, the fly ortholog of c-Fos, to control dendrite arborization. Additionally, in the Mushroom Bodies (MB) of both flies and the moth *Bombyx mori*, the transcription factor Hr38, a homolog of mammalian Nr4a proteins, is upregulated by neuronal activity, sensory experience, and ethanol exposure (Fujita, Nagata et al. 2013, Adhikari, Orozco et al. 2019), although the impact of Hr38 transcription in the developing brain has yet to be characterized.

The high-throughput approaches, such as RNA sequencing, have also benefitted the study of invertebrate models. In *Drosophila*, activity-dependent changes to transcriptomic profiles have been investigated at both the CNS-wide and tissue-specific levels, the latter including dopaminergic and circadian-related cell populations (Chen, Rahman et al. 2016). The findings revealed several key differences between mammalian and fly ARGs. Specifically, the *Drosophila* ARGs were significantly longer than their mammalian counterparts and functionally less likely to be classified as transcription factors. In a developmental study looking at how chronic upregulation of synaptic activity, achieved by rearing in constant light, alters the transcriptome in LNvs of the larval visual circuit, the resulting differentially expressed (DE) genes are enriched in functional categories related to transcriptional regulation, morphogenesis, and lipid metabolism/trafficking. Two of these, the lipophorin receptors LpR1 and LpR2, are significantly upregulated by activity and are potentially involved in the enhanced lipid shuttling induced by homeostatic responses towards chronic elevation of input activity (Yin, Gibbs et al. 2018).

Outlook: Given the rapidly evolving technologies, the logical next step for molecular studies related to dendrite plasticity is to generate cell-type specific multi-omics datasets that provide a comprehensive view of molecular pathways involved in synapse development and plasticity. These newly developed methods will be indispensable for addressing some of the current challenges and questions, including how neurons transform early phase information like synaptic activity and common IEGs into highly divergent late-phase responses, which are known to largely cell-type specific (Heinz and Bloodgood 2020). Several recent studies have already shown the potential of these approaches. For example, by analyzing single cell transcriptomes in the mouse brain during early postnatal development, Stroud and colleagues reveal that AP1-type transcription factors coordinate activation of a large array of cell-specific enhancer elements in an activity-dependent fashion (Stroud, Yang et al. 2020). Rodent barrel cortex synapses following whisker trimming, a classical paradigm discussed in Section 1, have been examined by the mass-spectrometry (MS)-based proteomics analysis. Here, reduced sensory stimulation has little impact on abundant postsynaptic proteins, such as PSD-95 and Gephyrin, but causes changes mostly to molecules implicated in dendrite spine structural maturation and synaptic strength, including glutamate receptors and proteins involved in proteasomal-dependent protein degradation (Butko, Savas et al. 2013). A related study used a specialized version of MS proteomics called BONCAT to specifically label the nascent proteome following neuronal stimulation. After pharmacologically-induced homeostatic scaling in cultured hippocampal neurons, the nascent synaptic proteome profile at 24hr post-manipulation differs from that at 2hr post-manipulation, although the functional classes broadly overlap (Schanzenbacher, Langer et al. 2018).

Lastly, in the *Xenopus* optic tectum system, visual experience produced strong changes in the RNA processing- and chromatin regulation-related proteins, a subset of which were functionally validated for their impact on cellular and behavioral plasticity (Liu, McClatchy et al. 2018).

2.3 Neuron-glia Interaction Regulates Dendritic Structural Plasticity

The heterogeneity and complexity of dendritic structural plasticity is largely determined by the intrinsic factors associated with different cell types and developmental stages, which we discussed in the previous section. At the same time, how a neuron or circuit responds to sensory experience or alterations in neural activity is strongly influenced by its cellular environment. Apart from synaptic partners, elements like the extracellular matrix, neighboring glia cells, as well as long-range neuromodulatory and network inputs, may also modify neurons' behaviors. In addition, recent studies indicate that structural changes induced by sensory deprivation are not limited to neurons, as the effect can be observed in glia and extracellular components as well (McRae, Rocco et al. 2007, Barrera, Chu et al. 2013, Chu, Abraham et al. 2018). These findings are consistent with the notion that sensory experience influences multiple cell types in the brain to elicit a coordinated response. Inspired by this concept and enabled by many technical advances, recent studies have started to reveal the significance of non-neuronal contributions to experience-dependent plasticity.

Glia have long been recognized as a critical component of the nervous system for their roles in providing neurons with metabolic support, neurotransmitter precursors and ion buffering. Studies over the past three decades have further revealed glia as active partners for neurons in synaptic transmission and essential modulators of synaptic structure and function in both invertebrate and vertebrate model systems (Eroglu and Barres 2010, Freeman 2015). When gliogenesis is inhibited genetically, mice show altered synaptogenesis, massive neuronal loss, and largely reduced motor output (Tsai, Li et al. 2012, Schreiner, Romanelli et al. 2015). In addition, neuron-glia crosstalk is crucial for neuroprotection and is implicated in human neurological diseases (Neniskyte and Gross 2017). Amongst the glial cells serving distinct roles in the nervous system, astrocytes and microglia have been directly linked to synapse development and plasticity, and both are considered integral parts of 'tripartite' or 'quad-partite' synapses (Perea, Navarrete et al. 2009, Schafer and Stevens 2013). As ramified cells, they extend numerous fine processes to the perisynaptic region, which monitor and influence local synaptic activity and structure (Panatier, Vallee et al. 2011). While there are many exciting new studies supporting the function of glia in regulating physiological and behavioral output of neural circuits, we will focus our discussion in the following sections on the role of astrocytes and microglia in circuit development and structural plasticity.

2.3.1 Astrocytes regulate excitatory and inhibitory synapse formation and maturation

Astrocytes constitute almost one third of cells in human brains and affect many aspects of neural development and function in both vertebrate and invertebrate CNS [reviewed by (Freeman 2015, Allen and Eroglu 2017). Using a purified neuron astrocyte co-culture system, Ben Barres' group performed a series of pioneering studies that revealed essential roles of astrocytes in promoting synapse formation and maturation (Meyer-Franke, Kaplan et al. 1995, Pfrieger and Barres 1997). In recent years, molecular studies helped identify a number of glia-derived secreted molecules as either synaptogenic or anti-synaptogenic factors, which are responsible for fine-tuning synapse formation, pruning and maintenance (Allen and Eroglu 2017). Astrocyte-secreted thrombospondins 1–5 (TSP1–5) were the first group of factors found by the co-culture studies. Through their interactions with the neuronally expressed Gabapentin receptor $\alpha2\delta$-1, TSPs initiate excitatory synapse formation within *in vitro* and *in vivo* models (Christopherson, Ullian et al. 2005, Eroglu, Allen et al. 2009). Later studies identified additional glial secreted factors as regulators for various aspects of excitatory synapse formation, including cholesterol transported by apolipoprotein E (APOE), glypicans 4 and 6, chondroitin sulfate proteoglycans (CSPGs), Transforming Growth factor (TGF)-β and Tumor necrosis factor (TNF)-α (Mauch, Nagler et al. 2001, Stellwagen and Malenka 2006, Frischknecht, Heine et al. 2009, Pyka, Wetzel et al. 2011, Allen, Bennett et al. 2012, Fuentes-Medel, Ashley et al. 2012). Additionally, one of the most well-characterized synaptogenic factors secreted by astrocytes is Hevin (Kucukdereli, Allen et al. 2011, Singh, Stogsdill et al. 2016). Hevin acts as a bridging factor between presynaptic Neurexin-1α and dendritic Neuroligin-1 during the assembly of glutamatergic synapses and serves critical functions in the formation and plasticity of thalamocortical connections in the developing visual cortex. Notably, astrocytes also release SPARC (Secreted Protein Acidic and Rich in Cysteine), which acts as a specific antagonist of Hevin induced synaptogenesis. While Hevin knockout mice show a reduced number of excitatory synapses in the superior colliculus,

SPARC mutant mice exhibit enhanced synaptogenesis in the same brain region, supporting their cooperative functions in tuning the number of excitatory synapses during mammalian cortical development (Kucukdereli, Allen et al. 2011).

Early studies also showed that astrocytes influence GABAergic inhibitory synapse formation in neuron cultures (Elmariah, Oh et al. 2005). However, the specific factors involved were not identified and whether and how astrocyte regulate inhibition *in vivo* is unclear. To address these questions, a recent study employed a chemico-genetic proximity labeling technique to identify the proteome enriched at astrocyte-neuron junctions in the primary visual cortex and revealed the role of neuronal cell adhesion molecule (NRCAM) in regulating inhibitory synapse formation. The study demonstrated that the astrocytic NRCAM interacts with the NRCAM-gephyrin complex on inhibitory postsynapses. Eliminating NRCAM from astrocytes reduces the number and function of inhibitory synapses, while having only minor effects on excitatory synapses (Takano, Wallace et al. 2020).

Taken together, these recent studies demonstrate that astrocytes play an integral role in controlling excitatory and inhibitory synapse formation and maturation. Importantly, a diverse set of astrocytic factors with specialized functions in synapse development has been uncovered. It is likely that the differential timing and patterns of their expression are determining factors that support the proper initiation and progression of synapse development in a brain region- or circuit-specific manner.

2.3.2 Astrocytes control circuit development and plasticity

Apart from influencing synaptogenesis, astrocytes are also involved in experience-dependent circuit refinement. As discussed earlier in this chapter, a classic model for studying developmental synaptic plasticity is ocular dominance plasticity (ODP) in the mammalian visual cortex. In wild-type animals, monocular deprivation during a critical developmental period causes the rearrangement of the binocular zone, which leads to the strengthening of the input from the open eye and the weakening of the input from the closed eye (Wiesel and Hubel 1963). While there are numerous studies illustrating neuronal signaling pathways required for the ODP, recent studies also indicate critical glial contributions, a part of which is conducted through astrocytic release of the synaptogenic protein Hevin. Unlike their wild type siblings, Hevin knockout mice fail to exhibit the monocular deprivation-induced shift, while the postnatal rescue of Hevin expression, specifically in astrocytes of the visual cortex, completely restores ODP, supporting a critical function of astrocyte-secreted proteins in the refinement of thalamocortical circuits (Risher, Patel et al. 2014, Singh, Stogsdill et al. 2016).

Experience-dependent synapse elimination is a critical process to ensure proper establishment and refinement of circuit connectivity (Sanes and Lichtman 1999). Astrocytes have been shown to directly and indirectly mediate synapse elimination (reviewed by (Chung, Allen et al. 2015)) . Using an *in vitro* engulfment assay and *in vivo* analysis of the developing retinogeniculate system, Chung *et al* demonstrated astrocytes' ability to engulf synapses (Chung, Clarke et al. 2013). This action requires the MEGF10 and MERTK phagocytic pathways and is activity dependent. Mice deficient in both pathways fail to refine retinogeniculate connections and retain ectopic synapses with reduced functionality. Importantly, astrocytes continuously engulf both excitatory and inhibitory synapses in the adult mouse brain, likely contributing to synaptic remodeling in the mature nervous system. In *Drosophila* central neurons, a similar phenomenon is observed during metamorphosis, when larval astrocytes transform into phagocytes and mediate large-scale circuit rewiring in the pupal neuropil (Tasdemir-Yilmaz and Freeman 2014). Specifically, the developmental elimination of the MB neuron axons are performed by astrocyte engulfment through activation of Draper, a fly homolog of MEGF10, as well as Crk/Mbc/dCed-12 signaling pathways. These studies demonstrate an evolutionarily conserved function of astrocytes in synaptic pruning and remodeling.

Another conserved function of astrocytes in developmental plasticity is its involvement in regulating critical period closure, shown by two recent publications studying *Drosophila* motor circuit and mouse visual circuit. Using optogenetic manipulations, Ackerman and colleagues define a critical period in the developing *Drosophila* motor circuit, 8 hours after larval hatching, during which period the motor neuron dendrite morphology can be readily modified by changes in neural activity. Furthermore, through genetic screens, the authors identified both cellular and molecular substrates regulating the closure of this critical period, which involves direct interactions between astrocyte-derived Neuroligin and dendritic localized Neurexin, as well as changes in dendrite microtubule dynamics (Ackerman, Perez-Catalan et al. 2021). Studies performed in mouse visual circuit showed a similar function of astrocyte in critical period closure (Ribot, Breton et al. 2021). Here, the authors found that injecting immature astrocytes into the primary visual cortex (V1) of adult mice (P100) reopens the critical period for ODP in the mature circuit. By comparing the expression profiles of immature and mature astrocytes, Ribot *et al* found that a developmental upregulation of astrocyte connexin signaling inhibits the expression of matrix metalloproteinase 9

(MMP9), an extracellular matrix–degrading enzyme. This promotes interneuron maturation and triggers the closure of critical period in the visual cortex. Together, both studies provide support for a function of astrocytes in coordinating circuit maturation and regulating the duration of critical periods.

2.3.3 Microglia regulate synaptic pruning and experience-dependent plasticity

Microglia are the resident macrophages of the CNS, constituting approximately 10% of brain cells. Similar to astrocytes, microglia send processes to infiltrate the neuropil regions and serve critical functions in regulating synapse development and pruning. Additionally, as immune cells, microglia can assume a wide range of morphologies in response to changes in neuronal activity and migrate and proliferate under inflammatory conditions (Lawson, Perry et al. 1990).

Under normal physiological conditions, microglia remain in the resting state. Using transgenic mice expressing EGFP specifically in microglia (CX3CR1-GFP mice) and 2-photon live imaging, microglia are found to be constantly monitoring the microenvironment in the presynaptic region and surveying neuronal and synaptic activity, through extending and retracting their processes (Weinhard, di Bartolomei et al. 2018). To understand their function in neural plasticity, researchers generated mice specifically depleted of microglia and identified deficits in multiple learning tasks and a significant reduction in motor-learning-dependent synapse formation. Most of these deficits can be recapitulated by Cre-dependent removal of BDNF directly from microglia, supporting a specific role for microglia-secreted BDNF in synapse formation and learning-dependent structural plasticity (Parkhurst, Yang et al. 2013).

An important function of microglia in the healthy brain is mediating synaptic pruning, a critical process that helps remove excessive or weak synapses during circuit refinement and experience-dependent plasticity. During postnatal developmental, microglia prune synapses through signaling mediated by the CX3CR1 receptor and complement receptor, CR3 (Paolicelli, Bolasco et al. 2011, Xavier, Menezes et al. 2014). Due to inappropriate synaptic pruning, CX3CR1 KO mice showed a transient increase in the density of immature spines in hippocampal CA1 pyramidal neurons (Schafer, Lehrman et al. 2012). A similar delay in synapse maturation was observed in the barrel cortex of mice with CX3CR1 deficiency (Hoshiko, Arnoux et al. 2012).

Another set of molecules implicated in microglia-mediated synaptic pruning is the classical complement proteins C1q and C3, localized to a subset of immature synapses, and the complement receptor 3 (CR3), expressed in resident microglia. Because microglia can sense neuronal communication and synaptic activity, less active presynaptic inputs are preferentially eliminated through a process mediated by the neuronal release of C1q and C3 (Stevens, Allen et al. 2007, Schafer, Lehrman et al. 2012). In the mouse visual system, C1q and its upstream regulator TGF-β as well as C3 are required for proper refinement of the retinogeniculate system (Bialas and Stevens 2013). Microglial engulfment of synapses is decreased in C3 and CR3 KO mice, consistent with the hypothesis that the complement proteins, such as C1q and C3, are activity-dependent "eat-me" signals that tag the less active synapses for targeted engulfment by phagocytic microglia (Hoshiko, Arnoux et al. 2012).

To evaluate microglial function in experience-dependent plasticity, researchers characterized microglial interactions with synapses during normal and altered sensory experience in the visual cortex of juvenile mice. In response to monocular deprivation during the critical period, microglia rapidly altered their morphology and synaptic interactions in the binocular zone of the visual cortex (Tremblay, Lowery et al. 2010). Notably, disrupting the purinergic P2Y12 receptor alters the microglial response to monocular deprivation and abrogates ocular dominance plasticity. A recent study in the somatosensory system demonstrated similar morphological changes in microglia upon sensory deprivation induced by whisker trimming (Kalambogias, Chen et al. 2020). These findings suggest that microglia actively contribute to the experience-dependent modification or elimination of a specific subset of synapses in the healthy brain (Sipe, Lowery et al. 2016).

Outlook: Glial function in circuit development, refinement and experience-dependent plasticity has been a subject of intensive research throughout the past two decades in both invertebrate and vertebrate systems. These findings indicate that not only do glia provide neuronal networks with essential structural and metabolic support, but they also modulate synaptic activity and plasticity during circuit formation and provide neuroprotection and modulation throughout the animal's lifetime. Additionally, although not described here, the significant glial involvement in regulating neurophysiology, animal behavior, as well as learning and memory are well demonstrated (Fields, Araque et al. 2014, Perea, Sur et al. 2014, Akther and Hirase 2022).

Many molecular pathways underlying neuron-glia crosstalk and their impacts on synapse development have been identified. As described above, the various glial-derived factors include secreted, membrane-bound and intracellular molecules (Summarized in Figure 2.1). For instance, Hevin, Sparc and TNF-α are secreted by astrocytes and modulate synapse number by

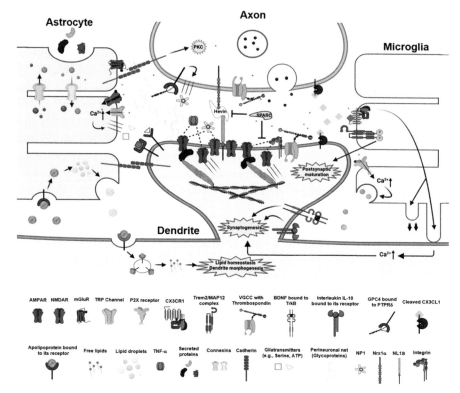

Figure 2.1 Synaptogenesis is governed by intercellular interactions between neurons and glia. Bidirectional signaling between astrocytes and microglia with proximal axon terminals and dendrites aids in the development and maturation of synapses. At this prototypical central glutamatergic synapse, neuron–glia interactions come in the form of physical contacts, such as by cell adhesion molecules, as well as secreted factors, including Hevin, Sparc, and the glycoprotein-based perineuronal network. Both microglia and astrocytes can detect nearby neuronal activity changes *via* calcium ion channels and neurotransmitter receptors and respond by releasing their own transmitters and secreted proteins in an activity-dependent manner.

interacting with glutamate receptors (i.e., AMPAR, NMDAR) and Neurexin-Neuroligin complexes directly (Jones, Bernardinelli et al. 2011). The release of these secreted molecules is often controlled by extracellular ligands or calcium entry. Stimulation of both metabotropic and ionotropic receptors, calcium channels and receptor tyrosine kinases induces astrocytes and microglia to release gliotransmitters, growth factors, and apolipoproteins (Gee and Keller 2005, Agulhon, Petravicz et al. 2008, Araque, Carmignoto et al. 2014, Yin, Spillman et al. 2021). Intracellular signaling within glia also controls these events through processes such as lipid trafficking/metabolism and Connexin-based communication between different astrocytic processes.

Finally, glia-neuron cell adhesion molecule interactions and a widely distributed glycoprotein-based perisynaptic net reinforce the structural integrity of the quadripartite synapse and regulate synaptic plasticity (Tewari, Chaunsali et al. 2022).

A number of open questions remain to be addressed in this field. There are several important areas demand further explorations, including how neurons and different types of glia communicate with each other during physiological and pathological conditions, as well as the molecular and functional heterogeneity of astrocytes and microglia (Khakh and Sofroniew 2015, Grabert, Michoel et al. 2016, Lawal, Ulloa Severino et al. 2022). In addition, both astrocytes and microglia infiltrate neuropil and cover specific territories. How their morphologies are intrinsically defined and modified by neural activity are not well understood. Recent advances in single-cell transcriptome analysis and high-resolution cellular and functional imaging in behaving animals, in combination with comparative studies using different animal models and human samples, will greatly aid researchers in solving these important questions in neurobiology (Li, Khankan et al. 2019, Farhy-Tselnicker, Boisvert et al. 2021).

2.4 Dendritic Structural Plasticity and Neurodevelopmental Disorders

Sensory experience interacts with genetic programs to shape and refine neural circuits underlying the cognitive functions of the brain. Human and animal studies suggest that altered states of neural plasticity during development are closely linked to a large spectrum of neurodevelopmental disorders. In this section, we will summarize the efforts and main findings elucidating the cellular and molecular basis of some of these disorders. While Fragile X Syndrome (FXS), Rett Syndrome and Angelman Syndrome are associated with monogenetic deficits, a large gene network has been linked to the highly prevalent autism spectrum disorders (ASD). To better understand the disease mechanisms and develop methods for detection and treatment of these complex diseases, many innovative technologies and experimental paradigms have been employed, which we will also touch upon in this section.

2.4.1 Fragile X syndrome

Fragile X Syndrome (FXS) is a common inherited cause of intellectual disability, characterized by behavioral abnormalities such as hyperactivity, emotional dysregulation, and learning deficits (Reviewed by (Garber, Visootsak et al. 2008, Hagerman, Berry-Kravis et al. 2017)). FXS is a monogenic condition caused by the expansion of CGG triplicates in the 5' UTR region of the Fragile X messenger ribonucleoprotein 1 (FMR1) gene. The result is a hypermethylated state of the *FMR1* promoter region which leads to a strong reduction or complete absence of the protein product, Fragile X Mental Retardation Protein (FMRP). The main function of FMRP is to regulate synapse-specific gene expression through inhibiting translation until the appropriate neuronal signals ease this suppression (Garber, Visootsak et al. 2008). Due to the diversity of its mRNA targets, the neuropathological outcome of FXS is complex. In *FMR1* knockout mice used to model FXS, cellular phenotypes, including structural and dynamic phenotypes of dendrite spines, are readily observed. In barrel cortex pyramidal neurons of the mutant mice, the dynamic period of spine formation and elimination is protracted and immature dendrite filopodia fail to transition into stable mushroom-type spines as they would normally (Cruz-Martin, Crespo et al. 2010, Pan, Aldridge et al. 2010).

One of the most critical molecular changes associated with FXS is the sustained and upregulated mGluR-dependent LTD. In wild type animals, stimulation of mGluRs leads to the disinhibition of translation by FMRP withdrawal (Huber, Gallagher et al. 2002). In FMRP knockout animals, there is a continuous production of LTD-related proteins. Moreover, lack of FMRP also leads to perturbations of multiple transcription-independent signaling networks and cellular pathways. These include altered mTOR signaling and autophagy (Sharma, Hoeffer et al. 2010, Yan, Porch et al. 2018), activity-dependent translocation of mRNA granules to the dendrite (Antar, Afroz et al. 2004, Dictenberg, Swanger et al. 2008), increased ribosomal stalling (Darnell, Van Driesche et al. 2011), and cap-dependent translational initiation by the eIF4E complex (Napoli, Mercaldo et al. 2008)

In terms of factors responsible for altered postsynaptic structural plasticity associated with FXS, the activity-induced transcription factor MEF2 is implicated by recent studies. In FMR1 knockout mice, the dysregulation of Mef2 prevents PSD-95 degradation and reduces synapse elimination (Pfeiffer, Zang et al. 2010, Tsai, Wilkerson et al. 2017). The immediate early gene Arc has also been associated with FXS pathogenesis, where rapid Arc translation is observed (Park, Park et al. 2008). Furthermore, PSD-95 appears to be a common factor found in several studies. Its mRNA stability and translational activity are controlled by the level of bound FMRP (Todd, Mack et al. 2003, Muddashetty, Kelic et al. 2007, Zalfa, Eleuteri et al. 2007, Nalavadi, Muddashetty et al. 2012). Lastly, cofilin, a negative regulator of actin polymerization, has been linked to the disruption of dendrite spine morphology, glutamatergic signaling and sensory processing in somatosensory cortical neurons in an FXS mouse model (Pyronneau, He et al. 2017).

2.4.2 Angelman syndrome

Angelman Syndrome (AS) is another neurodevelopmental disorder which causes intellectual disability, hyperactivity, severe impairment of speech, and atypical mood and disposition. The disease also features irregularities in motor control and seizures (Margolis, Sell et al. 2015). Most AS cases are associated with the improper neural expression of the maternally inherited Ubiquitin Protein Ligase E3a (UBE3A) gene, encoding the Ubiquitin ligase E6-associated protein (E6AP), which directs ubiquitinated targets for proteasomal degradation. The severity of AS symptoms occurs along a gradient that reflects its genetic etiology, including several genetic abnormalities linked to deletion, and/ or methylation, of the 15q11-q13 chromosomal region that contains the E6AP locus, as well as E6AP loss-of-function mutations (Khatri and Man 2019).

Due to the large span of its protein interactions, E6AP exerts a broad effect on cellular functions, similar to the case with FMRP. Investigations of the mechanisms for the pathophysiology of AS, including defects in chronic and acute activity-dependent plasticity, have relied on mouse models as well as *in vitro* systems. In the visual cortex of E6AP knockout mice, a reduction in pyramidal neuron basal dendrite spines is observed (Yashiro, Riday et al. 2009). In addition, the E6AP-/- neurons lack normal experience-dependent maturation and have a reduced capacity for cortical plasticity, demonstrated by a mild response towards an extended period of sensory deprivation (Sato and Stryker 2010). One likely underlying molecular component is the level and activity of the immediate early gene Arc. Normally, neuronal stimulation leads to decreased Arc levels, attenuating AMPA receptor internalization and thus increasing the density of AMPA receptor inserted in the postsynaptic membrane (Greer, Hanayama et al. 2010). In the AS knockout mouse model, Arc is not degraded, leading to a host of intracellular events, including reduced CaMKII activity, persistent interaction of PSD-95 with Arc, and consequently failure of PSD-95 to associate with other postsynaptic proteins such as TrkB (Weeber, Jiang et al. 2003, Cao, Rioult-Pedotti et al. 2013). Despite a possible role for controlling Arc protein levels directly, there is evidence indicating that E6AP does not physically interact with Arc. Instead, it prevents Arc transcription (Kuhnle, Mothes et al. 2013). Additionally, studies have identified other E6AP targets, such as Ephexin5, a RhoA GEF, whose proteolysis promotes excitatory synapse formation in young postnatal mice (Margolis, Salogiannis et al. 2010).

2.4.3 Rett syndrome

Rett Syndrome (RTT), like FSX and AS, is characterized by a spectrum of cognitive and motor deficits that appear early in development (reviewed by (Chahrour and Zoghbi 2007, Xu, Miller et al. 2014, Nakai, Takumi et al. 2018)). Despite reaching normal developmental checkpoints, such as walking and first word use, RTT individuals experience a regression in these learned skills. There is a concurrent deceleration in growth rate, including in head and brain expansion, which leads to microcephaly. Additional symptoms include social and emotional deficits, sleeping and breathing disruptions, and seizures. Physical health deteriorates later in life, commonly due to heart problems and severely restricted mobility. The syndromic features seen in RTT patients are due to deficits in the Methyl-CpG Binding Protein 2 (*Mecp2*) gene, which codes for a transcriptional regulator, and are recapitulated in Mecp2 mouse models. Protein levels of Mecp2, which is found in many cells but is enriched in neurons, rise during early postnatal development, regulating gene expression by binding to methylated DNA promoter regions and recruiting chromatin remodeling complexes and corepressors (Chahrour and Zoghbi 2007).

The neuropathology of RTT has long been known to arise, in part, from abnormal dendrite morphology and motility. In both postmortem RTT tissue (Armstrong, Dunn et al. 1995) and young postnatal Mecp2 mutant mice (Belichenko, Belichenko et al. 2009, Belichenko, Wright et al. 2009, Nguyen, Du et al. 2012), there are notable changes in dendrite spine density, motility, as well as dendrite branching pattern and complexity. This observation is seen in multiple brain regions, including visual and somatosensory cortex and hippocampus, as well as in primary hippocampal cultures (Chao, Zoghbi et al. 2007, Baj, Patrizio et al. 2014). Additional studies have directly linked these morphological aberrations to neurophysiological defects that include both reduced spontaneous excitatory drive *in vitro* and blunted evoked neurotransmission *in vivo* (Chao, Zoghbi et al. 2007, Lee, Tsytsarev et al. 2017).

The additive effect of these structural alterations to the dendrite and functional consequences to neurotransmission can lead to instances of abnormal plasticity. One clear example is the extension of the ocular dominance plasticity period in Mecp2-deficient mice, where Mecp2 is deleted specifically in PV[+] interneurons (Kuhlman, Olivas et al. 2013, Banerjee, Rikhye et al. 2016). Although the molecular basis for this permissive plasticity could be due to any number of genes whose transcripts are regulated by Mecp2, one factor thought to be at the forefront of both the cause and treatment, is BDNF. Many reports have provided evidence to support the link between BDNF and dendrite morphology, as well as synaptic maturation and plasticity (Poo 2001, Tyler, Alonso et al. 2002). Current models, based on a variety of techniques such as chromatin immunoprecipitation, reporter assays and phosphorylation-dependent immunoblotting, propose that the Mecp2-BDNF pathway begins after depolarization, such as by visual sensory experience, induces CaMKII-dependent Mecp2 phosphorylation, dissociating its corepressors from the BDNF promoter and potentiation its expression (Chen, Chang et al. 2003, Martinowich, Hattori et al. 2003, Zhou, Hong et al. 2006). Consistently, reduced BDNF and impaired activity induced BDNF trafficking and release have been tied to RTT syndrome itself, including simplified dendrite arbors and neurological deficits mimicking RTT pathology (Chang, Khare et al. 2006, Wang, Chan et al. 2006, Ogier, Wang et al. 2007, Li, Calfa et al. 2012, Xu, Miller et al. 2014). Finally, neuronal and behavioral symptoms can be ameliorated by modulating dysfunction at the level of both Mecp2 and BDNF. Such examples include phenotypic rescue by BDNF overexpression in both Mecp2 knockout mice and hippocampal cultures subjected to shRNA mediated Mecp2 knockdown (Chang, Khare et al. 2006, Larimore, Chapleau et al. 2009). Therapies based on synthetic BDNF-like ligands have even been developed and show promise for reducing RTT symptoms *in vivo* (Massa, Yang et al. 2010, Schmid, Yang et al. 2012, Simmons, Belichenko et al. 2013, Kajiya, Takeshita et al. 2014).

2.4.4 Autism and complex neurodevelopmental disorders

In contrast to the three monogenic neurodevelopmental disorders detailed above (summarized in Figure 2.2), other neurological disorders have a more complicated etiology, which vastly complicates the pathology of the disease. Intellectual disability (ID), autism spectrum disorders (ASD) as well as psychiatric illnesses with a developmental component, such as schizophrenia (SZ), have been linked to dozens or even hundreds of genes (Ebert and Greenberg 2013, Parenti, Rabaneda et al. 2020). Interestingly, these disorders are often comorbid with each other or additional neurological symptoms, such as seizures.

Perhaps the most representative of these complex, polygenic disorders is ASD. Characterized by impaired social interaction, repetitive behaviors and narrowed interests, ASDs may be caused by spontaneous germline mutations or have a syndromic basis where, for example, an individual with FXS

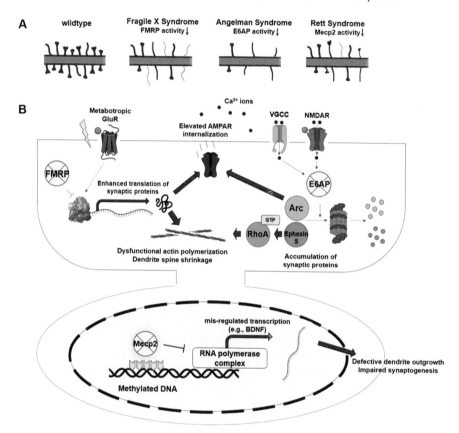

Figure 2.2　Cellular and molecular features of select monogenic neurodevelopmental disorders. (A) Stereotypical changes in dendrite and spine morphology for FXS, AS, and RTT, which include reduction of spine density and maturity. Although not pictured, RTT is also characterized by a reduced dendrite arbor complexity. **(B)** FXS, AS, and RTT arise from deficiencies of single genes. FXS results from FMRP mutations, which lead to upregulated translation of synaptic proteins. E6AP mutation reduces activity-dependent protein degradation and causes AS. Loss of Mecp2 activity observed in RTT results in unchecked transcription of synaptic proteins, such as BDNF, and impairs synapse formation and plasticity, as well as dendrite arborization.

will also be diagnosed with Autism (Ebert and Greenberg 2013). FXS, RTT and AS can all potentially result in an ASD diagnosis. In addition to these, Timothy Syndrome, stemming from dysfunctional activity of the *CACNA1C*-coding voltage-gated calcium channel, and Tuberous Sclerosis, caused by mutations in the TSC1 and TSC2 translational regulatory proteins, are common culprits of syndrome-based ASD cases ((Barrett and Tsien 2008,

Pasca, Portmann et al. 2011) and reviewed by (Han and Sahin 2011, Bhat, Dao et al. 2012)). In contrast to these more readily understood forms, there is also a great deal of evidence pointing to the Neurexin-Neuroligin cell-adhesion molecules as well as the SHANK class of PSD scaffolding proteins as the causative genes in non-syndromic instances (reviewed by (Ebert and Greenberg 2013)). One commonality between many of these genes of interest is that not only are they regulators of activity-dependent developmental plasticity, but also that their function or localization are themselves regulated by neuronal activity. For example, overexpression of Neuroligin in cultured rodent neurons results in elevated excitatory synapse numbers and enhanced NMDA receptor transmission and CaMKII activity (Chubykin, Atasoy et al. 2007).

Given the extreme heterogeneity of these neurodevelopmental disorders, online databases have been established to foster a more coherent understanding of the genetic causes for conditions like ASD and SZ (gene.sfari. org, szdb.org). SFARI Gene is one such resource which uploads candidate ASD-implicated genes from the literature as well as information on copy number variants (CNV) and genetic mouse models of ASD. The contribution of each gene is also weighted by providing a score which correlates to the strength of the experimental evidence. Gene scores are amenable to change based on new findings and heavily benefit from feedback from the research community.

2.4.5 New paradigms and technologies accelerate research on neurodevelopmental disorders

The study of developmental disorders, including those that are neurological and neuropsychiatric in origin, has undergone a transformation in the past few decades due to the implementation of genome-wide association studies, disease modeling using rodents and other animals, rational drug design, and other groundbreaking techniques. More recently, the invention of optogenetics and the discovery and rapid spread of CRISPR-based genomic editing has immensely helped to gain additional traction in cellular and genetic modeling of biological diseases. Two new technologies that have experienced a radical expansion in their use is human induced-pluripotent stem cells (iPSCs) and the related organoids (Ardhanareeswaran, Mariani et al. 2017, Shou, Liang et al. 2020). The advances made, and the tremendous potential still to be exploited, stems from the ability to directly model human disease in a human-specific biological context. The advantages of this system include bypassing the relative scarcity of patients for a given condition and confinement to postmortem samples, fine-tuned controls over the genetic background of the tissue and generation of a completely new biological sample in several months, comparable to the amount of time taken to develop a new mouse line. The final section below will highlight how this technology has already made influential discoveries with respect to neurodevelopmental disorders, both monogenic in nature like Rett Syndrome or complex and polygenic like the autism spectrum disorders.

The information gleaned from iPSC-based research has been especially productive in studies related to Rett Syndrome (RTT). Multiple studies have demonstrated that iPSC-derived neurons from RTT individuals, or those containing *Mecp2* mutations, have similar cellular anatomical abnormalities as those seen *in vivo*. These include decreased excitatory synapse number and synaptic immaturity, as well as reduced dendrite arbor complexity and spine number (Muotri, Marchetto et al. 2010, Cheung, Horvath et al. 2011, Kim, Hysolli et al. 2011, Livide, Patriarchi et al. 2015, Tang, Kim et al. 2016) The opposite effect was also observed in cells containing the *Mecp2* duplication (Nageshappa, Carromeu et al. 2016). Using this approach, researchers were able to reproduce Mecp2-dependent BDNF expression and TRPC channel opening, corroborating earlier reports of their involvement in RTT using traditional models (Griesi-Oliveira, Acab et al. 2015).

Similar iPSC studies have also revealed activity-dependent changes at the synapse and are used to model the rare Timothy Syndrome (TS). iPSCs taken from TS individuals harboring a mutation in the *CACNA1C*, a gene encoding a calcium channel, reproduce the phenotypes seen in TS model mouse primary cortical neurons. Specifically, KCl-induced depolarization is followed by dendritic retraction, in contrast to the extension events in wildtype neurons (Krey, Pasca et al. 2013, Simms and Zamponi 2014). This atypical response is accompanied by abnormal calcium signaling and altered electrophysiology. Additionally, both studies reported large deviations in activity-dependent gene expression, particularly among constituents of the cAMP- and CREB-signaling pathways (Pasca, Portmann et al. 2011, Tian, Voineagu et al. 2014).

iPSC-based approaches are especially useful in polygenic disorders, such as autism or neuropsychiatric disease, where there are potentially hundreds of genetic mutations and polymorphisms that combinatorically shape the etiology and the severity of the disease ((Ratanatharathorn, Koenen et al. 2021) and reviewed in (Rylaarsdam and Guemez-Gamboa 2019)). In ASDs, for example, mutations at these varied loci, such as the synaptic scaffold protein gene *SHANK3*, lead to dendritic phenotypes, such as reduced complexity and length of dendrite fields, as well as decreased dendrite spine densities

(Darville, Poulet et al. 2016, Yi, Danko et al. 2016, Grunwald, Stock et al. 2019). In a second study, tissues developed from ASD patient-derived iPSCs had a disproportionate expansion of GABAergic interneurons and inhibitory synapses, lending support to the excitatory-inhibitory balance hypothesis of ASD (Mariani, Coppola et al. 2015). This approach has also been used to show that Bipolar Disorder (BD) patient-derived iPSCs produce neural stem cells which fail to completely differentiate into mature neurons, a defect which could be rescued by a WNT-signaling agonist (Madison, Zhou et al. 2015).

Finally, a particularly promising subset of iPSC research uses these induced cells to create miniature brains, termed cerebral organoids, which are layered, 3-dimensional organs with differentiated neuronal subtypes (reviewed by (Shou, Liang et al. 2020)). Organoids hold a great advantage over other model systems due to their enhanced ability to trace and analyze cellular lineages during organ development. For example, a recent study demonstrated that mutations at several loci, in isolation, abolish the normal synchronous development between excitatory and inhibitory cortical neurons, which results in physiological defects (Paulsen, Velasco et al. 2022). Additionally, although still in its infancy, i.e., cerebral organoids are still an anatomically simplified version of actual brains, the technology may be able to overcome the challenge of translating findings from isolated cellular environments to meaningful functionality in a native, *in vivo* system. Such problems have been encountered before, including the seemingly contradictory results of how Mecp2 alters BDNF levels in cell culture vs. living animals (Chahrour and Zoghbi 2007). Together with other tools like scRNA sequencing, organoids will inform us how activity-dependent changes during development impact not just the immediate downstream neuron, but also other circuit components and supporting cells, such as astrocytes and microglia.

Outlook: As a whole, the field of research focused on neurodevelopmental disorders with dendritic underpinnings has made incredible progress over the years. What initially began as observations of behavioral abnormalities and gross anatomical changes in patients evolved into a more detailed perspective of deficits at the cellular, molecular, and genetic levels (Nakai, Takumi et al. 2018). One of the many remaining obstacles is integrating information collected on any given disease, which goes beyond the causative protein(s) and the cellular compartment or cell types occupied and affected by it. While complex disorders, such as autism and schizophrenia, have the most diverse genetic and environmental etiologies, even monogenic disorders may be characterized by a spectrum of cellular and molecular deficits. Such is the case with Rett Syndrome where a single defective transcriptional repressor leads to dysregulated expression for potentially thousands of genes (Boxer, Renthal et al. 2020). Therefore, recently developed technologies including multi-omics assays, patient-derived iPSCs and organoid-based lineage and neural circuit studies will be indispensable for elevating neurodevelopmental disease research to the next level. This shift may also advance the therapeutic sphere for neurological disorders, which has faced a disproportionate number of failures and hardships in the current era of research (Craven 2011).

Acknowledgements

We thank Anna Grigsby-Brown and Jun Yin for helpful discussions and comments on the manuscript. This work is supported by the Intramural Research Program of National Institute of Neurological Disorders and Stroke, National Institutes of Health. Project number 1ZIANS003137.

References

Abdolahi, S., A. Zare-Chahoki, F. Noorbakhsh and A. Gorji (2022). "A Review of Molecular Interplay between Neurotrophins and miRNAs in Neuropsychological Disorders." Mol Neurobiol **59**(10): 6260–6280.

Ackerman, S. D., N. A. Perez-Catalan, M. R. Freeman and C. Q. Doe (2021). "Astrocytes close a motor circuit critical period." Nature **592**(7854): 414–420.

Adhikari, P., D. Orozco, H. Randhawa and F. W. Wolf (2019). "Mef2 induction of the immediate early gene Hr38/Nr4a is terminated by Sirt1 to promote ethanol tolerance." Genes Brain Behav **18**(3): e12486.

Agulhon, C., J. Petravicz, A. B. McMullen, E. J. Sweger, S. K. Minton, S. R. Taves, K. B. Casper, T. A. Fiacco and K. D. McCarthy (2008). "What is the role of astrocyte calcium in neurophysiology?" Neuron **59**(6): 932–946.

Aizawa, H., S. C. Hu, K. Bobb, K. Balakrishnan, G. Ince, I. Gurevich, M. Cowan and A. Ghosh (2004). "Dendrite development regulated by CREST, a calcium-regulated transcriptional activator." Science **303**(5655): 197–202.

Akther, S. and H. Hirase (2022). "Assessment of astrocytes as a mediator of memory and learning in rodents." Glia **70**(8): 1484–1505.

Allen, N. J., M. L. Bennett, L. C. Foo, G. X. Wang, C. Chakraborty, S. J. Smith and B. A. Barres (2012). "Astrocyte glypicans 4 and 6 promote formation of excitatory synapses via GluA1 AMPA receptors." Nature **486**(7403): 410–414.

Allen, N. J. and C. Eroglu (2017). "Cell Biology of Astrocyte-Synapse Interactions." Neuron **96**(3): 697–708.

Alvarez, V. A. and B. L. Sabatini (2007). "Anatomical and physiological plasticity of dendritic spines." Annu Rev Neurosci **30**: 79–97.

Antar, L. N., R. Afroz, J. B. Dictenberg, R. C. Carroll and G. J. Bassell (2004). "Metabotropic glutamate receptor activation regulates fragile x mental retardation protein and FMR1 mRNA localization differentially in dendrites and at synapses." J Neurosci **24**(11): 2648–2655.

Araque, A., G. Carmignoto, P. G. Haydon, S. H. Oliet, R. Robitaille and A. Volterra (2014). "Gliotransmitters travel in time and space." Neuron **81**(4): 728–739.

Ardhanareeswaran, K., J. Mariani, G. Coppola, A. Abyzov and F. M. Vaccarino (2017). "Human induced pluripotent stem cells for modelling neurodevelopmental disorders." Nat Rev Neurol **13**(5): 265–278.

Armstrong, D., J. K. Dunn, B. Antalffy and R. Trivedi (1995). "Selective dendritic alterations in the cortex of Rett syndrome." J Neuropathol Exp Neurol **54**(2): 195–201.

Baj, G., A. Patrizio, A. Montalbano, M. Sciancalepore and E. Tongiorgi (2014). "Developmental and maintenance defects in Rett syndrome neurons identified by a new mouse staging system in vitro." Front Cell Neurosci **8**: 18.

Banerjee, A., R. V. Rikhye, V. Breton-Provencher, X. Tang, C. Li, K. Li, C. A. Runyan, Z. Fu, R. Jaenisch and M. Sur (2016). "Jointly reduced inhibition and excitation underlies circuit-wide changes in cortical processing in Rett syndrome." Proc Natl Acad Sci U S A **113**(46): E7287–E7296.

Barbagallo, B., A. Philbrook, D. Touroutine, N. Banerjee, D. Oliver, C. M. Lambert and M. M. Francis (2017). "Excitatory neurons sculpt GABAergic neuronal connectivity in the C. elegans motor circuit." Development **144**(10): 1807–1819.

Barrera, K., P. Chu, J. Abramowitz, R. Steger, R. L. Ramos and J. C. Brumberg (2013). "Organization of myelin in the mouse somatosensory barrel cortex and the effects of sensory deprivation." Dev Neurobiol **73**(4): 297–314.

Barrett, C. F. and R. W. Tsien (2008). "The Timothy syndrome mutation differentially affects voltage- and calcium-dependent inactivation of CaV1.2 L-type calcium channels." Proc Natl Acad Sci U S A **105**(6): 2157–2162.

Belichenko, N. P., P. V. Belichenko and W. C. Mobley (2009). "Evidence for both neuronal cell autonomous and nonautonomous effects of methyl-CpG-binding protein 2 in the cerebral cortex of female mice with Mecp2 mutation." Neurobiol Dis **34**(1): 71–77.

Belichenko, P. V., E. E. Wright, N. P. Belichenko, E. Masliah, H. H. Li, W. C. Mobley and U. Francke (2009). "Widespread changes in dendritic and axonal morphology in Mecp2-mutant mouse models of Rett syndrome: evidence for disruption of neuronal networks." J Comp Neurol **514**(3): 240–258.

Bhat, S., D. T. Dao, C. E. Terrillion, M. Arad, R. J. Smith, N. M. Soldatov and T. D. Gould (2012). "CACNA1C (Cav1.2) in the pathophysiology of psychiatric disease." Prog Neurobiol **99**(1): 1–14.

Bialas, A. R. and B. Stevens (2013). "TGF-beta signaling regulates neuronal C1q expression and developmental synaptic refinement." Nat Neurosci **16**(12): 1773–1782.

Biever, A., C. Glock, G. Tushev, E. Ciirdaeva, T. Dalmay, J. D. Langer and E. M. Schuman (2020). "Monosomes actively translate synaptic mRNAs in neuronal processes." Science **367**(6477).

Bloodgood, B. L., N. Sharma, H. A. Browne, A. Z. Trepman and M. E. Greenberg (2013). "The activity-dependent transcription factor NPAS4 regulates domain-specific inhibition." Nature **503**(7474): 121–125.

Borges, S. and M. Berry (1978). "The effects of dark rearing on the development of the visual cortex of the rat." J Comp Neurol **180**(2): 277–300.

Boxer, L. D., W. Renthal, A. W. Greben, T. Whitwam, A. Silberfeld, H. Stroud, E. Li, M. G. Yang, B. Kinde, E. C. Griffith, B. Bonev and M. E. Greenberg (2020). "MeCP2 Represses the Rate of Transcriptional Initiation of Highly Methylated Long Genes." Mol Cell **77**(2): 294–309 e299.

Butko, M. T., J. N. Savas, B. Friedman, C. Delahunty, F. Ebner, J. R. Yates, 3rd and R. Y. Tsien (2013). "In vivo quantitative proteomics of somatosensory cortical synapses shows which protein levels are modulated by sensory deprivation." Proc Natl Acad Sci U S A **110**(8): E726–735.

Cajigas, I. J., G. Tushev, T. J. Will, S. tom Dieck, N. Fuerst and E. M. Schuman (2012). "The local transcriptome in the synaptic neuropil revealed by deep sequencing and high-resolution imaging." Neuron **74**(3): 453–466.

Cao, C., M. S. Rioult-Pedotti, P. Migani, C. J. Yu, R. Tiwari, K. Parang, M. R. Spaller, D. J. Goebel and J. Marshall (2013). "Impairment of TrkB-PSD-95 signaling in Angelman syndrome." PLoS Biol **11**(2): e1001478.

Carvell, G. E. and D. J. Simons (1996). "Abnormal tactile experience early in life disrupts active touch." J Neurosci **16**(8): 2750–2757.

Chahrour, M. and H. Y. Zoghbi (2007). "The story of Rett syndrome: from clinic to neurobiology." Neuron **56**(3): 422–437.

Chang, J. Y., Y. Nakahata, Y. Hayano and R. Yasuda (2019). "Mechanisms of Ca(2+)/calmodulin-dependent kinase II activation in single dendritic spines." Nat Commun **10**(1): 2784.

Chang, J. Y., P. Parra-Bueno, T. Laviv, E. M. Szatmari, S. R. Lee and R. Yasuda (2017). "CaMKII Autophosphorylation Is Necessary for Optimal Integration of Ca(2+) Signals during LTP Induction, but Not Maintenance." Neuron **94**(4): 800–808 e804.

Chang, Q., G. Khare, V. Dani, S. Nelson and R. Jaenisch (2006). "The disease progression of Mecp2 mutant mice is affected by the level of BDNF expression." Neuron **49**(3): 341–348.

Chao, H. T., H. Y. Zoghbi and C. Rosenmund (2007). "MeCP2 controls excitatory synaptic strength by regulating glutamatergic synapse number." Neuron **56**(1): 58–65.

Chen, C. C. and J. C. Brumberg (2021). "Sensory Experience as a Regulator of Structural Plasticity in the Developing Whisker-to-Barrel System." Front Cell Neurosci **15**: 770453.

Chen, C. C., R. Steger and J. C. Brumberg (2009). "Barrels come of age: Barrels XXI meeting report." Somatosens Mot Res **26**(1): 25–30.

Chen, C. C., D. Tam and J. C. Brumberg (2012). "Sensory deprivation differentially impacts the dendritic development of pyramidal versus non-pyramidal neurons in layer 6 of mouse barrel cortex." Brain Struct Funct **217**(2): 435–446.

Chen, S. X., P. K. Tari, K. She and K. Haas (2010). "Neurexin-neuroligin cell adhesion complexes contribute to synaptotropic dendritogenesis via growth stabilization mechanisms in vivo." Neuron **67**(6): 967–983.

Chen, W. G., Q. Chang, Y. Lin, A. Meissner, A. E. West, E. C. Griffith, R. Jaenisch and M. E. Greenberg (2003). "Derepression of BDNF transcription involves calcium-dependent phosphorylation of MeCP2." Science **302**(5646): 885–889.

Chen, X., R. Rahman, F. Guo and M. Rosbash (2016). "Genome-wide identification of neuronal activity-regulated genes in Drosophila." Elife **5**.

Cheung, A. Y., L. M. Horvath, D. Grafodatskaya, P. Pasceri, R. Weksberg, A. Hotta, L. Carrel and J. Ellis (2011). "Isolation of MECP2-null Rett Syndrome patient hiPS cells and isogenic controls through X-chromosome inactivation." Hum Mol Genet **20**(11): 2103–2115.

Christopherson, K. S., E. M. Ullian, C. C. Stokes, C. E. Mullowney, J. W. Hell, A. Agah, J. Lawler, D. F. Mosher, P. Bornstein and B. A. Barres (2005). "Thrombospondins are astrocyte-secreted proteins that promote CNS synaptogenesis." Cell **120**(3): 421–433.

Chu, P., R. Abraham, K. Budhu, U. Khan, N. De Marco Garcia and J. C. Brumberg (2018). "The Impact of Perineuronal Net Digestion Using Chondroitinase ABC on the Intrinsic Physiology of Cortical Neurons." Neuroscience **388**: 23–35.

Chubykin, A. A., D. Atasoy, M. R. Etherton, N. Brose, E. T. Kavalali, J. R. Gibson and T. C. Sudhof (2007). "Activity-dependent validation of excitatory versus inhibitory synapses by neuroligin-1 versus neuroligin-2." Neuron **54**(6): 919–931.

Chung, W. S., N. J. Allen and C. Eroglu (2015). "Astrocytes Control Synapse Formation, Function, and Elimination." Cold Spring Harb Perspect Biol **7**(9): a020370.

Chung, W. S., L. E. Clarke, G. X. Wang, B. K. Stafford, A. Sher, C. Chakraborty, J. Joung, L. C. Foo, A. Thompson, C. Chen, S. J. Smith and B. A. Barres (2013). "Astrocytes mediate synapse elimination through MEGF10 and MERTK pathways." Nature **504**(7480): 394–400.

Cohn, J. A., E. R. Cebul, G. Valperga, L. Brose, M. de Bono, M. G. Heiman and J. T. Pierce (2020). "Long-term activity drives dendritic branch elaboration of a C. elegans sensory neuron." Dev Biol **461**(1): 66–74.

Costa, J. F., M. Dines and R. Lamprecht (2020). "The Role of Rac GTPase in Dendritic Spine Morphogenesis and Memory." Front Synaptic Neurosci **12**: 12.

Craven, R. (2011). "The risky business of drug development in neurology." Lancet Neurol **10**(2): 116–117.

Cruz-Martin, A., M. Crespo and C. Portera-Cailliau (2010). "Delayed stabilization of dendritic spines in fragile X mice." J Neurosci **30**(23): 7793–7803.

Darnell, J. C., S. J. Van Driesche, C. Zhang, K. Y. Hung, A. Mele, C. E. Fraser, E. F. Stone, C. Chen, J. J. Fak, S. W. Chi, D. D. Licatalosi, J. D. Richter and R. B. Darnell (2011). "FMRP stalls ribosomal translocation on mRNAs linked to synaptic function and autism." Cell **146**(2): 247–261.

Darville, H., A. Poulet, F. Rodet-Amsellem, L. Chatrousse, J. Pernelle, C. Boissart, D. Heron, C. Nava, A. Perrier, M. Jarrige, F. Coge, M. J. Millan, T. Bourgeron, M. Peschanski, R. Delorme and A. Benchoua (2016). "Human Pluripotent Stem Cell-derived Cortical Neurons for High Throughput Medication Screening in Autism: A Proof of Concept Study in SHANK3 Haploinsufficiency Syndrome." EBioMedicine **9**: 293–305.

Del Rio, T. and M. B. Feller (2006). "Early retinal activity and visual circuit development." Neuron **52**(2): 221–222.

Dictenberg, J. B., S. A. Swanger, L. N. Antar, R. H. Singer and G. J. Bassell (2008). "A direct role for FMRP in activity-dependent dendritic mRNA transport links filopodial-spine morphogenesis to fragile X syndrome." Dev Cell **14**(6): 926–939.

Dong, W., R. H. Lee, H. Xu, S. Yang, K. G. Pratt, V. Cao, Y. K. Song, A. Nurmikko and C. D. Aizenman (2009). "Visual avoidance in Xenopus tadpoles is correlated with the maturation of visual responses in the optic tectum." J Neurophysiol **101**(2): 803–815.

Dong, X., K. Shen and H. E. Bulow (2015). "Intrinsic and extrinsic mechanisms of dendritic morphogenesis." Annu Rev Physiol **77**: 271–300.

Donlin-Asp, P. G., C. Polisseni, R. Klimek, A. Heckel and E. M. Schuman (2021). "Differential regulation of local mRNA dynamics and translation following long-term potentiation and depression." Proc Natl Acad Sci U S A **118**(13).

Duman, J. G., F. A. Blanco, C. A. Cronkite, Q. Ru, K. C. Erikson, S. Mulherkar, A. B. Saifullah, K. Firozi and K. F. Tolias (2021). "Rac-maninoff and Rho-vel: The symphony of Rho-GTPase signaling at excitatory synapses." Small GTPases: 1–34.

Ebert, D. H. and M. E. Greenberg (2013). "Activity-dependent neuronal signalling and autism spectrum disorder." Nature **493**(7432): 327–337.

Elmariah, S. B., E. J. Oh, E. G. Hughes and R. J. Balice-Gordon (2005). "Astrocytes regulate inhibitory synapse formation via Trk-mediated modulation of postsynaptic GABAA receptors." J Neurosci **25**(14): 3638–3650.

Eroglu, C., N. J. Allen, M. W. Susman, N. A. O'Rourke, C. Y. Park, E. Ozkan, C. Chakraborty, S. B. Mulinyawe, D. S. Annis, A. D. Huberman, E. M. Green, J. Lawler, R. Dolmetsch, K. C. Garcia, S. J. Smith, Z. D. Luo, A. Rosenthal, D. F. Mosher and B. A. Barres (2009). "Gabapentin receptor alpha2delta-1 is a neuronal thrombospondin receptor responsible for excitatory CNS synaptogenesis." Cell **139**(2): 380–392.

Eroglu, C. and B. A. Barres (2010). "Regulation of synaptic connectivity by glia." Nature **468**(7321): 223–231.

Fagiolini, M., J. M. Fritschy, K. Low, H. Mohler, U. Rudolph and T. K. Hensch (2004). "Specific GABAA circuits for visual cortical plasticity." Science **303**(5664): 1681–1683.

Farhy-Tselnicker, I., M. M. Boisvert, H. Liu, C. Dowling, G. A. Erikson, E. Blanco-Suarez, C. Farhy, M. N. Shokhirev, J. R. Ecker and N. J. Allen (2021). "Activity-dependent modulation of synapse-regulating genes in astrocytes." Elife **10**.

Feller, M. B. (2009). "Retinal waves are likely to instruct the formation of eye-specific retinogeniculate projections." Neural Dev **4**: 24.

Fields, R. D., A. Araque, H. Johansen-Berg, S. S. Lim, G. Lynch, K. A. Nave, M. Nedergaard, R. Perez, T. Sejnowski and H. Wake (2014). "Glial biology in learning and cognition." Neuroscientist **20**(5): 426–431.

Forrest, M. P., E. Parnell and P. Penzes (2018). "Dendritic structural plasticity and neuropsychiatric disease." Nat Rev Neurosci **19**(4): 215–234.

Fox, K. and R. O. Wong (2005). "A comparison of experience-dependent plasticity in the visual and somatosensory systems." Neuron **48**(3): 465–477.

Freeman, M. R. (2015). "Drosophila Central Nervous System Glia." Cold Spring Harb Perspect Biol **7**(11).

Frischknecht, R., M. Heine, D. Perrais, C. I. Seidenbecher, D. Choquet and E. D. Gundelfinger (2009). "Brain extracellular matrix affects AMPA receptor lateral mobility and short-term synaptic plasticity." Nat Neurosci **12**(7): 897–904.

Fu, M. and Y. Zuo (2011). "Experience-dependent structural plasticity in the cortex." Trends Neurosci **34**(4): 177–187.

Fuentes-Medel, Y., J. Ashley, R. Barria, R. Maloney, M. Freeman and V. Budnik (2012). "Integration of a retrograde signal during synapse formation by glia-secreted TGF-beta ligand." Curr Biol **22**(19): 1831–1838.

Fujita, N., Y. Nagata, T. Nishiuchi, M. Sato, M. Iwami and T. Kiya (2013). "Visualization of neural activity in insect brains using a conserved immediate early gene, Hr38." Curr Biol **23**(20): 2063–2070.

Gao, M., K. Sossa, L. Song, L. Errington, L. Cummings, H. Hwang, D. Kuhl, P. Worley and H. K. Lee (2010). "A specific requirement of Arc/Arg3.1 for visual experience-induced homeostatic synaptic plasticity in mouse primary visual cortex." J Neurosci **30**(21): 7168–7178.

Garber, K. B., J. Visootsak and S. T. Warren (2008). "Fragile X syndrome." Eur J Hum Genet **16**(6): 666–672.

Gee, J. R. and J. N. Keller (2005). "Astrocytes: regulation of brain homeostasis via apolipoprotein E." Int J Biochem Cell Biol **37**(6): 1145–1150.

Gerges, N. Z., D. S. Backos and J. A. Esteban (2004). "Local control of AMPA receptor trafficking at the postsynaptic terminal by a small GTPase of the Rab family." J Biol Chem **279**(42): 43870–43878.

Gordon, J. A. and M. P. Stryker (1996). "Experience-dependent plasticity of binocular responses in the primary visual cortex of the mouse." J Neurosci **16**(10): 3274–3286.

Govek, E. E., S. E. Newey and L. Van Aelst (2005). "The role of the Rho GTPases in neuronal development." Genes Dev **19**(1): 1–49.

Grabert, K., T. Michoel, M. H. Karavolos, S. Clohisey, J. K. Baillie, M. P. Stevens, T. C. Freeman, K. M. Summers and B. W. McColl (2016). "Microglial brain region-dependent diversity and selective regional sensitivities to aging." Nat Neurosci **19**(3): 504–516.

Greer, P. L., R. Hanayama, B. L. Bloodgood, A. R. Mardinly, D. M. Lipton, S. W. Flavell, T. K. Kim, E. C. Griffith, Z. Waldon, R. Maehr, H. L.

Ploegh, S. Chowdhury, P. F. Worley, J. Steen and M. E. Greenberg (2010). "The Angelman Syndrome protein Ube3A regulates synapse development by ubiquitinating arc." Cell **140**(5): 704–716.

Griesi-Oliveira, K., A. Acab, A. R. Gupta, D. Y. Sunaga, T. Chailangkarn, X. Nicol, Y. Nunez, M. F. Walker, J. D. Murdoch, S. J. Sanders, T. V. Fernandez, W. Ji, R. P. Lifton, E. Vadasz, A. Dietrich, D. Pradhan, H. Song, G. L. Ming, X. Gu, G. Haddad, M. C. Marchetto, N. Spitzer, M. R. Passos-Bueno, M. W. State and A. R. Muotri (2015). "Modeling non-syndromic autism and the impact of TRPC6 disruption in human neurons." Mol Psychiatry **20**(11): 1350–1365.

Grueber, W. B. and Y. N. Jan (2004). "Dendritic development: lessons from Drosophila and related branches." Curr Opin Neurobiol **14**(1): 74–82.

Grunwald, L. M., R. Stock, K. Haag, S. Buckenmaier, M. C. Eberle, D. Wildgruber, H. Storchak, M. Kriebel, S. Weissgraeber, L. Mathew, Y. Singh, M. Loos, K. W. Li, U. Kraushaar, A. J. Fallgatter and H. Volkmer (2019). "Comparative characterization of human induced pluripotent stem cells (hiPSC) derived from patients with schizophrenia and autism." Transl Psychiatry **9**(1): 179.

Haas, K., J. Li and H. T. Cline (2006). "AMPA receptors regulate experience-dependent dendritic arbor growth in vivo." Proc Natl Acad Sci U S A **103**(32): 12127–12131.

Hafner, A. S., P. G. Donlin-Asp, B. Leitch, E. Herzog and E. M. Schuman (2019). "Local protein synthesis is a ubiquitous feature of neuronal pre- and postsynaptic compartments." Science **364**(6441).

Hagerman, R. J., E. Berry-Kravis, H. C. Hazlett, D. B. Bailey, Jr., H. Moine, R. F. Kooy, F. Tassone, I. Gantois, N. Sonenberg, J. L. Mandel and P. J. Hagerman (2017). "Fragile X syndrome." Nat Rev Dis Primers **3**: 17065.

Han, J. M. and M. Sahin (2011). "TSC1/TSC2 signaling in the CNS." FEBS Lett **585**(7): 973–980.

Hanover, J. L., Z. J. Huang, S. Tonegawa and M. P. Stryker (1999). "Brain-derived neurotrophic factor overexpression induces precocious critical period in mouse visual cortex." J Neurosci **19**(22): RC40.

Hartwig, C. L., J. Worrell, R. B. Levine, M. Ramaswami and S. Sanyal (2008). "Normal dendrite growth in Drosophila motor neurons requires the AP-1 transcription factor." Dev Neurobiol **68**(10): 1225–1242.

Hayashi-Takagi, A., S. Yagishita, M. Nakamura, F. Shirai, Y. I. Wu, A. L. Loshbaugh, B. Kuhlman, K. M. Hahn and H. Kasai (2015). "Labelling and optical erasure of synaptic memory traces in the motor cortex." Nature **525**(7569): 333–338.

He, H. Y., W. Shen, M. Hiramoto and H. T. Cline (2016). "Experience-Dependent Bimodal Plasticity of Inhibitory Neurons in Early Development." Neuron **90**(6): 1203–1214.

Heinz, D. A. and B. L. Bloodgood (2020). "Mechanisms that communicate features of neuronal activity to the genome." Curr Opin Neurobiol **63**: 131–136.

Hensch, T. K., M. Fagiolini, N. Mataga, M. P. Stryker, S. Baekkeskov and S. F. Kash (1998). "Local GABA circuit control of experience-dependent plasticity in developing visual cortex." Science **282**(5393): 1504–1508.

Herring, B. E. and R. A. Nicoll (2016). "Kalirin and Trio proteins serve critical roles in excitatory synaptic transmission and LTP." Proc Natl Acad Sci U S A **113**(8): 2264–2269.

Hiramoto, M. and H. T. Cline (2014). "Optic flow instructs retinotopic map formation through a spatial to temporal to spatial transformation of visual information." Proc Natl Acad Sci U S A **111**(47): E5105–5113.

Hofer, S. B., T. D. Mrsic-Flogel, T. Bonhoeffer and M. Hubener (2009). "Experience leaves a lasting structural trace in cortical circuits." Nature **457**(7227): 313–317.

Holtmaat, A., L. Wilbrecht, G. W. Knott, E. Welker and K. Svoboda (2006). "Experience-dependent and cell-type-specific spine growth in the neocortex." Nature **441**(7096): 979–983.

Hong, Y. K., S. Park, E. Y. Litvina, J. Morales, J. R. Sanes and C. Chen (2014). "Refinement of the retinogeniculate synapse by bouton clustering." Neuron **84**(2): 332–339.

Hoshiko, M., I. Arnoux, E. Avignone, N. Yamamoto and E. Audinat (2012). "Deficiency of the microglial receptor CX3CR1 impairs postnatal functional development of thalamocortical synapses in the barrel cortex." J Neurosci **32**(43): 15106–15111.

Huang, Z. J., A. Kirkwood, T. Pizzorusso, V. Porciatti, B. Morales, M. F. Bear, L. Maffei and S. Tonegawa (1999). "BDNF regulates the maturation of inhibition and the critical period of plasticity in mouse visual cortex." Cell **98**(6): 739–755.

Hubel, D. H. and T. N. Wiesel (1963). "Receptive Fields of Cells in Striate Cortex of Very Young, Visually Inexperienced Kittens." J Neurophysiol **26**: 994–1002.

Huber, K. M., S. M. Gallagher, S. T. Warren and M. F. Bear (2002). "Altered synaptic plasticity in a mouse model of fragile X mental retardation." Proc Natl Acad Sci U S A **99**(11): 7746–7750.

Huberman, A. D., D. Stellwagen and B. Chapman (2002). "Decoupling eye-specific segregation from lamination in the lateral geniculate nucleus." J Neurosci **22**(21): 9419–9429.

Ifrim, M. F., K. R. Williams and G. J. Bassell (2015). "Single-Molecule Imaging of PSD-95 mRNA Translation in Dendrites and Its Dysregulation in a Mouse Model of Fragile X Syndrome." J Neurosci **35**(18): 7116–7130.

Impey, S., M. Davare, A. Lesiak, D. Fortin, H. Ando, O. Varlamova, K. Obrietan, T. R. Soderling, R. H. Goodman and G. A. Wayman (2010). "An activity-induced microRNA controls dendritic spine formation by regulating Rac1-PAK signaling." Mol Cell Neurosci **43**(1): 146–156.

Iwai, Y., M. Fagiolini, K. Obata and T. K. Hensch (2003). "Rapid critical period induction by tonic inhibition in visual cortex." J Neurosci **23**(17): 6695–6702.

Jan, Y. N. and L. Y. Jan (2010). "Branching out: mechanisms of dendritic arborization." Nat Rev Neurosci **11**(5): 316–328.

Jin, Y. and Y. B. Qi (2018). "Building stereotypic connectivity: mechanistic insights into structural plasticity from C. elegans." Curr Opin Neurobiol **48**: 97–105.

Jones, E. V., Y. Bernardinelli, Y. C. Tse, S. Chierzi, T. P. Wong and K. K. Murai (2011). "Astrocytes control glutamate receptor levels at developing synapses through SPARC-beta-integrin interactions." J Neurosci **31**(11): 4154–4165.

Ju, W., W. Morishita, J. Tsui, G. Gaietta, T. J. Deerinck, S. R. Adams, C. C. Garner, R. Y. Tsien, M. H. Ellisman and R. C. Malenka (2004). "Activity-dependent regulation of dendritic synthesis and trafficking of AMPA receptors." Nat Neurosci **7**(3): 244–253.

Kajiya, M., K. Takeshita, M. Kittaka, S. Matsuda, K. Ouhara, K. Takeda, T. Takata, M. Kitagawa, T. Fujita, H. Shiba and H. Kurihara (2014). "BDNF mimetic compound LM22A-4 regulates cementoblast differentiation via the TrkB-ERK/Akt signaling cascade." Int Immunopharmacol **19**(2): 245–252.

Kalambogias, J., C. C. Chen, S. Khan, T. Son, R. Wercberger, C. Headlam, C. Lin and J. C. Brumberg (2020). "Development and sensory experience dependent regulation of microglia in barrel cortex." J Comp Neurol **528**(4): 559–573.

Kanamori, T., M. I. Kanai, Y. Dairyo, K. Yasunaga, R. K. Morikawa and K. Emoto (2013). "Compartmentalized calcium transients trigger dendrite pruning in Drosophila sensory neurons." Science **340**(6139): 1475–1478.

Kaneko, M. and M. P. Stryker (2017). "Homeostatic plasticity mechanisms in mouse V1." Philos Trans R Soc Lond B Biol Sci **372**(1715).

Katz, L. C. and C. J. Shatz (1996). "Synaptic activity and the construction of cortical circuits." Science **274**(5290): 1133–1138.

Keller, A. and G. C. Carlson (1999). "Neonatal whisker clipping alters intracortical, but not thalamocortical projections, in rat barrel cortex." J Comp Neurol **412**(1): 83–94.

Khakh, B. S. and M. V. Sofroniew (2015). "Diversity of astrocyte functions and phenotypes in neural circuits." Nat Neurosci **18**(7): 942–952.

Khatri, N. and H. Y. Man (2019). "The Autism and Angelman Syndrome Protein Ube3A/E6AP: The Gene, E3 Ligase Ubiquitination Targets and Neurobiological Functions." Front Mol Neurosci **12**: 109.

Kim, K. Y., E. Hysolli and I. H. Park (2011). "Neuronal maturation defect in induced pluripotent stem cells from patients with Rett syndrome." Proc Natl Acad Sci U S A **108**(34): 14169–14174.

Knott, G. W., C. Quairiaux, C. Genoud and E. Welker (2002). "Formation of dendritic spines with GABAergic synapses induced by whisker stimulation in adult mice." Neuron **34**(2): 265–273.

Koleske, A. J. (2013). "Molecular mechanisms of dendrite stability." Nat Rev Neurosci **14**(8): 536–550.

Kossel, A., S. Lowel and J. Bolz (1995). "Relationships between dendritic fields and functional architecture in striate cortex of normal and visually deprived cats." J Neurosci **15**(5 Pt 2): 3913–3926.

Krey, J. F., S. P. Pasca, A. Shcheglovitov, M. Yazawa, R. Schwemberger, R. Rasmusson and R. E. Dolmetsch (2013). "Timothy syndrome is associated with activity-dependent dendritic retraction in rodent and human neurons." Nat Neurosci **16**(2): 201–209.

Kucukdereli, H., N. J. Allen, A. T. Lee, A. Feng, M. I. Ozlu, L. M. Conatser, C. Chakraborty, G. Workman, M. Weaver, E. H. Sage, B. A. Barres and C. Eroglu (2011). "Control of excitatory CNS synaptogenesis by astrocyte-secreted proteins Hevin and SPARC." Proc Natl Acad Sci U S A **108**(32): E440–449.

Kuhlman, S. J., N. D. Olivas, E. Tring, T. Ikrar, X. Xu and J. T. Trachtenberg (2013). "A disinhibitory microcircuit initiates critical-period plasticity in the visual cortex." Nature **501**(7468): 543–546.

Kuhnle, S., B. Mothes, K. Matentzoglu and M. Scheffner (2013). "Role of the ubiquitin ligase E6AP/UBE3A in controlling levels of the synaptic protein Arc." Proc Natl Acad Sci U S A **110**(22): 8888–8893.

Lacar, B., S. B. Linker, B. N. Jaeger, S. R. Krishnaswami, J. J. Barron, M. J. E. Kelder, S. L. Parylak, A. C. M. Paquola, P. Venepally, M. Novotny, C. O'Connor, C. Fitzpatrick, J. A. Erwin, J. Y. Hsu, D. Husband, M. J. McConnell, R. Lasken and F. H. Gage (2016). "Nuclear RNA-seq of single neurons reveals molecular signatures of activation." Nat Commun **7**: 11022.

Larimore, J. L., C. A. Chapleau, S. Kudo, A. Theibert, A. K. Percy and L. Pozzo-Miller (2009). "Bdnf overexpression in hippocampal neurons prevents dendritic atrophy caused by Rett-associated MECP2 mutations." Neurobiol Dis **34**(2): 199–211.

Lawal, O., F. P. Ulloa Severino and C. Eroglu (2022). "The role of astrocyte structural plasticity in regulating neural circuit function and behavior." Glia **70**(8): 1467–1483.

Lawson, L. J., V. H. Perry, P. Dri and S. Gordon (1990). "Heterogeneity in the distribution and morphology of microglia in the normal adult mouse brain." Neuroscience **39**(1): 151–170.

Lee, K. F., C. Soares, J. P. Thivierge and J. C. Beique (2016). "Correlated Synaptic Inputs Drive Dendritic Calcium Amplification and Cooperative Plasticity during Clustered Synapse Development." Neuron **89**(4): 784–799.

Lee, L. J., V. Tsytsarev and R. S. Erzurumlu (2017). "Structural and functional differences in the barrel cortex of Mecp2 null mice." J Comp Neurol **525**(18): 3951–3961.

Lee, S. J., Y. Escobedo-Lozoya, E. M. Szatmari and R. Yasuda (2009). "Activation of CaMKII in single dendritic spines during long-term potentiation." Nature **458**(7236): 299–304.

Lefebvre, J. L., J. R. Sanes and J. N. Kay (2015). "Development of dendritic form and function." Annu Rev Cell Dev Biol **31**: 741–777.

Lemieux, M., S. Labrecque, C. Tardif, E. Labrie-Dion, E. Lebel and P. De Koninck (2012). "Translocation of CaMKII to dendritic microtubules supports the plasticity of local synapses." J Cell Biol **198**(6): 1055–1073.

Lendvai, B., E. A. Stern, B. Chen and K. Svoboda (2000). "Experience-dependent plasticity of dendritic spines in the developing rat barrel cortex in vivo." Nature **404**(6780): 876–881.

LeVay, S., T. N. Wiesel and D. H. Hubel (1980). "The development of ocular dominance columns in normal and visually deprived monkeys." J Comp Neurol **191**(1): 1–51.

Li, J., R. R. Khankan, C. Caneda, M. I. Godoy, M. S. Haney, M. C. Krawczyk, M. C. Bassik, S. A. Sloan and Y. Zhang (2019). "Astrocyte-to-astrocyte contact and a positive feedback loop of growth factor signaling regulate astrocyte maturation." Glia **67**(8): 1571–1597.

Li, W., G. Calfa, J. Larimore and L. Pozzo-Miller (2012). "Activity-dependent BDNF release and TRPC signaling is impaired in hippocampal neurons of Mecp2 mutant mice." Proc Natl Acad Sci U S A **109**(42): 17087–17092.

Li, Z., C. D. Aizenman and H. T. Cline (2002). "Regulation of rho GTPases by crosstalk and neuronal activity in vivo." Neuron **33**(5): 741–750.

Li, Z., L. Van Aelst and H. T. Cline (2000). "Rho GTPases regulate distinct aspects of dendritic arbor growth in Xenopus central neurons in vivo." Nat Neurosci **3**(3): 217–225.

Lin, Y., B. L. Bloodgood, J. L. Hauser, A. D. Lapan, A. C. Koon, T. K. Kim, L. S. Hu, A. N. Malik and M. E. Greenberg (2008). "Activity-dependent regulation of inhibitory synapse development by Npas4." Nature **455**(7217): 1198–1204.

Lisman, J., H. Schulman and H. Cline (2002). "The molecular basis of CaMKII function in synaptic and behavioural memory." Nat Rev Neurosci **3**(3): 175–190.

Liu, H. H., D. B. McClatchy, L. Schiapparelli, W. Shen, J. R. Yates, 3rd and H. T. Cline (2018). "Role of the visual experience-dependent nascent proteome in neuronal plasticity." Elife **7**.

Liu, X. F., P. K. Tari and K. Haas (2009). "PKM zeta restricts dendritic arbor growth by filopodial and branch stabilization within the intact and awake developing brain." J Neurosci **29**(39): 12229–12235.

Livide, G., T. Patriarchi, M. Amenduni, S. Amabile, D. Yasui, E. Calcagno, C. Lo Rizzo, G. De Falco, C. Ulivieri, F. Ariani, F. Mari, M. A. Mencarelli, J. W. Hell, A. Renieri and I. Meloni (2015). "GluD1 is a common altered player in neuronal differentiation from both MECP2-mutated and CDKL5-mutated iPS cells." Eur J Hum Genet **23**(2): 195–201.

Lohmann, C. and T. Bonhoeffer (2008). "A role for local calcium signaling in rapid synaptic partner selection by dendritic filopodia." Neuron **59**(2): 253–260.

Lu, H. E., H. D. MacGillavry, N. A. Frost and T. A. Blanpied (2014). "Multiple spatial and kinetic subpopulations of CaMKII in spines and dendrites as resolved by single-molecule tracking PALM." J Neurosci **34**(22): 7600–7610.

Lucic, V., G. J. Greif and M. B. Kennedy (2008). "Detailed state model of CaMKII activation and autophosphorylation." Eur Biophys J **38**(1): 83–98.

Ma, X. M., D. D. Kiraly, E. D. Gaier, Y. Wang, E. J. Kim, E. S. Levine, B. A. Eipper and R. E. Mains (2008). "Kalirin-7 is required for synaptic structure and function." J Neurosci **28**(47): 12368–12382.

Madison, J. M., F. Zhou, A. Nigam, A. Hussain, D. D. Barker, R. Nehme, K. van der Ven, J. Hsu, P. Wolf, M. Fleishman, C. O'Dushlaine, S. Rose, K. Chambert, F. H. Lau, T. Ahfeldt, E. H. Rueckert, S. D. Sheridan, D. M. Fass, J. Nemesh, T. E. Mullen, L. Daheron, S. McCarroll, P. Sklar,

R. H. Perlis and S. J. Haggarty (2015). "Characterization of bipolar disorder patient-specific induced pluripotent stem cells from a family reveals neurodevelopmental and mRNA expression abnormalities." Mol Psychiatry **20**(6): 703–717.

Maffei, A., S. B. Nelson and G. G. Turrigiano (2004). "Selective reconfiguration of layer 4 visual cortical circuitry by visual deprivation." Nat Neurosci **7**(12): 1353–1359.

Majdan, M. and C. J. Shatz (2006). "Effects of visual experience on activity-dependent gene regulation in cortex." Nat Neurosci **9**(5): 650–659.

Majewska, A. and M. Sur (2003). "Motility of dendritic spines in visual cortex in vivo: changes during the critical period and effects of visual deprivation." Proc Natl Acad Sci U S A **100**(26): 16024–16029.

Malpel, S., A. Klarsfeld and F. Rouyer (2002). "Larval optic nerve and adult extra-retinal photoreceptors sequentially associate with clock neurons during Drosophila brain development." Development **129**(6): 1443–1453.

Malun, D. and P. C. Brunjes (1996). "Development of olfactory glomeruli: temporal and spatial interactions between olfactory receptor axons and mitral cells in opossums and rats." J Comp Neurol **368**(1): 1–16.

Mameli, M., B. Balland, R. Lujan and C. Luscher (2007). "Rapid synthesis and synaptic insertion of GluR2 for mGluR-LTD in the ventral tegmental area." Science **317**(5837): 530–533.

Margolis, S. S., J. Salogiannis, D. M. Lipton, C. Mandel-Brehm, Z. P. Wills, A. R. Mardinly, L. Hu, P. L. Greer, J. B. Bikoff, H. Y. Ho, M. J. Soskis, M. Sahin and M. E. Greenberg (2010). "EphB-mediated degradation of the RhoA GEF Ephexin5 relieves a developmental brake on excitatory synapse formation." Cell **143**(3): 442–455.

Margolis, S. S., G. L. Sell, M. A. Zbinden and L. M. Bird (2015). "Angelman Syndrome." Neurotherapeutics **12**(3): 641–650.

Mariani, J., G. Coppola, P. Zhang, A. Abyzov, L. Provini, L. Tomasini, M. Amenduni, A. Szekely, D. Palejev, M. Wilson, M. Gerstein, E. L. Grigorenko, K. Chawarska, K. A. Pelphrey, J. R. Howe and F. M. Vaccarino (2015). "FOXG1-Dependent Dysregulation of GABA/Glutamate Neuron Differentiation in Autism Spectrum Disorders." Cell **162**(2): 375–390.

Marie, H., W. Morishita, X. Yu, N. Calakos and R. C. Malenka (2005). "Generation of silent synapses by acute in vivo expression of CaMKIV and CREB." Neuron **45**(5): 741–752.

Martinowich, K., D. Hattori, H. Wu, S. Fouse, F. He, Y. Hu, G. Fan and Y. E. Sun (2003). "DNA methylation-related chromatin remodeling in activity-dependent BDNF gene regulation." Science **302**(5646): 890–893.

Massa, S. M., T. Yang, Y. Xie, J. Shi, M. Bilgen, J. N. Joyce, D. Nehama, J. Rajadas and F. M. Longo (2010). "Small molecule BDNF mimetics activate TrkB signaling and prevent neuronal degeneration in rodents." J Clin Invest **120**(5): 1774–1785.

Mauch, D. H., K. Nagler, S. Schumacher, C. Goritz, E. C. Muller, A. Otto and F. W. Pfrieger (2001). "CNS synaptogenesis promoted by glia-derived cholesterol." Science **294**(5545): 1354–1357.

Maxwell, M. A. and G. E. Muscat (2006). "The NR4A subgroup: immediate early response genes with pleiotropic physiological roles." Nucl Recept Signal **4**: e002.

McCurry, C. L., J. D. Shepherd, D. Tropea, K. H. Wang, M. F. Bear and M. Sur (2010). "Loss of Arc renders the visual cortex impervious to the effects of sensory experience or deprivation." Nat Neurosci **13**(4): 450–457.

McRae, P. A., M. M. Rocco, G. Kelly, J. C. Brumberg and R. T. Matthews (2007). "Sensory deprivation alters aggrecan and perineuronal net expression in the mouse barrel cortex." J Neurosci **27**(20): 5405–5413.

McVicker, D. P., M. M. Millette and E. W. Dent (2015). "Signaling to the microtubule cytoskeleton: an unconventional role for CaMKII." Dev Neurobiol **75**(4): 423–434.

Meyer-Franke, A., M. R. Kaplan, F. W. Pfrieger and B. A. Barres (1995). "Characterization of the signaling interactions that promote the survival and growth of developing retinal ganglion cells in culture." Neuron **15**(4): 805–819.

Miller, S., M. Yasuda, J. K. Coats, Y. Jones, M. E. Martone and M. Mayford (2002). "Disruption of dendritic translation of CaMKIIalpha impairs stabilization of synaptic plasticity and memory consolidation." Neuron **36**(3): 507–519.

Morales, B., S. Y. Choi and A. Kirkwood (2002). "Dark rearing alters the development of GABAergic transmission in visual cortex." J Neurosci **22**(18): 8084–8090.

Muddashetty, R. S., S. Kelic, C. Gross, M. Xu and G. J. Bassell (2007). "Dysregulated metabotropic glutamate receptor-dependent translation of AMPA receptor and postsynaptic density-95 mRNAs at synapses in a mouse model of fragile X syndrome." J Neurosci **27**(20): 5338–5348.

Muotri, A. R., M. C. Marchetto, N. G. Coufal, R. Oefner, G. Yeo, K. Nakashima and F. H. Gage (2010). "L1 retrotransposition in neurons is modulated by MeCP2." Nature **468**(7322): 443–446.

Murakoshi, H., H. Wang and R. Yasuda (2011). "Local, persistent activation of Rho GTPases during plasticity of single dendritic spines." Nature **472**(7341): 100–104.

Murphy, T. H., P. F. Worley and J. M. Baraban (1991). "L-type voltage-sensitive calcium channels mediate synaptic activation of immediate early genes." Neuron **7**(4): 625–635.

Nadif Kasri, N., A. Nakano-Kobayashi, R. Malinow, B. Li and L. Van Aelst (2009). "The Rho-linked mental retardation protein oligophrenin-1 controls synapse maturation and plasticity by stabilizing AMPA receptors." Genes Dev **23**(11): 1289–1302.

Nadif Kasri, N., A. Nakano-Kobayashi and L. Van Aelst (2011). "Rapid synthesis of the X-linked mental retardation protein OPHN1 mediates mGluR-dependent LTD through interaction with the endocytic machinery." Neuron **72**(2): 300–315.

Nageshappa, S., C. Carromeu, C. A. Trujillo, P. Mesci, I. Espuny-Camacho, E. Pasciuto, P. Vanderhaeghen, C. M. Verfaillie, S. Raitano, A. Kumar, C. M. Carvalho, C. Bagni, M. B. Ramocki, B. H. Araujo, L. B. Torres, J. R. Lupski, H. Van Esch and A. R. Muotri (2016). "Altered neuronal network and rescue in a human MECP2 duplication model." Mol Psychiatry **21**(2): 178–188.

Nakahata, Y. and R. Yasuda (2018). "Plasticity of Spine Structure: Local Signaling, Translation and Cytoskeletal Reorganization." Front Synaptic Neurosci **10**: 29.

Nakai, N., T. Takumi, J. Nakai and M. Sato (2018). "Common Defects of Spine Dynamics and Circuit Function in Neurodevelopmental Disorders: A Systematic Review of Findings From in Vivo Optical Imaging of Mouse Models." Front Neurosci **12**: 412.

Nalavadi, V. C., R. S. Muddashetty, C. Gross and G. J. Bassell (2012). "Dephosphorylation-induced ubiquitination and degradation of FMRP in dendrites: a role in immediate early mGluR-stimulated translation." J Neurosci **32**(8): 2582–2587.

Napoli, I., V. Mercaldo, P. P. Boyl, B. Eleuteri, F. Zalfa, S. De Rubeis, D. Di Marino, E. Mohr, M. Massimi, M. Falconi, W. Witke, M. Costa-Mattioli, N. Sonenberg, T. Achsel and C. Bagni (2008). "The fragile X syndrome protein represses activity-dependent translation through CYFIP1, a new 4E-BP." Cell **134**(6): 1042–1054.

Neniskyte, U. and C. T. Gross (2017). "Errant gardeners: glial-cell-dependent synaptic pruning and neurodevelopmental disorders." Nat Rev Neurosci **18**(11): 658–670.

Nguyen, M. V., F. Du, C. A. Felice, X. Shan, A. Nigam, G. Mandel, J. K. Robinson and N. Ballas (2012). "MeCP2 is critical for maintaining mature neuronal networks and global brain anatomy during late stages of postnatal brain development and in the mature adult brain." J Neurosci **32**(29): 10021–10034.

Nithianantharajah, J. and A. J. Hannan (2006). "Enriched environments, experience-dependent plasticity and disorders of the nervous system." Nat Rev Neurosci **7**(9): 697–709.

Ogier, M., H. Wang, E. Hong, Q. Wang, M. E. Greenberg and D. M. Katz (2007). "Brain-derived neurotrophic factor expression and respiratory function improve after ampakine treatment in a mouse model of Rett syndrome." J Neurosci **27**(40): 10912–10917.

Oswald, M. C., P. S. Brooks, M. F. Zwart, A. Mukherjee, R. J. West, C. N. Giachello, K. Morarach, R. A. Baines, S. T. Sweeney and M. Landgraf (2018). "Reactive oxygen species regulate activity-dependent neuronal plasticity in Drosophila." Elife **7**.

Pan, F., G. M. Aldridge, W. T. Greenough and W. B. Gan (2010). "Dendritic spine instability and insensitivity to modulation by sensory experience in a mouse model of fragile X syndrome." Proc Natl Acad Sci U S A **107**(41): 17768–17773.

Panatier, A., J. Vallee, M. Haber, K. K. Murai, J. C. Lacaille and R. Robitaille (2011). "Astrocytes are endogenous regulators of basal transmission at central synapses." Cell **146**(5): 785–798.

Paolicelli, R. C., G. Bolasco, F. Pagani, L. Maggi, M. Scianni, P. Panzanelli, M. Giustetto, T. A. Ferreira, E. Guiducci, L. Dumas, D. Ragozzino and C. T. Gross (2011). "Synaptic pruning by microglia is necessary for normal brain development." Science **333**(6048): 1456–1458.

Parenti, I., L. G. Rabaneda, H. Schoen and G. Novarino (2020). "Neurodevelopmental Disorders: From Genetics to Functional Pathways." Trends Neurosci **43**(8): 608–621.

Park, S., J. M. Park, S. Kim, J. A. Kim, J. D. Shepherd, C. L. Smith-Hicks, S. Chowdhury, W. Kaufmann, D. Kuhl, A. G. Ryazanov, R. L. Huganir, D. J. Linden and P. F. Worley (2008). "Elongation factor 2 and fragile X mental retardation protein control the dynamic translation of Arc/Arg3.1 essential for mGluR-LTD." Neuron **59**(1): 70–83.

Parkhurst, C. N., G. Yang, I. Ninan, J. N. Savas, J. R. Yates, 3rd, J. J. Lafaille, B. L. Hempstead, D. R. Littman and W. B. Gan (2013). "Microglia promote learning-dependent synapse formation through brain-derived neurotrophic factor." Cell **155**(7): 1596–1609.

Pasca, S. P., T. Portmann, I. Voineagu, M. Yazawa, A. Shcheglovitov, A. M. Pasca, B. Cord, T. D. Palmer, S. Chikahisa, S. Nishino, J. A. Bernstein, J. Hallmayer, D. H. Geschwind and R. E. Dolmetsch (2011). "Using iPSC-derived neurons to uncover cellular phenotypes associated with Timothy syndrome." Nat Med **17**(12): 1657–1662.

Paulsen, B., S. Velasco, A. J. Kedaigle, M. Pigoni, G. Quadrato, A. J. Deo, X. Adiconis, A. Uzquiano, R. Sartore, S. M. Yang, S. K. Simmons, P. Symvoulidis, K. Kim, K. Tsafou, A. Podury, C. Abbate, A. Tucewicz, S. N. Smith, A. Albanese, L. Barrett, N. E. Sanjana, X. Shi, K. Chung, K. Lage, E. S. Boyden, A. Regev, J. Z. Levin and P. Arlotta (2022). "Autism genes converge on asynchronous development of shared neuron classes." Nature **602**(7896): 268–273.

Penn, A. A., P. A. Riquelme, M. B. Feller and C. J. Shatz (1998). "Competition in retinogeniculate patterning driven by spontaneous activity." Science **279**(5359): 2108–2112.

Perea, G., M. Navarrete and A. Araque (2009). "Tripartite synapses: astrocytes process and control synaptic information." Trends Neurosci **32**(8): 421–431.

Perea, G., M. Sur and A. Araque (2014). "Neuron-glia networks: integral gear of brain function." Front Cell Neurosci **8**: 378.

Pfeiffer, B. E., T. Zang, J. R. Wilkerson, M. Taniguchi, M. A. Maksimova, L. N. Smith, C. W. Cowan and K. M. Huber (2010). "Fragile X mental retardation protein is required for synapse elimination by the activity-dependent transcription factor MEF2." Neuron **66**(2): 191–197.

Pfrieger, F. W. and B. A. Barres (1997). "Synaptic efficacy enhanced by glial cells in vitro." Science **277**(5332): 1684–1687.

Poo, M. M. (2001). "Neurotrophins as synaptic modulators." Nat Rev Neurosci **2**(1): 24–32.

Pyka, M., C. Wetzel, A. Aguado, M. Geissler, H. Hatt and A. Faissner (2011). "Chondroitin sulfate proteoglycans regulate astrocyte-dependent synaptogenesis and modulate synaptic activity in primary embryonic hippocampal neurons." Eur J Neurosci **33**(12): 2187–2202.

Pyronneau, A., Q. He, J. Y. Hwang, M. Porch, A. Contractor and R. S. Zukin (2017). "Aberrant Rac1-cofilin signaling mediates defects in dendritic spines, synaptic function, and sensory perception in fragile X syndrome." Sci Signal **10**(504).

Qiu, Z. and A. Ghosh (2008). "A calcium-dependent switch in a CREST-BRG1 complex regulates activity-dependent gene expression." Neuron **60**(5): 775–787.

Rajgor, D., T. M. Sanderson, M. Amici, G. L. Collingridge and J. G. Hanley (2018). "NMDAR-dependent Argonaute 2 phosphorylation regulates miRNA activity and dendritic spine plasticity." EMBO J **37**(11).

Rangamani, P., M. G. Levy, S. Khan and G. Oster (2016). "Paradoxical signaling regulates structural plasticity in dendritic spines." Proc Natl Acad Sci U S A **113**(36): E5298–5307.

Ratanatharathorn, A., K. C. Koenen, L. B. Chibnik, M. G. Weisskopf, J. W. Rich-Edwards and A. L. Roberts (2021). "Polygenic risk for autism, attention-deficit hyperactivity disorder, schizophrenia, major depressive disorder, and neuroticism is associated with the experience of childhood abuse." Mol Psychiatry **26**(5): 1696–1705.

Redmond, L., A. H. Kashani and A. Ghosh (2002). "Calcium regulation of dendritic growth via CaM kinase IV and CREB-mediated transcription." Neuron **34**(6): 999–1010.

Rial Verde, E. M., J. Lee-Osbourne, P. F. Worley, R. Malinow and H. T. Cline (2006). "Increased expression of the immediate-early gene arc/arg3.1 reduces AMPA receptor-mediated synaptic transmission." Neuron **52**(3): 461–474.

Ribot, J., R. Breton, C. F. Calvo, J. Moulard, P. Ezan, J. Zapata, K. Samama, M. Moreau, A. P. Bemelmans, V. Sabatet, F. Dingli, D. Loew, C. Milleret, P. Billuart, G. Dallerac and N. Rouach (2021). "Astrocytes close the mouse critical period for visual plasticity." Science **373**(6550): 77–81.

Richter, J. D. and E. Klann (2009). "Making synaptic plasticity and memory last: mechanisms of translational regulation." Genes Dev **23**(1): 1–11.

Risher, W. C., S. Patel, I. H. Kim, A. Uezu, S. Bhagat, D. K. Wilton, L. J. Pilaz, J. Singh Alvarado, O. Y. Calhan, D. L. Silver, B. Stevens, N. Calakos, S. H. Soderling and C. Eroglu (2014). "Astrocytes refine cortical connectivity at dendritic spines." Elife **3**.

Rosenthal, J. S., J. Yin, J. Lei, A. Sathyamurthy, J. Short, C. Long, E. Spillman, C. Sheng and Q. Yuan (2021). "Temporal regulation of nicotinic acetylcholine receptor subunits supports central cholinergic synapse development in Drosophila." Proc Natl Acad Sci U S A **118**(23).

Ruthazer, E. S., C. J. Akerman and H. T. Cline (2003). "Control of axon branch dynamics by correlated activity in vivo." Science **301**(5629): 66–70.

Rylaarsdam, L. and A. Guemez-Gamboa (2019). "Genetic Causes and Modifiers of Autism Spectrum Disorder." Front Cell Neurosci **13**: 385.

Sanes, J. R. and J. W. Lichtman (1999). "Development of the vertebrate neuromuscular junction." Annu Rev Neurosci **22**: 389–442.

Sato, M. and M. P. Stryker (2010). "Genomic imprinting of experience-dependent cortical plasticity by the ubiquitin ligase gene Ube3a." Proc Natl Acad Sci U S A **107**(12): 5611–5616.

Scarnati, M. S., R. Kataria, M. Biswas and K. G. Paradiso (2018). "Active presynaptic ribosomes in the mammalian brain, and altered transmitter release after protein synthesis inhibition." Elife **7**.

Schafer, D. P., E. K. Lehrman, A. G. Kautzman, R. Koyama, A. R. Mardinly, R. Yamasaki, R. M. Ransohoff, M. E. Greenberg, B. A. Barres and B. Stevens (2012). "Microglia sculpt postnatal neural circuits in an activity and complement-dependent manner." Neuron **74**(4): 691–705.

Schafer, D. P. and B. Stevens (2013). "Phagocytic glial cells: sculpting synaptic circuits in the developing nervous system." Curr Opin Neurobiol **23**(6): 1034–1040.

Schanzenbacher, C. T., J. D. Langer and E. M. Schuman (2018). "Time- and polarity-dependent proteomic changes associated with homeostatic scaling at central synapses." Elife **7**.

Schmid, D. A., T. Yang, M. Ogier, I. Adams, Y. Mirakhur, Q. Wang, S. M. Massa, F. M. Longo and D. M. Katz (2012). "A TrkB small molecule partial agonist rescues TrkB phosphorylation deficits and improves respiratory function in a mouse model of Rett syndrome." J Neurosci **32**(5): 1803–1810.

Schreiner, B., E. Romanelli, P. Liberski, B. Ingold-Heppner, B. Sobottka-Brillout, T. Hartwig, V. Chandrasekar, H. Johannssen, H. U. Zeilhofer, A. Aguzzi, F. Heppner, M. Kerschensteiner and B. Becher (2015). "Astrocyte Depletion Impairs Redox Homeostasis and Triggers Neuronal Loss in the Adult CNS." Cell Rep **12**(9): 1377–1384.

Shalizi, A., B. Gaudilliere, Z. Yuan, J. Stegmuller, T. Shirogane, Q. Ge, Y. Tan, B. Schulman, J. W. Harper and A. Bonni (2006). "A calcium-regulated MEF2 sumoylation switch controls postsynaptic differentiation." Science **311**(5763): 1012–1017.

Sharma, A., C. A. Hoeffer, Y. Takayasu, T. Miyawaki, S. M. McBride, E. Klann and R. S. Zukin (2010). "Dysregulation of mTOR signaling in fragile X syndrome." J Neurosci **30**(2): 694–702.

Shen, W., J. S. Da Silva, H. He and H. T. Cline (2009). "Type A GABA-receptor-dependent synaptic transmission sculpts dendritic arbor structure in Xenopus tadpoles in vivo." J Neurosci **29**(15): 5032–5043.

Shieh, P. B., S. C. Hu, K. Bobb, T. Timmusk and A. Ghosh (1998). "Identification of a signaling pathway involved in calcium regulation of BDNF expression." Neuron **20**(4): 727–740.

Shou, Y., F. Liang, S. Xu and X. Li (2020). "The Application of Brain Organoids: From Neuronal Development to Neurological Diseases." Front Cell Dev Biol **8**: 579659.

Silva, A. J., J. H. Kogan, P. W. Frankland and S. Kida (1998). "CREB and memory." Annu Rev Neurosci **21**: 127–148.

Simmons, D. A., N. P. Belichenko, T. Yang, C. Condon, M. Monbureau, M. Shamloo, D. Jing, S. M. Massa and F. M. Longo (2013). "A small molecule TrkB ligand reduces motor impairment and neuropathology in R6/2 and BACHD mouse models of Huntington's disease." J Neurosci **33**(48): 18712–18727.

Simms, B. A. and G. W. Zamponi (2014). "Neuronal voltage-gated calcium channels: structure, function, and dysfunction." Neuron **82**(1): 24–45.

Sin, W. C., K. Haas, E. S. Ruthazer and H. T. Cline (2002). "Dendrite growth increased by visual activity requires NMDA receptor and Rho GTPases." Nature **419**(6906): 475–480.

Singh, A. P., K. VijayRaghavan and V. Rodrigues (2010). "Dendritic refinement of an identified neuron in the Drosophila CNS is regulated by neuronal activity and Wnt signaling." Development **137**(8): 1351–1360.

Singh, S. K., J. A. Stogsdill, N. S. Pulimood, H. Dingsdale, Y. H. Kim, L. J. Pilaz, I. H. Kim, A. C. Manhaes, W. S. Rodrigues, Jr., A. Pamukcu, E. Enustun, Z. Ertuz, P. Scheiffele, S. H. Soderling, D. L. Silver, R. R. Ji, A. E. Medina and C. Eroglu (2016). "Astrocytes Assemble Thalamocortical Synapses by Bridging NRX1alpha and NL1 via Hevin." Cell **164**(1–2): 183–196.

Sipe, G. O., R. L. Lowery, M. E. Tremblay, E. A. Kelly, C. E. Lamantia and A. K. Majewska (2016). "Microglial P2Y12 is necessary for synaptic plasticity in mouse visual cortex." Nat Commun **7**: 10905.

Smith, G. B., A. J. Heynen and M. F. Bear (2009). "Bidirectional synaptic mechanisms of ocular dominance plasticity in visual cortex." Philos Trans R Soc Lond B Biol Sci **364**(1515): 357–367.

Smith, S. L. and J. T. Trachtenberg (2007). "Experience-dependent binocular competition in the visual cortex begins at eye opening." Nat Neurosci **10**(3): 370–375.

Smith, W. B., S. R. Starck, R. W. Roberts and E. M. Schuman (2005). "Dopaminergic stimulation of local protein synthesis enhances surface expression of GluR1 and synaptic transmission in hippocampal neurons." Neuron **45**(5): 765–779.

Soderling, S. H., E. S. Guire, S. Kaech, J. White, F. Zhang, K. Schutz, L. K. Langeberg, G. Banker, J. Raber and J. D. Scott (2007). "A WAVE-1 and

WRP signaling complex regulates spine density, synaptic plasticity, and memory." J Neurosci **27**(2): 355–365.

Spiegel, I., A. R. Mardinly, H. W. Gabel, J. E. Bazinet, C. H. Couch, C. P. Tzeng, D. A. Harmin and M. E. Greenberg (2014). "Npas4 regulates excitatory-inhibitory balance within neural circuits through cell-type-specific gene programs." Cell **157**(5): 1216–1229.

Sprecher, S. G., A. Cardona and V. Hartenstein (2011). "The Drosophila larval visual system: high-resolution analysis of a simple visual neuropil." Dev Biol **358**(1): 33–43.

Staiger, J. F., I. Flagmeyer, D. Schubert, K. Zilles, R. Kotter and H. J. Luhmann (2004). "Functional diversity of layer IV spiny neurons in rat somatosensory cortex: quantitative morphology of electrophysiologically characterized and biocytin labeled cells." Cereb Cortex **14**(6): 690–701.

Stankiewicz, T. R. and D. A. Linseman (2014). "Rho family GTPases: key players in neuronal development, neuronal survival, and neurodegeneration." Front Cell Neurosci **8**: 314.

Stellwagen, D. and R. C. Malenka (2006). "Synaptic scaling mediated by glial TNF-alpha." Nature **440**(7087): 1054–1059.

Stellwagen, D. and C. J. Shatz (2002). "An instructive role for retinal waves in the development of retinogeniculate connectivity." Neuron **33**(3): 357–367.

Stevens, B., N. J. Allen, L. E. Vazquez, G. R. Howell, K. S. Christopherson, N. Nouri, K. D. Micheva, A. K. Mehalow, A. D. Huberman, B. Stafford, A. Sher, A. M. Litke, J. D. Lambris, S. J. Smith, S. W. John and B. A. Barres (2007). "The classical complement cascade mediates CNS synapse elimination." Cell **131**(6): 1164–1178.

Stroud, H., M. G. Yang, Y. N. Tsitohay, C. P. Davis, M. A. Sherman, S. Hrvatin, E. Ling and M. E. Greenberg (2020). "An Activity-Mediated Transition in Transcription in Early Postnatal Neurons." Neuron **107**(5): 874–890 e878.

Sun, Y. J., J. S. Espinosa, M. S. Hoseini and M. P. Stryker (2019). "Experience-dependent structural plasticity at pre- and postsynaptic sites of layer 2/3 cells in developing visual cortex." Proc Natl Acad Sci U S A **116**(43): 21812–21820.

Suzuki, S., H. Zhou, J. F. Neumaier and T. A. Pham (2007). "Opposing functions of CREB and MKK1 synergistically regulate the geometry of dendritic spines in visual cortex." J Comp Neurol **503**(5): 605–617.

Takano, T., J. T. Wallace, K. T. Baldwin, A. M. Purkey, A. Uezu, J. L. Courtland, E. J. Soderblom, T. Shimogori, P. F. Maness, C. Eroglu and

S. H. Soderling (2020). "Chemico-genetic discovery of astrocytic control of inhibition in vivo." Nature **588**(7837): 296–302.

Tang, X., J. Kim, L. Zhou, E. Wengert, L. Zhang, Z. Wu, C. Carromeu, A. R. Muotri, M. C. Marchetto, F. H. Gage and G. Chen (2016). "KCC2 rescues functional deficits in human neurons derived from patients with Rett syndrome." Proc Natl Acad Sci U S A **113**(3): 751–756.

Tasdemir-Yilmaz, O. E. and M. R. Freeman (2014). "Astrocytes engage unique molecular programs to engulf pruned neuronal debris from distinct subsets of neurons." Genes Dev **28**(1): 20–33.

Tatavarty, V., M. F. Ifrim, M. Levin, G. Korza, E. Barbarese, J. Yu and J. H. Carson (2012). "Single-molecule imaging of translational output from individual RNA granules in neurons." Mol Biol Cell **23**(5): 918–929.

Tewari, B. P., L. Chaunsali, C. E. Prim and H. Sontheimer (2022). "A glial perspective on the extracellular matrix and perineuronal net remodeling in the central nervous system." Front Cell Neurosci **16**: 1022754.

Tian, N. and D. R. Copenhagen (2003). "Visual stimulation is required for refinement of ON and OFF pathways in postnatal retina." Neuron **39**(1): 85–96.

Tian, Y., I. Voineagu, S. P. Pasca, H. Won, V. Chandran, S. Horvath, R. E. Dolmetsch and D. H. Geschwind (2014). "Alteration in basal and depolarization induced transcriptional network in iPSC derived neurons from Timothy syndrome." Genome Med **6**(10): 75.

Todd, P. K., K. J. Mack and J. S. Malter (2003). "The fragile X mental retardation protein is required for type-I metabotropic glutamate receptor-dependent translation of PSD-95." Proc Natl Acad Sci U S A **100**(24): 14374–14378.

Trachtenberg, J. T., B. E. Chen, G. W. Knott, G. Feng, J. R. Sanes, E. Welker and K. Svoboda (2002). "Long-term in vivo imaging of experience-dependent synaptic plasticity in adult cortex." Nature **420**(6917): 788–794.

Tremblay, M. E., R. L. Lowery and A. K. Majewska (2010). "Microglial interactions with synapses are modulated by visual experience." PLoS Biol **8**(11): e1000527.

Tripodi, M., J. F. Evers, A. Mauss, M. Bate and M. Landgraf (2008). "Structural homeostasis: compensatory adjustments of dendritic arbor geometry in response to variations of synaptic input." PLoS Biol **6**(10): e260.

Tropea, D., A. K. Majewska, R. Garcia and M. Sur (2010). "Structural dynamics of synapses in vivo correlate with functional changes during experience-dependent plasticity in visual cortex." J Neurosci **30**(33): 11086–11095.

Tropea, D., A. Van Wart and M. Sur (2009). "Molecular mechanisms of experience-dependent plasticity in visual cortex." Philos Trans R Soc Lond B Biol Sci **364**(1515): 341–355.

Tsai, H. H., H. Li, L. C. Fuentealba, A. V. Molofsky, R. Taveira-Marques, H. Zhuang, A. Tenney, A. T. Murnen, S. P. Fancy, F. Merkle, N. Kessaris, A. Alvarez-Buylla, W. D. Richardson and D. H. Rowitch (2012). "Regional astrocyte allocation regulates CNS synaptogenesis and repair." Science **337**(6092): 358–362.

Tsai, N. P., J. R. Wilkerson, W. Guo and K. M. Huber (2017). "FMRP-dependent Mdm2 dephosphorylation is required for MEF2-induced synapse elimination." Hum Mol Genet **26**(2): 293–304.

Tu, S., M. W. Akhtar, R. M. Escorihuela, A. Amador-Arjona, V. Swarup, J. Parker, J. D. Zaremba, T. Holland, N. Bansal, D. R. Holohan, K. Lopez, S. D. Ryan, S. F. Chan, L. Yan, X. Zhang, X. Huang, A. Sultan, S. R. McKercher, R. Ambasudhan, H. Xu, Y. Wang, D. H. Geschwind, A. J. Roberts, A. V. Terskikh, R. A. Rissman, E. Masliah, S. A. Lipton and N. Nakanishi (2017). "NitroSynapsin therapy for a mouse MEF2C haplo-insufficiency model of human autism." Nat Commun **8**(1): 1488.

Tyler, W. J., M. Alonso, C. R. Bramham and L. D. Pozzo-Miller (2002). "From acquisition to consolidation: on the role of brain-derived neurotrophic factor signaling in hippocampal-dependent learning." Learn Mem **9**(5): 224–237.

Udagawa, T., S. A. Swanger, K. Takeuchi, J. H. Kim, V. Nalavadi, J. Shin, L. J. Lorenz, R. S. Zukin, G. J. Bassell and J. D. Richter (2012). "Bidirectional control of mRNA translation and synaptic plasticity by the cytoplasmic polyadenylation complex." Mol Cell **47**(2): 253–266.

Van der Loos, H. and T. A. Woolsey (1973). "Somatosensory cortex: structural alterations following early injury to sense organs." Science **179**(4071): 395–398.

Vaughn, J. E. (1989). "Fine structure of synaptogenesis in the vertebrate central nervous system." Synapse **3**(3): 255–285.

Vaughn, J. E., R. P. Barber and T. J. Sims (1988). "Dendritic development and preferential growth into synaptogenic fields: a quantitative study of Golgi-impregnated spinal motor neurons." Synapse **2**(1): 69–78.

Volkmar, F. R. and W. T. Greenough (1972). "Rearing complexity affects branching of dendrites in the visual cortex of the rat." Science **176**(4042): 1445–1447.

Wang, G. Y., L. C. Liets and L. M. Chalupa (2001). "Unique functional properties of on and off pathways in the developing mammalian retina." J Neurosci **21**(12): 4310–4317.

Wang, H., S. A. Chan, M. Ogier, D. Hellard, Q. Wang, C. Smith and D. M. Katz (2006). "Dysregulation of brain-derived neurotrophic factor expression and neurosecretory function in Mecp2 null mice." J Neurosci **26**(42): 10911–10915.

Watson, J. R., D. Owen and H. R. Mott (2017). "Cdc42 in actin dynamics: An ordered pathway governed by complex equilibria and directional effector handover." Small GTPases **8**(4): 237–244.

Weeber, E. J., Y. H. Jiang, Y. Elgersma, A. W. Varga, Y. Carrasquillo, S. E. Brown, J. M. Christian, B. Mirnikjoo, A. Silva, A. L. Beaudet and J. D. Sweatt (2003). "Derangements of hippocampal calcium/calmodulin-dependent protein kinase II in a mouse model for Angelman mental retardation syndrome." J Neurosci **23**(7): 2634–2644.

Weinhard, L., G. di Bartolomei, G. Bolasco, P. Machado, N. L. Schieber, U. Neniskyte, M. Exiga, A. Vadisiute, A. Raggioli, A. Schertel, Y. Schwab and C. T. Gross (2018). "Microglia remodel synapses by presynaptic trogocytosis and spine head filopodia induction." Nat Commun **9**(1): 1228.

Weller, W. L. and J. I. Johnson (1975). "Barrels in cerebral cortex altered by receptor disruption in newborn, but not in five-day-old mice (Cricetidoe and Muridae)." Brain Res **83**(3): 504–508.

West, A. E. and M. E. Greenberg (2011). "Neuronal activity-regulated gene transcription in synapse development and cognitive function." Cold Spring Harb Perspect Biol **3**(6).

Whitford, K. L., P. Dijkhuizen, F. Polleux and A. Ghosh (2002). "Molecular control of cortical dendrite development." Annu Rev Neurosci **25**: 127–149.

Wiesel, T. N. and D. H. Hubel (1963). "Effects of Visual Deprivation on Morphology and Physiology of Cells in the Cats Lateral Geniculate Body." J Neurophysiol **26**: 978–993.

Wiesel, T. N. and D. H. Hubel (1963). "Single-Cell Responses in Striate Cortex of Kittens Deprived of Vision in One Eye." J Neurophysiol **26**: 1003–1017.

Withers, G. S. and W. T. Greenough (1989). "Reach training selectively alters dendritic branching in subpopulations of layer II-III pyramids in rat motor-somatosensory forelimb cortex." Neuropsychologia **27**(1): 61–69.

Wong, R. O. and A. Ghosh (2002). "Activity-dependent regulation of dendritic growth and patterning." Nat Rev Neurosci **3**(10): 803–812.

Woolsey, T. A., M. L. Dierker and D. F. Wann (1975). "Mouse SmI cortex: qualitative and quantitative classification of golgi-impregnated barrel neurons." Proc Natl Acad Sci U S A **72**(6): 2165–2169.

Wu, B., C. Eliscovich, Y. J. Yoon and R. H. Singer (2016). "Translation dynamics of single mRNAs in live cells and neurons." Science **352**(6292): 1430–1435.

Wu, G., R. Malinow and H. T. Cline (1996). "Maturation of a central glutamatergic synapse." Science **274**(5289): 972–976.

Wu, G. Y. and H. T. Cline (1998). "Stabilization of dendritic arbor structure in vivo by CaMKII." Science **279**(5348): 222–226.

Wu, J. I., J. Lessard, I. A. Olave, Z. Qiu, A. Ghosh, I. A. Graef and G. R. Crabtree (2007). "Regulation of dendritic development by neuron-specific chromatin remodeling complexes." Neuron **56**(1): 94–108.

Xavier, A. L., J. R. Menezes, S. A. Goldman and M. Nedergaard (2014). "Fine-tuning the central nervous system: microglial modelling of cells and synapses." Philos Trans R Soc Lond B Biol Sci **369**(1654): 20130593.

Xie, Z., M. E. Cahill and P. Penzes (2010). "Kalirin loss results in cortical morphological alterations." Mol Cell Neurosci **43**(1): 81–89.

Xie, Z., D. P. Srivastava, H. Photowala, L. Kai, M. E. Cahill, K. M. Woolfrey, C. Y. Shum, D. J. Surmeier and P. Penzes (2007). "Kalirin-7 controls activity-dependent structural and functional plasticity of dendritic spines." Neuron **56**(4): 640–656.

Xu, H., A. S. Khakhalin, A. V. Nurmikko and C. D. Aizenman (2011). "Visual experience-dependent maturation of correlated neuronal activity patterns in a developing visual system." J Neurosci **31**(22): 8025–8036.

Xu, X., E. C. Miller and L. Pozzo-Miller (2014). "Dendritic spine dysgenesis in Rett syndrome." Front Neuroanat **8**: 97.

Yan, J., M. W. Porch, B. Court-Vazquez, M. V. L. Bennett and R. S. Zukin (2018). "Activation of autophagy rescues synaptic and cognitive deficits in fragile X mice." Proc Natl Acad Sci U S A **115**(41): E9707–E9716.

Yang, G., F. Pan and W. B. Gan (2009). "Stably maintained dendritic spines are associated with lifelong memories." Nature **462**(7275): 920–924.

Yap, E. L. and M. E. Greenberg (2018). "Activity-Regulated Transcription: Bridging the Gap between Neural Activity and Behavior." Neuron **100**(2): 330–348.

Yashiro, K., T. T. Riday, K. H. Condon, A. C. Roberts, D. R. Bernardo, R. Prakash, R. J. Weinberg, M. D. Ehlers and B. D. Philpot (2009). "Ube3a is required for experience-dependent maturation of the neocortex." Nat Neurosci **12**(6): 777–783.

Yi, F., T. Danko, S. C. Botelho, C. Patzke, C. Pak, M. Wernig and T. C. Sudhof (2016). "Autism-associated SHANK3 haploinsufficiency causes Ih channelopathy in human neurons." Science **352**(6286): aaf2669.

Yin, J., M. Gibbs, C. Long, J. Rosenthal, H. S. Kim, A. Kim, C. Sheng, P. Ding, U. Javed and Q. Yuan (2018). "Transcriptional Regulation of Lipophorin Receptors Supports Neuronal Adaptation to Chronic Elevations of Activity." Cell Rep **25**(5): 1181–1192 e1184.

Yin, J., E. Spillman, E. S. Cheng, J. Short, Y. Chen, J. Lei, M. Gibbs, J. S. Rosenthal, C. Sheng, Y. X. Chen, K. Veerasammy, T. Choetso, R. Abzalimov, B. Wang, C. Han, Y. He and Q. Yuan (2021). "Brain-specific lipoprotein receptors interact with astrocyte derived apolipoprotein and mediate neuron-glia lipid shuttling." Nat Commun **12**(1): 2408.

Yoon, Y. J., B. Wu, A. R. Buxbaum, S. Das, A. Tsai, B. P. English, J. B. Grimm, L. D. Lavis and R. H. Singer (2016). "Glutamate-induced RNA localization and translation in neurons." Proc Natl Acad Sci U S A **113**(44): E6877–E6886.

Younts, T. J., H. R. Monday, B. Dudok, M. E. Klein, B. A. Jordan, I. Katona and P. E. Castillo (2016). "Presynaptic Protein Synthesis Is Required for Long-Term Plasticity of GABA Release." Neuron **92**(2): 479–492.

Yuan, Q., Y. Xiang, Z. Yan, C. Han, L. Y. Jan and Y. N. Jan (2011). "Light-induced structural and functional plasticity in Drosophila larval visual system." Science **333**(6048): 1458–1462.

Zalfa, F., B. Eleuteri, K. S. Dickson, V. Mercaldo, S. De Rubeis, A. di Penta, E. Tabolacci, P. Chiurazzi, G. Neri, S. G. Grant and C. Bagni (2007). "A new function for the fragile X mental retardation protein in regulation of PSD-95 mRNA stability." Nat Neurosci **10**(5): 578–587.

Zhang, G., Z. Gao, S. Guan, Y. Zhu and J. H. Wang (2013). "Upregulation of excitatory neurons and downregulation of inhibitory neurons in barrel cortex are associated with loss of whisker inputs." Mol Brain **6**: 2.

Zhou, Z., E. J. Hong, S. Cohen, W. N. Zhao, H. Y. Ho, L. Schmidt, W. G. Chen, Y. Lin, E. Savner, E. C. Griffith, L. Hu, J. A. Steen, C. J. Weitz and M. E. Greenberg (2006). "Brain-specific phosphorylation of MeCP2 regulates activity-dependent Bdnf transcription, dendritic growth, and spine maturation." Neuron **52**(2): 255–269.

Zuo, Y., G. Yang, E. Kwon and W. B. Gan (2005). "Long-term sensory deprivation prevents dendritic spine loss in primary somatosensory cortex." Nature **436**(7048): 261–265.

3

Out with the Old, In with the New: Dendrite Degeneration and Regeneration

James I. Hertzler and Melissa M. Rolls

The Huck Institutes of the Life Sciences and Biochemistry and Molecular Biology, The Pennsylvania State University, USA

Abstract

Dendrites do not form macroscopic structures analogous to axons bundled into nerves. There has therefore been little investigation of how neurons respond to dendrite damage. Although in vertebrate animals, dendrites typically reside under bone in the central nervous system, they are damaged by trauma including stroke, traumatic brain injury, and seizure. Whether neurons can recover from irreversible dendrite damage in these scenarios is not yet known. However, acute removal of dendrites using laser microsurgery in model organisms has been used to probe responses of neurons to dendrite damage. After severing, the detached region of the dendrite undergoes stereotyped degeneration similar to Wallerian degeneration of axons. This degeneration is followed by robust regeneration of the dendrite arbor in *Caenorhabditis elegans* (worms), *Drosophila melanogaster* (flies), and *Danio rerio* (zebrafish). While little is known about the proteins that initiate dendrite regeneration, the core axon injury sensing pathway is not used. Some progress has been made on dissecting key cellular processes required for the outgrowth of new dendrites, but, overall, the molecular drivers of dendrite regeneration remain largely open to discovery. Here, we compare dendrite and axon regeneration and summarize what is known in the new field of dendrite regeneration.

3.1 Historical Perspective of Neuronal Regeneration

For most of human history, nerves were thought not to regenerate after injury (West, 1978). This prevailing view began to crumble when William

Cruikshank presented his findings on vagus nerve severing in dogs to the Royal Society in 1776. Much to his surprise, he found that if he waited for weeks rather than days after the surgery, the animal would completely recover (Cruikshank, 1795). As with many controversial findings, it took some time – 19 years – for this work to actually be published (Ochs, 1977). The same volume of the Philosophical Transactions of the Royal Society of London in which Cruikshank's work was finally published included John Haighton's work on vagus nerve transection (Haighton, 1795). Haighton made similar observations to Cruikshank: that recovery was possible, but only if weeks were allowed. The opening to his article makes it very clear that what was going on during this recovery process was poorly understood. It was debated whether the repair of nerves involved nervous tissue or instead some other bridging material; Haighton argued that it was nerve tissue (Haighton, 1795). Improvements in microscopy allowed the fibrous substance in nerves (axons) to be visualized better, and two camps emerged in the next century: those that thought repair was mediated by reusing the fibers in the part distal to transection, and those that thought new fibers emerged from the proximal part (Ochs, 1977; West, 1978). Note that although most of the body was accepted to be made up of cells by 1850, the intertwined networks of the nervous system meant it was not until the 1890s that it was generally accepted to be composed of individual cells (Shepherd, 1991). However, even before neurons were defined, Augustus Waller's careful microscopy and descriptions of frog and cat nerves after transection in the 1850s laid the foundation for understanding what happens inside nerves after injury. He described internal beading within the distal regions, and fibers extending in from the proximal side (Ochs, 1977). Although acceptance of these observations was not immediate, the basic model that fibers in cut-off pieces of the nerve degenerate and are replaced by growth from the proximal stump forms the framework for our understanding of nervous system regeneration.

Today, when we talk about regeneration in the nervous system, we primarily mean axon regeneration in the periphery. Early anatomists like Cruikshank and Haighton could identify individual nerves, perform surgeries to remove segments of them, and then track whether the animal recovered. Sprouting of fibers from the stump was observed by Waller, Cajal, and others, and this kept the cell body largely out of the picture. This is in contrast to most other tissues, where regeneration refers to rebuilding the tissue through addition of new cells. That most bilaterian animals do not add new neurons (at least in most areas of the nervous system) after early development (Ming and Song, 2011) supports the idea that neuronal regeneration is axon regeneration. However, there may be another conserved type of endogenous neuronal regeneration that we simply did not consider for historical and technical reasons: dendrite regeneration. Before we move on to considering the evidence that neurons may respond to dendrite injury in a manner similar to axon injury, let us first consider several variations on axon regeneration that are outside the original anatomical framework.

The competing model for the growth of fibers from the stump into the distal damaged nerve was that fibers (axons) in the distal piece contributed to recovery, perhaps by fusing with upstream segments. In fact, this type of repair has been observed in some invertebrates including earthworms, leeches, and crayfish (Neumann et al., 2019). This process has been best documented in the nematode *C. elegans*. In this animal, cut-off pieces of some axons can rejoin with the proximal axon to be reconnected to the cell body (Teoh et al., 2018). This type of regeneration involves plasma membrane fusion and can lead to functional recovery (Abay et al., 2017; Basu et al., 2017). However, it seems restricted to animals with few neurons, perhaps because fusion in a nerve with many axons would be difficult to accomplish without potentially disastrous connections between mismatched proximal and distal axons.

The other variation of axon regeneration that was not accessible to early anatomists was regeneration from a site other than the severed stump. In 2008, the Bradke lab used modern visualization methods to demonstrate that, after axons of cultured mouse hippocampal neurons were severed near the soma, the stump was not competent to reinitiate growth. Instead, a new axon emerged by converting a dendrite and growing out from it (Gomis-Ruth et al., 2008). Precedent for this observation came from studies in sea lampreys (Hall and Cohen, 1983; Hall et al., 1989), cats (MacDermid et al., 2002; MacDermid et al., 2004; Rose and Odlozinski, 1998), hamsters (Cho and So, 1992), and rats (Hoang et al., 2005). This ability to convert a dendrite into a regenerating axon after proximal axotomy seems broadly conserved as it also occurs in *Drosophila* (Stone et al., 2010). One interesting aspect of this type of regeneration is that the new axon typically emerges outside the nerve that would normally guide growth of axons regenerating from the stump. However, in slice culture, these axons can make synaptic connections (Gomis-Ruth et al., 2008). *In vivo* in *Drosophila*, the new axons wander, but if they happen to encounter the nerve that originally carried them, they grow in a directed manner along it (Rao and Rolls, 2017). The ability to track single cells after injury has revealed some unexpected variations on axon regeneration. Is it therefore possible that other types of nervous system regeneration remain to be discovered? One might imagine that, for many neuron types, loss of the receptive field via dendrite damage would be functionally as problematic as a severed axon. In that context, investigating regeneration of dendrites would seem as important as that of the axon.

3.2 Do Dendrites Get Damaged?

For the possibility of dendrite regeneration to be worth exploring, there should be scenarios where dendrites become damaged and regeneration might be useful. In vertebrate animals, dendrites are largely shielded by bone in the brain and spinal cord. One possible exception is the enteric nervous system, although these neurons have not been characterized enough at the cellular level to know whether they have dendrites. However, even under bone, dendrites have been shown to suffer acute injury in several clinically important scenarios. Traumatic brain injury (TBI) can result in dendrite beading (Gao and Chen, 2011; Gao et al., 2011) and loss of branches (Wang et al., 2016). Dendrite beading and degeneration have also been observed in human samples after surgical removal from epilepsy patients (Isokawa and Levesque, 1991) as well as in experimental kainate-induced seizure *in vivo* (Zeng et al., 2007) and in explants (Al-Noori and Swann, 2000). In fact, excessive electrical activity and neurite beading were linked over 100 years ago by Jean DeMoor (1898). Ischemia also causes dendrite beading and loss (Ji et al., 2021; Purpura et al., 1982). One model for dendritic sensitivity to epilepsy and ischemic stroke is that both conditions lead to high extracellular concentration of glutamate, which in turn activates NMDA receptors on dendrites and leads to massive calcium and sodium influx (Greenwood and Connolly, 2007; Verma et al., 2022).

Dendrite beading is used as a key hallmark of dendrite injury in part because it can be detected in fixed tissues by classic methods including Golgi staining. However, it is not as easy to interpret as, say, cutting out a section of nerve to initiate axon regeneration. Using live cell imaging of neurons in slice culture or *in vivo*, it has become possible to track individual dendrites after seizure or ischemia. These studies indicate that some level of dendrite beading is rapidly (minutes to several hours) reversible once normal activity or blood flow is restored (Murphy et al., 2008; Zeng et al., 2007). However, more global damage (Oliva et al., 2002) or repeated spreading depolarization after initial ischemia (Risher et al., 2010) can lead to irreversible beading and dendrite loss. Thus, it is likely that dendrites are acutely and irreversibly damaged in conditions that have a large impact on human health.

Dendrites also accumulate damage in long-term degenerative diseases including Alzheimer's (Anderton et al., 1998). However, whether regeneration plays a role in mitigating the effects of neurodegenerative disease has not yet even been determined for axons, so will be set aside for now in favor of acute injury scenarios.

3.3 Does Naturally Occurring Dendrite Damage Lead to Regeneration?

In the previous section, we identified TBI, stroke, and seizure as causes of dendrite damage. So, what are the cellular outcomes of this damage? Reversal of beading is one outcome that has been documented, and, at the other extreme, all of these types of trauma lead to cell death. The live imaging techniques that allowed rapid recovery to be observed are much more difficult on the longer timescales required to track the fate of individual neurons that suffer irreversible dendrite damage. The bottom line then is that, as far as we know, individual cells that have undergone dendrite beading without immediate recovery have not been tracked in mammals. One hint that neurons can recover from at least moderate dendrite damage was, however, published recently. Dendrite complexity was examined at different times after ischemic stroke in mice. Notably, 6–24 h after ischemia, dendrites of pyramidal neurons in the stroke penumbra lost length and complexity (Ji et al., 2021). In 4 days after ischemia, these changes were no longer detectable (Ji et al., 2021). Whether this partial loss and recovery of dendrite complexity is regeneration in the sense we mean for axons, or whether it is a larger scale version of normal dendrite plasticity, remains to be determined. But it does suggest that dendrite regrowth could be an important contributor to nervous system resilience in vertebrates.

If it is not definitively known whether dendrite regeneration happens in clinically relevant conditions, should we pursue it? First, because a phenomenon is technically difficult to observe does not mean it does not happen. One reason to think it may be important is the ability of dendrites to regenerate after controlled injury in invertebrate, and now vertebrate (Stone et al., 2022), model systems. Another reason is the existence of an active program of dendrite degeneration similar to Wallerian axon degeneration. That dendrites can be injured in the same manner as axons and also possess a similar method of injury-induced degeneration suggests that regenerative responses may also exist for both.

3.4 Dendrites have an active program of degeneration

Axon regeneration is preceded by Wallerian degeneration, an active process that clears away pieces of the axon no longer connected to the cell body.

It proceeds in a stereotyped stepwise manner. The basic framework for a molecular understanding of Wallerian degeneration has been pieced together relatively recently (Coleman and Hoke, 2020; Ding and Hammarlund, 2019; Figley and DiAntonio, 2020), even though the process itself was described in some detail in the 19th century. The central player in Wallerian degeneration is Sarm, which was linked to axon degeneration in 2012 (Osterloh et al., 2012). Sarm is an NAD hydrolase that becomes activated after axon injury to rapidly deplete NAD in the cut-off region (Essuman et al., 2017; Gerdts et al., 2015). Either NAD depletion or products of NAD hydrolysis, or both, lead to axon self-destruction (Coleman and Hoke, 2020; Ding and Hammarlund, 2019; Figley and DiAntonio, 2020). Nmnat, an enzyme in both the NAD synthesis and salvage pathways, acts as an axon survival factor by counteracting Sarm (Coleman and Hoke, 2020; Ding and Hammarlund, 2019; Figley and DiAntonio, 2020).

Does a degeneration program also exist for injured dendrites? Dendrite degeneration after injury morphologically resembles axon degeneration, in that there are discrete steps including beading before clearance (Tao and Rolls, 2011). Like axon degeneration, injury-induced dendrite degeneration is blocked by expression of Wlds (Tao and Rolls, 2011), an activated form of Nmnat, hinting that Sarm activation may also drive dendrite degeneration. Indeed, Sarm is required for injury-induced dendrite degeneration and degeneration induced by loss of Nmnat (Ji et al., 2022). There may be some differences between active axon and dendrite degeneration, for example, phosphatidylserine exposure is an important downstream mediator of Sarm activity in dendrites (Ji et al., 2022), but has not been placed downstream of Sarm in axon degeneration. In addition, the microtubule severing protein fidgetin plays a role in dendrite degeneration but not axon degeneration (Tao et al., 2016). However, it seems that dendrites have an active program of injury-induced degeneration, and the core machinery likely overlaps with that of axon degeneration.

3.5 Dendrites Can Regenerate After Controlled Injury

While it remains to be determined whether dendrites can regenerate after tissue-level damage induced by stroke, TBI or other trauma, after controlled dendrite removal, neurons can regrow a new arbor (Figure 3.1). This process has been best described in *Drosophila* dendritic arborization neurons. Although these are peripheral sensory neurons that innervate the body wall, they are polarized in many of the same ways that were initially described in mammalian central neurons (Rolls, 2011; Rolls and Jegla, 2015). For

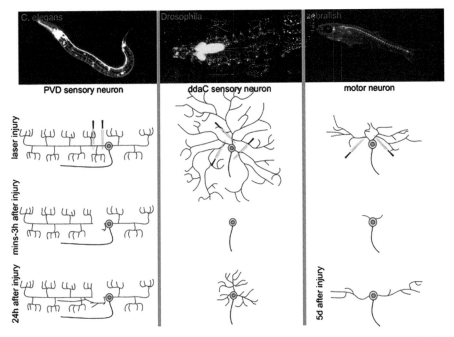

Figure 3.1 Model systems for studying dendrite regeneration. Laser microsurgery (indicated with light saber) has been used to sever dendrites and initiate regeneration in *C. elegans* (left), *Drosophila* larvae (middle), and zebrafish larvae (right). Sensory neurons in *C. elegans* initiate dendrite outgrowth followed by fusion. After complete removal of *Drosophila* sensory dendrites, a new arbor is grown. Similarly, severing dendrites of motor neurons in the zebrafish spinal cord is followed by outgrowth of dendrites until they reach approximately the same length. Times diagrammed for injury responses in each organism are shown at the left of the *C. elegans* column; the same times are shown for all organisms except the last time point for zebrafish (five days).

example, axons and dendrites have different arrangements of microtubules (Stone et al., 2008), dendrites contain Golgi outposts (Ye et al., 2007) and ribosomes (Hill et al., 2012), and the proximal axon houses a diffusion barrier organized by giant ankyrins (Jegla et al., 2016). Perhaps the most important broadly shared feature of these cells in the context of injury is their reliance upon dual leucine zipper kinase (DLK) to initiate axon regeneration. DLK was first identified as essential for axon regeneration in *C. elegans* (Hammarlund et al., 2009; Yan et al., 2009). It was then shown to be critical for axon injury signaling in *Drosophila* motor neurons (Xiong et al., 2010) and for response to peripheral axon injury in rodents (Shin et al., 2012). DLK is absolutely required to initiate axon regeneration in dendritic arborization neurons (Stone et al., 2014) and without DLK and its sister kinase

LZK, motor axon regeneration in zebrafish is eliminated (Adula et al., 2022). Because the *Drosophila* dendritic arborization neurons rely on the conserved core injury signaling machinery and have dendrites near the surface of the animal, they are an excellent model in which to study the response to dendrite injury.

The most complex class of dendritic arborization neurons, class IV, which includes the ddaC neuron, has been used as a model in which to investigate dendrite patterning, pruning, microtubule polarity, and regeneration in *Drosophila* larvae (Corty et al., 2009; Furusawa and Emoto, 2021; Singhania and Grueber, 2014). These neurons are nociceptors that are responsible for detecting oviposition by parasitoid wasps and initiating escape behavior (Hwang et al., 2007). They grow large arbors and display both stereotyped homotypic and heterotypic repulsion – that is, each neuron has a specific receptive field and avoids its own and the dendrites of neighboring neurons (Corty et al., 2009) to most efficiently provide the body with nociceptive capability. Laser surgery was first used to study the effect of dendrite removal in these cells in 2003 (Sugimura et al., 2003). Single dendrite branches were removed in young larvae and the newly empty area was filled in by growth from the stump or neighboring dendrites (Sugimura et al., 2003). This recovery was interpreted as a response to removal of growth inhibition rather than activation of an injury signal and subsequent regeneration. In support of this argument, removal of one branch from the simpler ddaE neuron, which does not exhibit the same type of tiling behavior as ddaC, did not trigger growth to fill the missing area (Sugimura et al., 2003). In 2014, laser microsurgery was used to remove the entire dendrite arbors from both ddaC and ddaE neurons and both cell types were able to regrow dendrite arbors (Stone et al., 2014 and Figure 3.1). For the ddaE cell, the injury was performed after final dendrite shape had been attained and these cells grew a new dendrite arbor of similar complexity, but quite different shape, to the initial arbor (Stone et al., 2014). ddaC neurons continue to add branches throughout larval life; so these cells were still undergoing shape change at the time of injury. They grew to recover their normal territory within four days (Stone et al., 2014 and Figure 3.2). Regeneration of ddaE and ddaC dendrites was corroborated by another group (Thompson-Peer et al., 2016) that also analyzed another type of sensory neuron, the class III ddaA cell, and found it too could regenerate dendrite branches after injury (Thompson-Peer et al., 2016). In these studies, injury initiated a change in cellular behavior, leading to the interpretation that dendrite regeneration is triggered by an injury signal analogous to axon regeneration. However, it is possible that the signal to initiate regeneration is removal of growth inhibition as proposed in

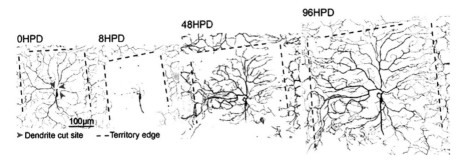

Figure 3.2 Dendrites of *Drosophila* ddaC sensory neurons regenerate to cover their receptive field after laser severing. *Drosophila* ddaC neurons have complex dendrite arbors that cover specific, tiled regions of the larval epidermis. When those dendrites are individually severed with a laser (first panel on left), they start to degenerate within a couple of hours, and most of the debris is cleared by 8 hours post dendrotomy (HPD) (second panel). By 4 HPD, regeneration has already been initiated and new small, branchy dendrites are emerging from the cell body. At 48 HPD the dendrites are long enough to reach the edges of the larval body segment (third panel). This regeneration of dendrites continues over a period of days until the dendrites fully cover the voided area at 96 HPD (fourth panel). Images to show the full dendrite arbor are assembled from multiple image tiles.

2003. In either case, these studies clearly demonstrated that, *in vivo*, mature, fully functional peripheral neurons can regrow dendrites in response to their removal.

Responses to dendrite injury have also been studied in another invertebrate, *C. elegans*. Most *C. elegans* neurons have simple, unbranched dendrites, but the PVD cell is a dramatic exception. This peripheral neuron, which, like *Drosophila* dendritic arborization neurons, innervates the body wall and responds to mechanical stimuli, has two large dendrite branches that elaborate a stereotyped branching pattern along the length of the organism (Tsalik et al., 2003). There is one neuron on each side of the animal, with quaternary branches reaching toward the dorsal and ventral midlines. Laser microsurgery of dendrites triggers dendrite outgrowth and subsequent fusion to repair the arbor (Oren-Suissa et al., 2017 and Figure 3.1). Axon repair by fusion also occurs in *C. elegans* as discussed in the first section. Thus, dendrite injury seems to initiate a regenerative response that is overtly similar to axon regeneration in *C. elegans*. Another injury paradigm has also suggested that *C. elegans* neurons sense and respond to dendrite injury. One key difference in this study was that the cell that was used, the ASJ sensory neuron, has a dendrite that terminates in a cilium rather than a branched dendrite arbor like PVD. Laser injury to the dendrite at the same time as the axon altered the axon regeneration program so that it no longer required DLK (Chung et al., 2016). Growth of dendrites was not tracked in this study, but may not be possible for ciliated dendrites as the cilium is likely irreplaceable.

In mice, neurons can survive laser-mediated dendrite severing, but cells have only been tracked for 3 h after injury; so regeneration capacity was not determined (Zhao et al., 2017). A recent study in zebrafish has, however, demonstrated that neurons can regrow dendrites after laser surgery in the spinal cord (Stone et al., 2022). Motor neuron dendrites were severed in young fish, and after one or both major branches were removed, regrowth was initiated. By about five days after injury, their former length was restored (Figure 3.1). Thus, the phenomenon of dendrite arbor regrowth after controlled injury has been observed in invertebrates and vertebrates. Therefore, animals may broadly share the capacity to regenerate dendrites just as they share a program of axon regeneration.

Whether regenerated dendrites can restore function to a circuit remained an open question until recently. In *Drosophila*, two earlier studies suggested that functional recovery occurs. Class III dendritic arborization neurons including ddaA normally respond to gentle touch, and action potential bursts were seen in extracellular field recordings when a probe was applied to the cuticle both near and far from the soma (Thompson-Peer et al., 2016). Recently balded (all dendrites removed) neurons showed no response, and neurons with regenerated dendrites had an attenuated but reasonable response to stimulus (Thompson-Peer et al., 2016). A similar paradigm was employed in class IV v'ada neurons in adult *Drosophila*. These neurons are chemically sensitive and display bursts of action potentials upon administration of an acid stimulus. Again, recently balded neurons did not respond to the stimulus, but after seven days, regenerated and uninjured dendrites were almost identical in their ability to transduce an acid stimulus to an action potential burst (DeVault et al., 2018). Note that these neurons that regenerated in the adult had smaller, more compact, dendrite arbors than uninjured counterparts, but their electrical response was identical (DeVault et al., 2018). In 2023, laser surgery was used to remove dendrites or axons of almost all Class IV neurons that innervate the dorsal surface of the animal. This large-scale axon or dendrite removal allowed standard functional assays using a heated probe to target the denervated region. Removal of dendrites strongly reduced the response to noxious heat, but, surprisingly, responsiveness was almost completely restored 24 hours after injury when new dendrite arbors were still small (Hertzler, Bernard, & Rolls, 2023). Functional recovery did not occur in a genetic background in which regenerative growth was blocked, confirming that it is dendrite regeneration that restores neuronal function to sensory dendrite arbors (Hertzler et al., 2023). It will be interesting to determine whether post-synaptic dendrites can be similarly restored.

3.6 The Molecular Program of Dendrite Regeneration is Distinct from that of Axon Regeneration

The basic process of dendrite regrowth after injury is visually similar to axon regeneration. After injury, cells that had previously attained a stable shape reinitiate massive outgrowth, either from the injured stump or another site. Dendrite regeneration therefore likely involves similar steps to axon regeneration including injury sensing, transcriptional reprogramming to a growth state, growth initiation and extension, and, finally, connecting with a target. It therefore seems possible that some of the machinery that controls axon regeneration could be used for dendrite regeneration. In particular, the injury signaling machinery is a good candidate for shared use. In the case of controlled laser axotomy, exactly the same type of injury can elicit axon and dendrite regeneration. As described above, DLK is at the core of axon injury sensing; so is it also involved in sensing dendrite injury? This question has been addressed in both *Drosophila* dendritic arborization neurons and the *C. elegans* PVD neuron. In *Drosophila*, DLK, as well as downstream kinase JNK, and transcription factor fos, are dispensable for dendrite regeneration (Stone et al., 2014). Importantly, axon injury assays were performed in the same cell type and genetic backgrounds, and DLK, JNK, and fos were required for axon regeneration (Stone et al., 2014). A transcriptional reporter for injury signaling initiated by DLK was robustly activated by axon injury, but not by dendrite injury, indicating that not only is the DLK kinase cascade not required for dendrite regeneration, it is not even activated by dendrite injury (Stone et al., 2014). Similarly, the *C. elegans* PVD neuron requires DLK signaling to initiate axon regeneration, but does not use it for dendrite regeneration (Brar et al., 2022). In addition, while elevation of cAMP by reducing levels of a phosphodiesterase improves axon regeneration in *C. elegans* (Ghosh-Roy et al., 2010), there is no effect on dendrite regeneration (Brar et al., 2022). While axon and dendrite regeneration share some broad requirements for growth machinery (see below), these pathways also do not completely converge at later steps. For example, spastin and atlastin are important for the growth phase of axon regeneration but not dendrite regeneration (Rao et al., 2016; Stone et al., 2012).

If different programs are activated by axon and dendrite injury, it is possible that these programs could interfere with one another. However, this does not seem to be the case. In the example of combined axon and dendrite injury in the ASJ neuron, injury to the dendrite actually enhances axon outgrowth (Chung et al., 2016). In *Drosophila* dendritic arborization neurons, removal of axons and dendrites together initiates regrowth of both types of processes simultaneously (Shorey et al., 2020).

3.7 Molecular Requirements for Dendrite Regeneration

If much of the core axon regeneration machinery is not used during dendrite regeneration, what do we know about the molecular requirements for dendrite regeneration? Dendrite regeneration seems likely to involve steps similar to axon injury. First, a physiological alteration like voltage change or buildup of a specific protein could signal injury (like activation of DLK in axon regeneration (Xiong et al., 2010)). Second, this signal could be transduced into a pathway that activates transcription factors and leads to pro-regenerative gene expression (similar to regeneration-associated gene (RAG) expression after axon injury (Mahar and Cavalli, 2018)). Finally, dendrite outgrowth would begin and involve microtubule activity and membrane addition (the importance of microtubule dynamics in dendrite regeneration already has experimental support (Feng et al., 2019)). Players in the early steps responsible for injury signal and transcriptional reprogramming have not yet been identified (Figure 3.4). This lack of information is striking in contrast to the breadth of knowledge in the field of axon regeneration. Hundreds to thousands of regeneration-associated genes (RAGs) have been shown to change levels after axon injury (Ma and Willis, 2015). There has been only one set of genes described as upregulated after dendrite injury in *Drosophila* (Hertzler et al., 2020). These genes encode kinetochore proteins, which connect microtubules to chromosomes during mitosis. In neurons, they suppress microtubule nucleation in dendrites, and absence of this suppression has a minor inhibitory effect on dendrite regeneration (Hertzler et al., 2020). However, upstream transcriptional regulators were not identified.

So far, our knowledge of proteins that influence dendrite regeneration is mainly limited to those that facilitate growth. These proteins fall broadly into those that seem more important for dendrite regeneration than other types of neurite outgrowth, and proteins broadly required for cell growth that have a shared role in axon and dendrite regeneration or dendrite development. A theme across both categories is the importance of interactions with surrounding cells.

Cytoskeletal regulators:

Cytoskeletal regulators are the main class of protein known to have a specific role in promoting dendrite regeneration. In *C. elegans*, the RAC GTPase

CED-10 and upstream guanine nucleotide exchange factor (GEF) Tiam-1 were recently demonstrated to be required for PVD dendrite, but not axon, regeneration (Brar et al., 2022). As previously mentioned, *C. elegans* dendrites initiate growth and reconnect dendrite stumps with their severed ends after injury, and CED-10 knockdown severely impairs both processes (Brar et al., 2022). Interestingly, both epidermal- and neuron-specific expression of the wild type gene in a null background rescues the phenotype, but in different ways. Re-expression in neurons rescued both reconnection and ectopic branching defects, while re-expression in epidermal cells only rescued the reconnection defect. This suggests that CED-10 has a cell-autonomous role in neurons for promoting regrowth and branching but also a non-autonomous role in neighboring epidermal cells to promote fusion of severed neurites. The RhoGEF TIAM-1 was found to be the upstream activator of CED-10 in this context; knockdown produced the same phenotypes and expression of a constitutively active version of CED-10 in the TIAM-1 null background rescued both branching and fusion phenotypes (Brar et al., 2022). It is not entirely clear how to extrapolate data on fusion of severed neuronal processes from worms to flies or vertebrates; however, it does illustrate well the ideas that epidermal-derived factors are important for regrowth of dendrites and that specific types of cytoskeletal regulation promote dendrite regeneration.

Cytoskeletal regulators that are specifically important for dendrite regeneration have also been identified in *Drosophila*. One of the most critical drivers of neuronal morphology, and regeneration, is the microtubule cytoskeleton. These long polymers of α-β tubulin heterodimers give neurons their shape and an ability to transport proteins to support the long axonal and dendritic processes. Microtubules have intrinsic polarity, and the plus end, where the β-tubulin subunit is exposed, is highly dynamic and undergoes rapid bouts of growth and shrinkage. Axonal microtubule polarity is typically plus-end-out (microtubule plus end oriented away from the soma) and dendrites are characterized by at least partial minus-end-out polarity (microtubule plus end toward the soma) (Baas and Lin, 2011; Rolls and Jegla, 2015). Because the arrangement of microtubules differs in axons and dendrites, it makes sense that microtubule regulators might be differentially important for the two types of regeneration. Uninjured *Drosophila* dendrites are almost exclusively populated by minus-end-out microtubules (Stone et al., 2008). During the first day of dendrite regeneration, growing dendrites have mixed, rather than minus-end-out, polarity, presumably for plus-end-out microtubules to promote growth. Minus-end-out polarity is restored after the second day of regeneration (Stone et al., 2014). Patronin, a microtubule minus end binding protein, helps microtubule minus ends grow into dendrites, and is critical for restoring minus-end-out polarity during regeneration (Feng et al., 2019). When Patronin is knocked down, not only is microtubule polarity disrupted, but outgrowth of new dendrites is strongly reduced (Feng et al., 2019). Patronin is also required for establishment of microtubule polarity in development, but developmental dendrite outgrowth is not obviously disrupted and relatively normal dendrite shape is obtained in uninjured Patronin knockdown neurons (Feng et al., 2019; Thyagarajan et al., 2022).

Nucleation of new microtubules has also been shown to be critical for dendrite regeneration in *Drosophila* peripheral neurons. The receptor tyrosine kinase (RTK) Ror was identified in a candidate screen to identify RTKs involved in dendrite regeneration (Nye et al., 2020). Rather than being involved in injury signaling, Ror seems to function constitutively to position microtubule nucleation sites in dendrites (Nye et al., 2020). Ror can itself act as a Wnt receptor (Green et al., 2014; Green et al., 2008; Ripp et al., 2018; Stricker et al., 2017) and acts in concert with three other Wnt receptors (frizzled, frizzled2, and arrow), as well as scaffolding proteins Dishevelled and Axin, to recruit nucleation sites to dendrite branch points (Nye et al., 2020; Weiner et al., 2020). Loss of Ror causes specific reductions in dendrite regeneration, but not dendrite outgrowth or axon regeneration (Nye et al., 2020). However, nucleation sites are reduced in uninjured as well as injured dendrites in Ror knockdown neurons (Nye et al., 2020) indicating that this pathway functions prior to injury. Adding to the evidence that regulation of microtubule nucleation is important for dendrite regeneration is the aforementioned paper showing a novel role for kinetochore proteins in neurons (Hertzler et al., 2020). Reduction of kinetochore proteins caused an increase in microtubule dynamics in dendrites, but not axons, and a deficit in dendrite, but not axon, regeneration (Hertzler et al., 2020). The ability to rescue both microtubule and regeneration phenotypes with partial reduction of γ-tubulin, the core microtubule nucleation protein, indicated that kinetochore proteins normally function to limit dendritic microtubule nucleation (Hertzler et al., 2020). Like Wnt signaling proteins, kinetochore protein function was not limited to injured neurons; microtubule phenotypes were observed in uninjured neurons although shape was normal (Hertzler et al., 2020). Dendrite regeneration may be more sensitive to partial depletion of specific proteins than developmental growth in general because more rapid outgrowth is required. During development, dendrites initially grow out in small animals and then expand as the animal grows. During regeneration, the entire area of a now much bigger animal needs to be recovered.

Together, these studies show that dendrite regeneration is particularly sensitive to alterations in microtubule minus end regulation. Developmental dendrite outgrowth seems more resilient to minus end disruption, perhaps because parallel pathways can compensate in this context. Axon regeneration also involves very rapid neurite outgrowth and is unaffected by loss of Ror or kinetochore proteins. In this case, the lack of minus-end-out microtubules in axons may be responsible for their resilience. While control of microtubule minus ends seems unlikely to fit the broad theme of regulation of regeneration by interactions with surrounding cells, it may actually not be an exception. The involvement of Ror and three other Wnt receptors suggests that microtubule nucleation, and thus dendrite regeneration, may require Wnt ligands to be secreted from surrounding cells.

Receptors for environmental cues:
Clear support for the idea that close interactions between dendrites and their environment facilitate regeneration derives from studies on the role of extra-cellular matrix (ECM) receptors. *Drosophila* dendritic arborization neurons elaborate dendrites on the basal surface of epithelial cells and require proper attachment with the ECM for patterning. Neuronal integrins interact with ECM secreted from epithelial cells during dendrite development in the larva (Han et al., 2012; Kim et al., 2012). A subset of dendritic arborization neurons undergoes dendrite pruning in the pupal stage and regrowth into the adult body wall (Shimono et al., 2009). This adult outgrowth is reduced when integrins are knocked down, as is injury-induced regeneration in the adult (DeVault et al., 2018). Moreover, dendrites preferentially regenerated into collagen-rich areas of the ECM in adult flies, and knockdown of matrix metalloproteinase 2, which remodels the ECM after eclosion (Yasunaga et al., 2010), preserved an ECM permissive to dendrite regrowth (DeVault et al., 2018). Consistent with a key role for dendrite-ECM interactions during dendrite development and regeneration, the Ret RTK works with integrins to promote ECM interactions during dendrite development of large class IV dendritic arborization neurons in the Drosophila larva (Soba et al., 2015). It is also important for regeneration of these same neurons after dendrite injury (Nye et al., 2020 and Figure 3.3). The output of these dendrite–ECM interactions has been suggested to be Rac1 control of actin localization (Soba et al., 2015). In *C. elegans* PVD neurons, Rac1 seems more important for dendrite regeneration than outgrowth (see above; Brar et al., 2022), while in class IV Drosophila neurons integrins/Ret acting through Rac1 are important for normal growth and regeneration.

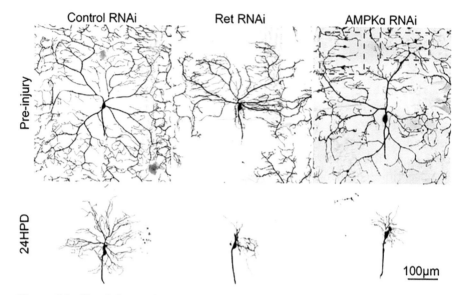

Figure 3.3   Knockdowns that cause dendrite morphology phenotypes usually corre-spond to defects in dendrite regeneration. While central regulators of dendrite injury sig-naling and regeneration have not been discovered, there are many proteins that play a role in dendrite morphogenesis and maintenance that also have a role in regeneration. With a control RNAi, dendrites regenerate robustly as early as 24 HPD (left). When Ret is knocked down, there are large gaps in the usually precisely tiled dendrite arbors due to lack of cell adhesion (middle, top). Regeneration after laser severing is also impaired when Ret is knocked down (middle, bottom). AMPKα is responsible for promoting oxidative phosphorylation in neurons, usually reliant on glycolysis, when carbohydrate energy is sparse. This is important for den-drite maintenance during late larval and pupal life of drosophila: when AMPKα is knocked down, dendrites bead and degenerate (right, top, with red dashed regions showing beading). That dendrite regeneration after laser injury is impaired in this knockdown as well suggests that the energy intensive process of regenerating dendrites relies on optimized glycolytic and oxidative phosphorylation energy production.

Cell growth and metabolism regulators:

So far, we have considered regulators of dendrite regeneration that seem to act through the cytoskeleton, either microtubules or actin. The other major class of proteins implicated in dendrite regeneration control cellular growth through membrane delivery, protein synthesis and metabolism. Both axon and dendrite regeneration require rapid neurite outgrowth, and so perhaps unsurprisingly the exocyst complex, which is important for post-Golgi ves-icle fusion with the plasma membrane, is strongly required for both (Swope et al., 2022). However, another membrane pathway, concentration of the endoplasmic reticulum near growing neurite tips, is exclusively used for

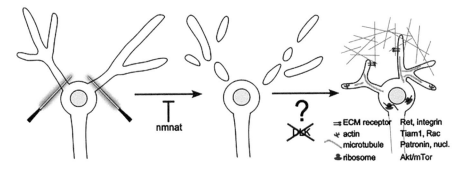

Figure 3.4   Overview of pathways that regulate dendrite degeneration and regeneration. After dendrite removal (left), severed regions undergo beading and then are cleared. Beading and clearance are delayed by expression of the NAD synthesis enzyme nmnat. It is not known what factors initiate regenerative dendrite outgrowth. However, the core DLK-mediated axon injury signaling pathway is not involved. During the growth phase of regeneration, interactions with the ECM through integrins and Ret are important. Akt signaling, likely acting through mTor-mediated increases in translation, is also important for growth. A requirement for Tiam1 and RAC in regeneration in *C. elegans* implicates the actin cytoskeleton, and in *Drosophila* microtubule nucleation (nucl.) and minus end growth mediated by Patronin seems particularly important for dendrite regeneration compared to other types of growth.

axon outgrowth (Rao et al., 2016); so it is not a given that seemingly general growth pathways will be equally used to regrow axons and dendrites.

Akt is a central player downstream of growth factor signaling and upstream of mTor to control cell survival, growth, and metabolism (Manning and Cantley, 2007). PTEN antagonizes Akt signaling (Worby and Dixon, 2014) and its knockout enhances axon regeneration in the mammalian central nervous system (CNS) (Park et al., 2010; Park et al., 2008). Extra Akt or reduced PTEN enhances axon and dendrite regeneration in *Drosophila* (Song et al., 2012) and the pathway also promotes developmental dendrite growth (Parrish et al., 2009). Although upstream regulators of Akt in dendritic arborization neurons have not been identified, the pathway is regulated by signals from epithelial cells. Expression of a microRNA, bantam, in epithelial cells dampens Akt activity in neurons (Parrish et al., 2009). AMPK is another broad regulator of cellular metabolism and growth (Inoki et al., 2012). Its reduction in *Drosophila* class IV dendritic arborization neurons leads to dendrite blebbing (Marzano et al., 2021; Swick et al., 2013) and gaps in coverage (Figure 3.3). Dendrite regeneration is reduced similarly to Akt knockdown in AMPK RNAi neurons (Figure 3.3). While it makes intuitive sense that proteins required generally for cell growth and metabolism would be important for dendrite regeneration (Figure 3.4), regeneration of PVD dendrites in

C. elegans is not affected in *Akt* mutants (Brar et al., 2022). Perhaps compensatory pathways make some cellular processes, cell types, or animals more resilient to reduction of broadly used growth pathways.

Beyond sensory dendrites:
All studies on molecular requirements for dendrite regeneration have so far been performed in peripheral neurons that have sensory, rather than post-synaptic, dendrites. How applicable are these findings likely to be to central neurons, whose dendrites contain synapses and are surrounded by glia and other neurons? This question has not been addressed, as it is much more difficult to access and manipulate dendrites in the CNS, but it seems likely that at least early steps of regeneration would be shared between sensory and post-synaptic dendrites. Injury would still need to be sensed, and outgrowth of new dendrites initiated. Forming synapses would be a late-stage, necessary addition intrinsic to central neurons that may involve neuron-to-neuron interaction that sensory dendrites do not require. Interactions with ECM, cytoskeletal organization, and regulation of cell growth pathways are all likely to be similarly important for regeneration of all types of dendrites.

Research has uncovered a plethora of proteins required for axon injury signaling, and many that promote both dendrite and axon regeneration. However, finding proteins required specifically for a dendrite injury response has been elusive, and so it remains unclear how similar axon and dendrite regenerations really are. More work is needed in this field to compare how axons and dendrites signal damage and respond in morphologically distinct ways.

3.8 Where We Stand with Dendrite Injury Responses

The study of axon regeneration is hundreds of years old. While there is also a long history that suggests that dendrites can be damaged in physiologically important scenarios, the discovery that neurons possess the capacity to regenerate dendrites de novo after acute cellular injury is very recent and relies on controlled delivery of dendrite damage. The laser injury paradigm used to perform dendrite microsurgery is less than 20 years old (Galbraith and Terasaki, 2003; Sugimura et al., 2003). Important work has since differentiated dendrite from axon regeneration (Brar et al., 2022; Nye et al., 2020; Rao et al., 2016; Stone et al., 2014; Stone et al., 2012); however, the major pathways and proteins that govern regeneration of dendrites have yet to be discovered (Figure 3.4).

Most work on dendrite regeneration has been in the optically friendly *Drosophila* and *C. elegans* model systems. A recently published paper demonstrates the first evidence of de novo dendrite regeneration in a vertebrate model system (Stone et al., 2022). Much of what is currently known about dendrite regeneration falls into two categories: factors that are required for a permissive extracellular environment, and factors that enhance cell growth (Figure 3.4). An extracellular space that does not inhibit growth is critical for regeneration of both axons (Yiu and He, 2006) and dendrites (DeVault et al., 2018). In both *Drosophila* and *C. elegans*, sensory neurons embedded in skin cells require interaction with the epithelial cells and/or ECM for both normal growth and regeneration (Brar et al., 2022; DeVault et al., 2018; Jiang et al., 2019; Liu et al., 2016; Oren-Suissa et al., 2017; Poe et al., 2017; Soba et al., 2015; Zou et al., 2016). On the intracellular side, for instance, Akt activation promotes dendrite regeneration (Song et al., 2012). Microtubule-related proteins have also been shown to have dendrite outgrowth and regeneration phenotypes when knocked down: if new microtubules cannot nucleate or grow from the minus end, dendrite outgrowth is significantly restricted (Feng et al., 2019; Hertzler et al., 2020; Nye et al., 2020).

However, much remains to be discovered about the actual signals and physiological changes that kick off dendrite regeneration. That dendrites of multiple neuron types in both vertebrates and invertebrates show regeneration and re-elaboration implies that a mechanism exists for sensing injury or incomplete function of the dendritic compartment, but it remains unknown how neurons sense this damage and which pathways are activated as a result. While transcriptional changes are almost certainly required, these transcription factors and genes involved have yet to be identified.

The biggest question to be answered is whether there exists a conserved dendrite regeneration pathway that is analogous to the DLK-mediated axon regeneration pathway. Many different neuron types have stereotyped dendrite arbors and extracellular interactions that may require transcription of different genes for their proper regeneration. However, as microscope technology and genetic tools continue to evolve in multiple model organisms, we can start to gain a clearer view (pun intended) of how neurons sense and respond to injury.

Acknowledgements

Work in our lab on projects related to dendrite regeneration is supported by the National Institutes of Health including grants GM085115 and NS117396. We are grateful to the members of the Rolls lab for discussions on neuronal injury responses, and to former lab members Alex Weiner, Matthew Shorey, and Chengye Feng for providing images used in Figure 3.1.

References

Abay, Z. C., Wong, M. Y., Teoh, J. S., Vijayaraghavan, T., Hilliard, M. A. and Neumann, B. (2017). Phosphatidylserine save-me signals drive functional recovery of severed axons in Caenorhabditis elegans. *Proc Natl Acad Sci U S A* **114**, E10196–E10205.

Adula, K. P., Shorey, M., Chauhan, V., Nassman, K., Chen, S. F., Rolls, M. M. and Sagasti, A. (2022). The MAP3Ks DLK and LZK direct diverse responses to axon damage in zebrafish peripheral neurons. *J Neurosci* **42**(32), 6195–210. doi:10.1523/JNEUROSCI.1395-21.2022

Al-Noori, S. and Swann, J. W. (2000). A role for sodium and chloride in kainic acid-induced beading of inhibitory interneuron dendrites. *Neuroscience* **101**, 337–48.

Anderton, B. H., Callahan, L., Coleman, P., Davies, P., Flood, D., Jicha, G. A., Ohm, T. and Weaver, C. (1998). Dendritic changes in Alzheimer's disease and factors that may underlie these changes. *Prog Neurobiol* **55**, 595–609.

Baas, P. W. and Lin, S. (2011). Hooks and comets: The story of microtubule polarity orientation in the neuron. *Dev Neurobiol* **71**, 403–18.

Basu, A., Dey, S., Puri, D., Das Saha, N., Sabharwal, V., Thyagarajan, P., Srivastava, P., Koushika, S. P. and Ghosh-Roy, A. (2017). let-7 miRNA controls CED-7 homotypic adhesion and EFF-1-mediated axonal self-fusion to restore touch sensation following injury. *Proc Natl Acad Sci U S A* **114**, E10206–E10215.

Brar, H. K., Dey, S., Bhardwaj, S., Pande, D., Singh, P., Dey, S. and Ghosh-Roy, A. (2022). Dendrite regeneration in C. elegans is controlled by the RAC GTPase CED-10 and the RhoGEF TIAM-1. *PLoS Genet* **18**, e1010127.

Cho, E. Y. and So, K. F. (1992). Characterization of the sprouting response of axon-like processes from retinal ganglion cells after axotomy in adult hamsters: a model using intravitreal implantation of a peripheral nerve. *J Neurocytol* **21**, 589–603.

Chung, S. H., Awal, M. R., Shay, J., McLoed, M. M., Mazur, E. and Gabel, C. V. (2016). Novel DLK-independent neuronal regeneration in Caenorhabditis elegans shares links with activity-dependent ectopic outgrowth. *Proc Natl Acad Sci U S A* **113**, E2852–60.

Coleman, M. P. and Hoke, A. (2020). Programmed axon degeneration: from mouse to mechanism to medicine. *Nat Rev Neurosci* **21**, 183–196.

Corty, M. M., Matthews, B. J. and Grueber, W. B. (2009). Molecules and mechanisms of dendrite development in Drosophila. *Development* **136**, 1049–61.

Cruikshank, W. (1795). VI. Experiments on the nerves, particularly on their reproduction; and on the spinal marrow of living animals. *Philos Trans R Soc Lond* **85**, 177–189.

DeMoor, J. (1898). La mecanisme et la signification de l'etat moniliforme des neurones. *Bulletin de la Societe de Medecine Mentale de Belgique*, 387–390.

DeVault, L., Li, T., Izabel, S., Thompson-Peer, K. L., Jan, L. Y. and Jan, Y. N. (2018). Dendrite regeneration of adult Drosophila sensory neurons diminishes with aging and is inhibited by epidermal-derived matrix metalloproteinase 2. *Genes Dev* **32**, 402–414.

Ding, C. and Hammarlund, M. (2019). Mechanisms of injury-induced axon degeneration. *Curr Opin Neurobiol* **57**, 171–178.

Essuman, K., Summers, D. W., Sasaki, Y., Mao, X., DiAntonio, A. and Milbrandt, J. (2017). The SARM1 Toll/Interleukin-1 Receptor Domain Possesses Intrinsic NAD(+) Cleavage Activity that Promotes Pathological Axonal Degeneration. *Neuron* **93**, 1334–1343 e5.

Feng, C., Thyagarajan, P., Shorey, M., Seebold, D. Y., Weiner, A. T., Albertson, R. M., Rao, K. S., Sagasti, A., Goetschius, D. J. and Rolls, M. M. (2019). Patronin-mediated minus end growth is required for dendritic microtubule polarity. *J Cell Biol* **218**, 2309–2328.

Figley, M. D. and DiAntonio, A. (2020). The SARM1 axon degeneration pathway: control of the NAD(+) metabolome regulates axon survival in health and disease. *Curr Opin Neurobiol* **63**, 59–66.

Furusawa, K. and Emoto, K. (2021). Spatiotemporal regulation of developmental neurite pruning: Molecular and cellular insights from Drosophila models. *Neurosci Res* **167**, 54–63.

Galbraith, J. A. and Terasaki, M. (2003). Controlled damage in thick specimens by multiphoton excitation. *Mol Biol Cell* **14**, 1808–17.

Gao, X. and Chen, J. (2011). Mild traumatic brain injury results in extensive neuronal degeneration in the cerebral cortex. *J Neuropathol Exp Neurol* **70**, 183–91.

Gao, X., Deng, P., Xu, Z. C. and Chen, J. (2011). Moderate traumatic brain injury causes acute dendritic and synaptic degeneration in the hippocampal dentate gyrus. *PLoS One* **6**, e24566.

Gerdts, J., Brace, E. J., Sasaki, Y., DiAntonio, A. and Milbrandt, J. (2015). SARM1 activation triggers axon degeneration locally via NAD(+) destruction. *Science* **348**, 453–7.

Ghosh-Roy, A., Wu, Z., Goncharov, A., Jin, Y. and Chisholm, A. D. (2010). Calcium and cyclic AMP promote axonal regeneration in Caenorhabditis elegans and require DLK-1 kinase. *J Neurosci* **30**, 3175–83.

Gomis-Ruth, S., Wierenga, C. J. and Bradke, F. (2008). Plasticity of polarization: changing dendrites into axons in neurons integrated in neuronal circuits. *Curr Biol* **18**, 992–1000.

Green, J., Nusse, R. and van Amerongen, R. (2014). The role of Ryk and Ror receptor tyrosine kinases in Wnt signal transduction. *Cold Spring Harb Perspect Biol* **6**.

Green, J. L., Kuntz, S. G. and Sternberg, P. W. (2008). Ror receptor tyrosine kinases: orphans no more. *Trends Cell Biol* **18**, 536–44.

Greenwood, S. M. and Connolly, C. N. (2007). Dendritic and mitochondrial changes during glutamate excitotoxicity. *Neuropharmacology* **53**, 891–8.

Haighton, J. (1795). VII. An experimental inquiry concerning the reproduction of nerves. *Philos Trans R Soc Lond* **85**, 190–201.

Hall, G. F. and Cohen, M. J. (1983). Extensive dendritic sprouting induced by close axotomy of central neurons in the lamprey. *Science* **222**, 518–21.

Hall, G. F., Poulos, A. and Cohen, M. J. (1989). Sprouts emerging from the dendrites of axotomized lamprey central neurons have axonlike ultrastructure. *J Neurosci* **9**, 588–99.

Hammarlund, M., Nix, P., Hauth, L., Jorgensen, E. M. and Bastiani, M. (2009). Axon regeneration requires a conserved MAP kinase pathway. *Science* **323**, 802–6.

Han, C., Wang, D., Soba, P., Zhu, S., Lin, X., Jan, L. Y. and Jan, Y. N. (2012). Integrins regulate repulsion-mediated dendritic patterning of drosophila sensory neurons by restricting dendrites in a 2D space. *Neuron* **73**, 64–78.

Hertzler, J. I., Bernard, A. R. and Rolls, M. M. (2023). Dendrite regeneration mediates functional recovery after complete dendrite removal. *Dev Biol*. doi:10.1016/j.ydbio.2023.03.001

Hertzler, J. I., Simonovitch, S. I., Albertson, R. M., Weiner, A. T., Nye, D. M. R. and Rolls, M. M. (2020). Kinetochore proteins suppress neuronal microtubule dynamics and promote dendrite regeneration. *Mol Biol Cell* **31**, 2125–2138.

Hill, S. E., Parmar, M., Gheres, K. W., Guignet, M. A., Huang, Y., Jackson, F. R. and Rolls, M. M. (2012). Development of dendrite polarity in Drosophila neurons. *Neural Dev* **7**, 34.

Hoang, T. X., Nieto, J. H. and Havton, L. A. (2005). Regenerating supernumerary axons are cholinergic and emerge from both autonomic and motor neurons in the rat spinal cord. *Neuroscience* **136**, 417–23.

Hwang, R. Y., Zhong, L., Xu, Y., Johnson, T., Zhang, F., Deisseroth, K. and Tracey, W. D. (2007). Nociceptive neurons protect Drosophila larvae from parasitoid wasps. *Curr Biol* **17**, 2105–16.

Inoki, K., Kim, J. and Guan, K. L. (2012). AMPK and mTOR in cellular energy homeostasis and drug targets. *Annu Rev Pharmacol Toxicol* **52**, 381–400.

Isokawa, M. and Levesque, M. F. (1991). Increased NMDA responses and dendritic degeneration in human epileptic hippocampal neurons in slices. *Neurosci Lett* **132**, 212–6.

Jegla, T., Nguyen, M. M., Feng, C., Goetschius, D. J., Luna, E., van Rossum, D. B., Kamel, B., Pisupati, A., Milner, E. S. and Rolls, M. M. (2016). Bilaterian Giant Ankyrins Have a Common Evolutionary Origin and Play a Conserved Role in Patterning the Axon Initial Segment. *PLoS Genet* **12**, e1006457.

Ji, H., Sapar, M. L., Sarkar, A., Wang, B. and Han, C. (2022). Phagocytosis and self-destruction break down dendrites of Drosophila sensory neurons at distinct steps of Wallerian degeneration. *Proc Natl Acad Sci U S A* **119**.

Ji, Y., Koch, D., Gonzalez Delgado, J., Gunther, M., Witte, O. W., Kessels, M. M., Frahm, C. and Qualmann, B. (2021). Poststroke dendritic arbor regrowth requires the actin nucleator Cobl. *PLoS Biol* **19**, e3001399.

Jiang, N., Rasmussen, J. P., Clanton, J. A., Rosenberg, M. F., Luedke, K. P., Cronan, M. R., Parker, E. D., Kim, H. J., Vaughan, J. C., Sagasti, A. et al. (2019). A conserved morphogenetic mechanism for epidermal ensheathment of nociceptive sensory neurites. *Elife* **8**.

Kim, M. E., Shrestha, B. R., Blazeski, R., Mason, C. A. and Grueber, W. B. (2012). Integrins establish dendrite-substrate relationships that promote dendritic self-avoidance and patterning in drosophila sensory neurons. *Neuron* **73**, 79–91.

Liu, X., Wang, X. and Shen, K. (2016). Receptor tyrosine phosphatase CLR-1 acts in skin cells to promote sensory dendrite outgrowth. *Dev Biol* **413**, 60–9.

Ma, T. C. and Willis, D. E. (2015). What makes a RAG regeneration associated? *Front Mol Neurosci* **8**, 43.

MacDermid, V., Neuber-Hess, M., Short, C. and Rose, P. K. (2002). Alterations to neuronal polarity following permanent axotomy: a quantitative analysis of changes to MAP2a/b and GAP-43 distributions in axotomized motoneurons in the adult cat. *J Comp Neurol* **450**, 318–33.

MacDermid, V. E., Neuber-Hess, M. S. and Rose, P. K. (2004). The temporal sequence of morphological and molecular changes in axotomized feline motoneurons leading to the formation of axons from the ends of dendrites. *J Comp Neurol* **468**, 233–50.

Mahar, M. and Cavalli, V. (2018). Intrinsic mechanisms of neuronal axon regeneration. *Nat Rev Neurosci* **19**, 323–337.

Manning, B. D. and Cantley, L. C. (2007). AKT/PKB signaling: navigating downstream. *Cell* **129**, 1261–74.

Marzano, M., Herzmann, S., Elsbroek, L., Sanal, N., Tarbashevich, K., Raz, E., Krahn, M. P. and Rumpf, S. (2021). AMPK adapts metabolism to developmental energy requirement during dendrite pruning in Drosophila. *Cell Rep* **37**, 110024.

Ming, G. L. and Song, H. (2011). Adult neurogenesis in the mammalian brain: significant answers and significant questions. *Neuron* **70**, 687–702.

Murphy, T. H., Li, P., Betts, K. and Liu, R. (2008). Two-photon imaging of stroke onset in vivo reveals that NMDA-receptor independent ischemic depolarization is the major cause of rapid reversible damage to dendrites and spines. *J Neurosci* **28**, 1756–72.

Neumann, B., Linton, C., Giordano-Santini, R. and Hilliard, M. A. (2019). Axonal fusion: An alternative and efficient mechanism of nerve repair. *Prog Neurobiol* **173**, 88–101.

Nye, D. M. R., Albertson, R. M., Weiner, A. T., Hertzler, J. I., Shorey, M., Goberdhan, D. C. I., Wilson, C., Janes, K. A. and Rolls, M. M. (2020). The receptor tyrosine kinase Ror is required for dendrite regeneration in Drosophila neurons. *PLoS Biol* **18**, e3000657.

Ochs, S. (1977). The early history of nerve regeneration beginning with Cruikshank's observations in 1776. *Med Hist* **21**, 261–74.

Oliva, A. A., Jr., Lam, T. T. and Swann, J. W. (2002). Distally directed dendrotoxicity induced by kainic Acid in hippocampal interneurons of green fluorescent protein-expressing transgenic mice. *J Neurosci* **22**, 8052–62.

Oren-Suissa, M., Gattegno, T., Kravtsov, V. and Podbilewicz, B. (2017). Extrinsic Repair of Injured Dendrites as a Paradigm for Regeneration by Fusion in Caenorhabditis elegans. *Genetics* **206**, 215–230.

Osterloh, J. M., Yang, J., Rooney, T. M., Fox, A. N., Adalbert, R., Powell, E. H., Sheehan, A. E., Avery, M. A., Hackett, R., Logan, M. A. et al. (2012). dSarm/Sarm1 is required for activation of an injury-induced axon death pathway. *Science* **337**, 481–4.

Park, K. K., Liu, K., Hu, Y., Kanter, J. L. and He, Z. (2010). PTEN/mTOR and axon regeneration. *Exp Neurol* **223**, 45–50.

Park, K. K., Liu, K., Hu, Y., Smith, P. D., Wang, C., Cai, B., Xu, B., Connolly, L., Kramvis, I., Sahin, M. et al. (2008). Promoting axon regeneration in the adult CNS by modulation of the PTEN/mTOR pathway. *Science* **322**, 963–6.

Parrish, J. Z., Xu, P., Kim, C. C., Jan, L. Y. and Jan, Y. N. (2009). The microRNA bantam functions in epithelial cells to regulate scaling growth of dendrite arbors in drosophila sensory neurons. *Neuron* **63**, 788–802.

Poe, A. R., Tang, L., Wang, B., Li, Y., Sapar, M. L. and Han, C. (2017). Dendritic space-filling requires a neuronal type-specific extracellular permissive signal in Drosophila. *Proc Natl Acad Sci U S A* **114**, E8062–E8071.

Purpura, D. P., Bodick, N., Suzuki, K., Rapin, I. and Wurzelmann, S. (1982). Microtubule disarray in cortical dendrites and neurobehavioral failure. I. Golgi and electron microscopic studies. *Brain Res* **281**, 287–97.

Rao, K., Stone, M. C., Weiner, A. T., Gheres, K. W., Zhou, C., Deitcher, D. L., Levitan, E. S. and Rolls, M. M. (2016). Spastin, atlastin, and ER relocalization are involved in axon but not dendrite regeneration. *Mol Biol Cell* **27**, 3245–3256.

Rao, K. S. and Rolls, M. M. (2017). Two Drosophila model neurons can regenerate axons from the stump or from a converted dendrite, with feedback between the two sites. *Neural Development* **12**.

Ripp, C., Loth, J., Petrova, I., Linnemannstons, K., Ulepic, M., Fradkin, L., Noordermeer, J. and Wodarz, A. (2018). Drosophila Ror is a nervous system-specific co-receptor for Wnt ligands. *Biol Open* **7**.

Risher, W. C., Ard, D., Yuan, J. and Kirov, S. A. (2010). Recurrent spontaneous spreading depolarizations facilitate acute dendritic injury in the ischemic penumbra. *J Neurosci* **30**, 9859–68.

Rolls, M. M. (2011). Neuronal polarity in Drosophila: Sorting out axons and dendrites. *Dev Neurobiol* **71**, 419–29.

Rolls, M. M. and Jegla, T. J. (2015). Neuronal polarity: an evolutionary perspective. *J Exp Biol* **218**, 572–80.

Rose, P. K. and Odlozinski, M. (1998). Expansion of the dendritic tree of motoneurons innervating neck muscles of the adult cat after permanent axotomy. *J Comp Neurol* **390**, 392–411.

Shepherd, G. M. (1991). Foundations of the neuron doctrine: Oxford University Press.

Shimono, K., Fujimoto, A., Tsuyama, T., Yamamoto-Kochi, M., Sato, M., Hattori, Y., Sugimura, K., Usui, T., Kimura, K. and Uemura, T. (2009). Multidendritic sensory neurons in the adult Drosophila abdomen:

origins, dendritic morphology, and segment- and age-dependent pro-grammed cell death. *Neural Dev* **4**, 37.

Shin, J. E., Cho, Y., Beirowski, B., Milbrandt, J., Cavalli, V. and Diantonio, A. (2012). Dual leucine zipper kinase is required for retrograde injury sig-naling and axonal regeneration. *Neuron* **74**, 1015–22.

Shorey, M., Stone, M. C., Mandel, J. and Rolls, M. M. (2020). Neurons sur-vive simultaneous injury to axons and dendrites and regrow both types of processes in vivo. *Dev Biol* **465**, 108–118.

Singhania, A. and Grueber, W. B. (2014). Development of the embryonic and larval peripheral nervous system of Drosophila. *Wiley Interdiscip Rev Dev Biol* **3**, 193–210.

Soba, P., Han, C., Zheng, Y., Perea, D., Miguel-Aliaga, I., Jan, L. Y. and Jan, Y. N. (2015). The Ret receptor regulates sensory neuron dendrite growth and integrin mediated adhesion. *Elife* **4**.

Song, Y., Ori-McKenney, K. M., Zheng, Y., Han, C., Jan, L. Y. and Jan, Y. N. (2012). Regeneration of Drosophila sensory neuron axons and den-drites is regulated by the Akt pathway involving Pten and microRNA bantam. *Genes Dev*.

Stone, M. C., Albertson, R. M., Chen, L. and Rolls, M. M. (2014). Dendrite injury triggers DLK-independent regeneration. *Cell Rep* **6**, 247–53.

Stone, M. C., Nguyen, M. M., Tao, J., Allender, D. L. and Rolls, M. M. (2010). Global up-regulation of microtubule dynamics and polarity reversal during regeneration of an axon from a dendrite. *Mol Biol Cell* **21**, 767–77.

Stone, M. C., Rao, K., Gheres, K. W., Kim, S., Tao, J., La Rochelle, C., Folker, C. T., Sherwood, N. T. and Rolls, M. M. (2012). Normal Spastin Gene Dosage Is Specifically Required for Axon Regeneration. *Cell Rep*.

Stone, M. C., Roegiers, F. and Rolls, M. M. (2008). Microtubules Have Opposite Orientation in Axons and Dendrites of Drosophila Neurons. *Mol Biol Cell* **19**, 4122–9.

Stone, M. C., Seebold, D. Y., Shorey, M., Kothe, G. O. and Rolls, M. M. (2022). Dendrite regeneration in the vertebrate spinal cord. *Dev Biol* **488**, 114–119.

Stricker, S., Rauschenberger, V. and Schambony, A. (2017). ROR-Family Receptor Tyrosine Kinases. *Curr Top Dev Biol* **123**, 105–142.

Sugimura, K., Yamamoto, M., Niwa, R., Satoh, D., Goto, S., Taniguchi, M., Hayashi, S. and Uemura, T. (2003). Distinct developmental modes and lesion-induced reactions of dendrites of two classes of Drosophila sen-sory neurons. *J Neurosci* **23**, 3752–60.

Swick, L. L., Kazgan, N., Onyenwoke, R. U. and Brenman, J. E. (2013). Isolation of AMP-activated protein kinase (AMPK) alleles required for neuronal maintenance in Drosophila melanogaster. *Biol Open* **2**, 1321–3.

Swope, R. D., Hertzler, J. I., Stone, M. C., Kothe, G. O. and Rolls, M. M. (2022). The exocyst complex is required for developmental and regenerative neurite growth in vivo. *Dev Biol* **492**, 1–13. doi:10.1016/j.ydbio.2022.09.005

Tao, J., Feng, C. and Rolls, M. M. (2016). The microtubule-severing protein fidgetin acts after dendrite injury to promote their degeneration. *J Cell Sci* **129**, 3274–81.

Tao, J. and Rolls, M. M. (2011). Dendrites have a rapid program of injury-induced degeneration that is molecularly distinct from developmental pruning. *J Neurosci* **31**, 5398–405.

Teoh, J. S., Wong, M. Y., Vijayaraghavan, T. and Neumann, B. (2018). Bridging the gap: axonal fusion drives rapid functional recovery of the nervous system. *Neural Regen Res* **13**, 591–594.

Thompson-Peer, K. L., DeVault, L., Li, T., Jan, L. Y. and Jan, Y. N. (2016). In vivo dendrite regeneration after injury is different from dendrite development. *Genes Dev* **30**, 1776–89.

Thyagarajan, P., Feng, C., Lee, D., Shorey, M. and Rolls, M. M. (2022). Microtubule polarity is instructive for many aspects of neuronal polarity. *Dev Biol*.

Tsalik, E. L., Niacaris, T., Wenick, A. S., Pau, K., Avery, L. and Hobert, O. (2003). LIM homeobox gene-dependent expression of biogenic amine receptors in restricted regions of the C. elegans nervous system. *Dev Biol* **263**, 81–102.

Verma, M., Lizama, B. N. and Chu, C. T. (2022). Excitotoxicity, calcium and mitochondria: a triad in synaptic neurodegeneration. *Transl Neurodegener* **11**, 3.

Wang, C. F., Zhao, C. C., Jiang, G., Gu, X., Feng, J. F. and Jiang, J. Y. (2016). The Role of Posttraumatic Hypothermia in Preventing Dendrite Degeneration and Spine Loss after Severe Traumatic Brain Injury. *Sci Rep* **6**, 37063.

Weiner, A. T., Lanz, M. C., Goetschius, D. J., Hancock, W. O. and Rolls, M. M. (2016). Kinesin-2 and Apc function at dendrite branch points to resolve microtubule collisions. *Cytoskeleton (Hoboken)* **73**, 35–44.

West, J. R. (1978). Early history of mammalian nerve regeneration. *Neuroscience and Behavioral Reviews* **2**, 27–32.

Worby, C. A. and Dixon, J. E. (2014). Pten. *Annu Rev Biochem* **83**, 641–69.

Xiong, X., Wang, X., Ewanek, R., Bhat, P., Diantonio, A. and Collins, C. A. (2010). Protein turnover of the Wallenda/DLK kinase regulates a retrograde response to axonal injury. *J Cell Biol* **191**, 211–23.

Yan, D., Wu, Z., Chisholm, A. D. and Jin, Y. (2009). The DLK-1 kinase promotes mRNA stability and local translation in C. elegans synapses and axon regeneration. *Cell* **138**, 1005–18.

Yasunaga, K., Kanamori, T., Morikawa, R., Suzuki, E. and Emoto, K. (2010). Dendrite reshaping of adult Drosophila sensory neurons requires matrix metalloproteinase-mediated modification of the basement membranes. *Dev Cell* **18**, 621–32.

Ye, B., Zhang, Y., Song, W., Younger, S. H., Jan, L. Y. and Jan, Y. N. (2007). Growing dendrites and axons differ in their reliance on the secretory pathway. *Cell* **130**, 717–29.

Yiu, G. and He, Z. (2006). Glial inhibition of CNS axon regeneration. *Nat Rev Neurosci* **7**, 617–27.

Zeng, L. H., Xu, L., Rensing, N. R., Sinatra, P. M., Rothman, S. M. and Wong, M. (2007). Kainate seizures cause acute dendritic injury and actin depolymerization in vivo. *J Neurosci* **27**, 11604–13.

Zhao, Z., Chen, S., Luo, Y., Li, J., Badea, S., Ren, C. and Wu, W. (2017). Time-lapse changes of in vivo injured neuronal substructures in the central nervous system after low energy two-photon nanosurgery. *Neural Regen Res* **12**, 751–756.

Zou, W., Shen, A., Dong, X., Tugizova, M., Xiang, Y. K. and Shen, K. (2016). A multi-protein receptor-ligand complex underlies combinatorial dendrite guidance choices in C. elegans. *Elife* **5**.

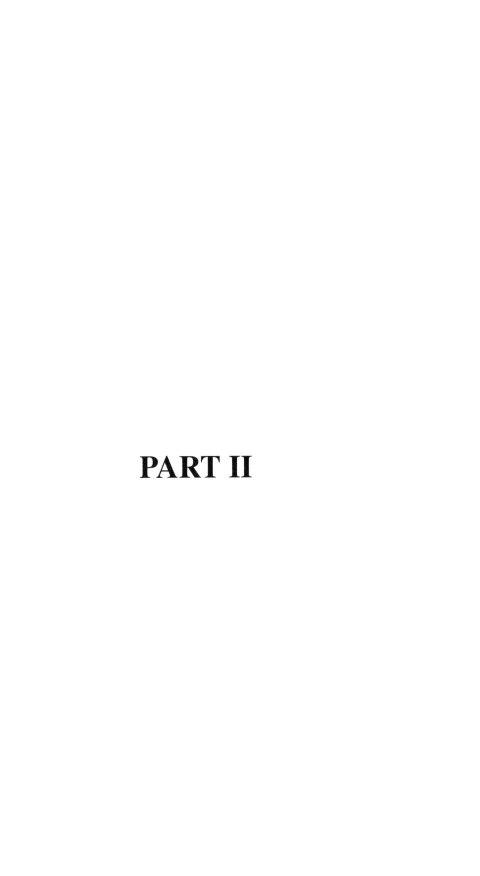

PART II

4

Constructing by Disposing: Regulation of Neuronal Morphogenesis by Phagocytosis

Hui Ji and Chun Han

Weill Institute for Cell and Molecular Biology and Department of Molecular Biology and Genetics, Cornell University, USA
Corresponding Email: chun.han@cornell.edu

Abstract

The construction of a functional nervous system involves not only the addition of new neurites or synapses but also the elimination of excessive or temporary structures. Being responsible for the trimming work, diverse phagocytes engulf apoptotic neurons, dissolve large pieces of axons or dendrites, or nibble away specific synapses. In these processes, phagocytes do not merely clean up the mess resulting from neuronal destruction. Instead, they are often responsible for killing the neurons or dismantling the excessive neurites/synapses. Thus, failure of phagocytosis can result in defects in neuronal morphology and connectivity. Phagocytosis of neurons is triggered by "eat-me" signals exposed on the neuronal surface. Engulfment receptors on phagocytes recognize these signals and promote cytoskeletal and transcriptional changes necessary for phagocytosis and other responses. Here, we review the experimental systems used to study phagocytosis during neuronal remodeling in both invertebrates and vertebrates and recent progress that sheds light on the molecular pathways underlying phagocytosis in the developing nervous system.

Main Text

To build functional neural circuits, neurons need to constantly interact with the surrounding tissues. Many steps in neuronal morphogenesis involve removing neurons or neuronal compartments that are no longer needed. The removal of unnecessary neuronal material is primarily carried out by resident phagocytes in both the central nervous system (CNS) and the peripheral nervous system (PNS). These resident phagocytes may perform other functions but can turn into phagocytic cells when they are presented with the material to be engulfed. Phagocytosis sculpts the nervous system at multiple scales – from elimination of dying neurons, large-scale remodeling of axons or dendritic arbors, to pruning of axonal/dendritic tips or synapses. Abnormal phagocytosis can have a profound impact on the development and homeostasis of the nervous system (Faust et al., 2021; Galloway et al., 2019; Neniskyte and Gross, 2017). In this chapter, we survey the neuronal morphogenic processes in which phagocytosis of neuronal structures has been observed and discuss the role of phagocytosis in the construction of mature neurons or neural circuits. We also review the molecular mechanisms underlying phagocytosis of neuronal structures. One focus is on a surface signal that labels degenerative compartments of neurons to trigger phagocytosis. The second focus is on the phagocytic receptors involved in recognizing the signal in diverse systems and the signaling downstream of receptor activation. Other topics that have been extensively reviewed elsewhere, such as the neuronal-intrinsic processes of prime neurons for degeneration, are not discussed in detail here.

4.1 Phagocytosis in Diverse Contexts of Neuronal Morphogenesis

4.1.1 Elimination of whole neurons

4.1.1.1 Elimination of neuronal corpses resulting from programmed cell death (PCD)

PCD, or apoptosis, is a common phenomenon in the development of the nervous system in both invertebrates and vertebrates (reviewed by Buss et al., 2006). By estimate, about half of the motoneurons produced during the embryonic development of the mouse (Lance-Jones, 1982), rat (Oppenheim, 1986), and chicken (Oppenheim et al., 1997) are lost. PCD serves a variety of adaptive functions in the nervous system, including adjusting cell numbers to control organ and tissue sizes (Cecconi et al., 1998; Rogulja-Ortmann et al., 2007), matching the numbers of neurons with their efferent targets and afferent inputs (reviewed by Buss et al., 2006), and eliminating defective cells resulting from developmental errors and noise (Baek et al., 2013; Clarke, 1992; Jiang and Reichert, 2012; Rogulja-Ortmann et al., 2007). During early morphogenesis of the neural tube and the brain in vertebrates, PCD regulates dynamic movement of cells and erases signaling centers (Nonomura et al., 2013; Offner et al., 2005). During metamorphosis in insects (Choi et al., 2006; Togane et al., 2012; Winbush and Weeks, 2011) and puberty in mammals (Forger, 2009), PCD removes certain anatomical structures of the post-embryonic CNS before the formation of the final adult structures. Apoptotic cells resulting from PCD are usually efficiently engulfed by tissue-resident phagocytes before rupture, preventing leakage of toxic materials and inflammatory damage to neighboring cells (Figure 4.1(A)) (reviewed by Fricker et al., 2018).

In *Drosophila*, three resident glial subtypes remove cell corpses in the CNS at both distinct and overlapping developmental stages. Cortex glia engulf apoptotic neurons from early embryogenesis to larval and pupal stages (Etchegaray et al., 2016; Kurant et al., 2008; McLaughlin et al., 2019; Nakano et al., 2019). Astrocyte-like glia and ensheathing glia engulf apoptotic neurons during metamorphosis (Hilu-Dadia et al., 2018). In vertebrates, microglia are the major phagocytes for clearing neuronal corpses. Microglia have been reported to engulf apoptotic neurons in the embryonic brain of zebrafish (Mazaheri et al., 2014) and in the developing and the mature CNS of mammals (Dalmau et al., 2003; Sierra et al., 2010). Other glial types can engulf apoptotic cells during development. For example, in the mouse PNS, satellite glial cell precursors remove apoptotic corpses in developing dorsal root ganglia (DRG) (Wu et al., 2009).

4.1.1.2 Phagocytosis of live neurons

Phagocytes can sometimes engulf stressed cells that are still alive. This type of cell execution, termed "phagoptosis" (Brown and Neher, 2012), is distinct from PCD, in that inhibiting phagocytosis in phagoptosis prevents cell death, while inhibiting phagocytosis in PCD results in accumulation of dead cells. Studies on *Caenorhabditis elegans* showed that loss-of-function (LOF) mutations in genes encoding engulfment receptors cause survival of neuronal precursors that are normally lost during development (Darland-Ransom et al., 2008; Hoeppner et al., 2001; Reddien et al., 2001). Similarly, studies in rats and monkeys showed that microglia engulf neural precursors to regulate the size of the precursor pool in the developing cerebral cortex (Cunningham et al., 2013). In addition, microglia kill and engulf differentiating neurons in the developing cerebellum and hippocampus of mice (Marin-Teva et al., 2004; Wakselman et al., 2008). Thus, killing extra neural precursors or neurons by phagocytosis is a conserved developmental mechanism to achieve the desired number of neurons in the mature nervous system.

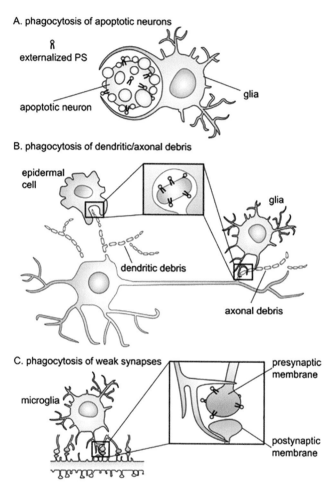

Figure 4.1   Phagocytosis in the developing nervous system. (A) In the CNS, resident phago-cytes (blue), such as astrocytes and microglia, engulf apoptotic neurons (orange). **(B)** Glia also engulf damaged or pruned neurites. In the PNS, amateur phagocytes that normally contact neuronal processes, such as epidermal cells in *Drosophila* and zebrafish skins, break down and clear degenerating neurites. **(C)** In the CNS, glia eliminate weak synapses by engulfing pre-and/or post-synaptic membranes. In all scenarios, phosphatidylserine (PS, pink) is externalized on the surface of the degenerative compartment of neurons to serve as an "eat-me" signal.

4.1.2 Large-scale remodeling of axons/dendrites during development

During development, neurons often make inappropriate, excessive, or tran-sient connections that must be eliminated as circuits mature. Pruning of selec-tive axonal and dendritic branches is an important aspect of neural circuit refinement (reviewed by Corty and Freeman, 2013; Luo and O'Leary, 2005). In some animals, the same neuron can belong to two different functional circuits at the juvenile and adult stages. The axonal and dendritic connections established for the juvenile stage need to be pruned before the construction of the adult circuits. For instance, holometabolous insects, such as *Drosophila*, undergo dramatic remodeling of many neuronal structures when transitioning from the larval stage to the adult stage (Watts et al., 2003; Williams and Truman, 2005a, b). In mammals, large-scale axon elimination precedes the generation of adult patterns of callosal, intracortical, and subcortical projections due to the reduced numbers of collaterals and targets in the adults (reviewed by O'Leary, 1992; O'Leary and Koester, 1993). Thus, phagocytotic removal of the pruned axons and dendrites is a shared mechanism in circuit remodeling in both invertebrates and vertebrates.

4.1.2.1 Axon pruning of *Drosophila* mushroom body (MB) γ-neurons

The *Drosophila* MB γ-neurons have been a popular model for studying developmental axon pruning. MBs in the *Drosophila* brain play an essential role in olfactory learning and memory (de Belle and Heisenberg, 1994; Heisenberg et al., 1985). Axons of MB γ neurons initially bifurcate into dorsal and medial lobes at the larval stage. Shortly after puparium formation, γ axons in the lobes are selectively pruned by local degeneration to retain only the main processes, which then project into the adult medial γ lobe without bifurcation (Lee et al., 1999; Watts et al., 2003). Astrocyte-like glia selectively invade MB axon lobes at the onset of metamorphosis and engulf degenerating axon fragments during pruning (Awasaki and Ito, 2004; Awasaki et al., 2006; Hakim et al., 2014; Tasdemir-Yilmaz and Freeman, 2014; Watts et al., 2004). In addition to clearing axonal debris, astrocyte-like glia also actively promote fragmentation of pruned axons (Figure 4.1(B)), as inhibition of glia-mediated phagocytosis suppresses axon breakdown (Awasaki and Ito, 2004; Awasaki et al., 2006; Hakim et al., 2014).

4.1.2.2 Dendrite pruning of *Drosophila* dendritic arborization (da) neurons

Dendritic arborization (da) neurons are somatosensory neurons that innervate the larval epidermis with free-ending dendrites. A subset of these neurons dies during metamorphosis, while others persist and remodel their dendritic arbors for the adult stage (Shimono et al., 2009). Among those that survive are dorsal class IV da (C4da) neurons (Shimono et al., 2009; Williams and Truman, 2005a). Because these neurons are close to the translucent body wall, they are particularly suitable for living imaging in the immobile pupa.

Soon after metamorphosis starts, C4da neurons undergo a series of degenerative events, including severing of proximal dendrites, thinning and beading of low-order branches, and dendrite fragmentation. Dendrite degeneration and clearance complete by 16–18 hours (hrs) after puparium formation (APF), while the cell bodies and axons remain (Han et al., 2014; Kuo et al., 2005; Lee et al., 2009; Williams and Truman, 2005a). The epidermal cells that directly contact da sensory dendrites function as the primary phagocytes responsible for clearing the pruned dendrites (Figure 4.1(B)) (Han et al., 2014). Rather than merely internalizing disintegrated dendrite pieces, epidermal cells also wrap degenerating dendrites to facilitate dendrite fragmentation (Han et al., 2014). Circulating phagocytic blood cells called plasmatocytes can also attack dendritic branches and contribute to dendrite fragmentation (Williams and Truman, 2005a); however, they are not required for the clearance of degenerating dendrites (Han et al., 2014). Phagocytic clearance of sensory neurites seems to be a conserved function of epidermal cells from insects to vertebrates, as zebrafish epidermal cells are also responsible for clearing degenerating sensory axons after injury (Rasmussen et al., 2015).

4.1.2.3 Axon removal at the mammalian neuromuscular junction (NMJ)

During development of the mammalian motor system, one motor neuron initially projects axonal branches to multiple muscle fibers, and each muscle fiber is innervated by axons from multiple motor neurons. Within the first several postnatal weeks, through a process of activity-dependent intercellular competition, only one "winning" motor input is left to innervate one muscle fiber, with "loser" axons and pre-synaptic terminals being eliminated (Colman et al., 1997; Walsh and Lichtman, 2003). The "losing" axonal branches withdraw by shedding membrane vesicles termed axosomes, resulting in large-scale elimination of axon branches (Bishop et al., 2004; Song et al., 2008). Special Schwann cells that ensheath the junctions play important roles in eliminating the "loser" synapses and axons. They phagocytose nerve terminals contacting the muscle fiber, thus promoting synaptic turnover (Smith et al., 2013) and engulf the axosomes shed by retracting axons (Song et al., 2008).

4.1.3 Activity-dependent elimination of short axon/dendrite segments or synapses

In addition to developmentally programmed large-scale pruning of axons and dendrites, neuronal remodeling may occur at restricted compartments, such as specific synapses and axon or dendrite tips. In this type of remodeling, neuronal activity usually plays an important role in defining the neuronal compartments to be eliminated (reviewed by Neniskyte and Gross, 2017).

4.1.3.1 Membrane shedding during *Drosophila* NMJ expansion

In the *Drosophila* larva, a motor neuron innervates a muscle fiber by elaborating a single axon arbor onto the muscle. At the NMJ, the axon arbor sheds presynaptic debris or ghost boutons (undifferentiated synaptic boutons) in an activity-dependent manner during normal synaptic growth (Fuentes-Medel et al., 2009). However, instead of eliminating arbors, as seen in the axonal removal of mammalian NMJs, this membrane shedding in *Drosophila* occurs while new arbors are being added at the NMJ. The shed material is cleared by both the glia and muscle cells that directly contact the axons: Glia invade the NMJ and mainly engulf small presynaptic debris, while post-synaptic muscles mainly engulf larger ghost boutons. The presynaptic debris is inhibitory to synaptic growth and expansion if left unengulfed (Fuentes-Medel et al., 2009).

4.1.3.2 Engulfment of worm sensory microvilli

The AFD neuron is one of the major thermosensory neurons in adult *C. elegans*. The neuron-receptive ending (NRE), the sensory structure of AFD, comprises actin-based microvilli and a single microtubule-based cilium, both embedded in the AMsh glial cell (Singhvi et al., 2016). In healthy adult worms, AFD neurons constantly shed fragments of the NRE, leaving pieces disconnected from the rest of the neuron (Raiders et al., 2021; Singhvi et al., 2016). A recent study found that AMsh glia actively engulf the NRE fragments. Perturbations of the glial engulfment led to defects in the NRE shape and the associated thermosensory behaviors of the animals (Raiders et al., 2021). Thus, constant glial engulfment of the NRE maintains tissue homeostasis and physiological functions of the AFD neuron.

4.1.3.3 Shedding of mammalian photoreceptor outer segments (POS)

In the mammalian retina, the light-sensitive outer segments of photoreceptor rods and cones are each composed of a stack of many hundreds of densely packed discs, which are formed by invaginated plasma membrane. The photoreceptors continuously renew their outer segments by shedding their aged tips (Young, 1967, 1971). Rods shed their membranes each morning at the onset of light, whereas cones shed their membranes at the onset of night (LaVail, 1976; Young, 1977). The membrane shedding precedes a burst of phagocytosis by the adjacent retinal pigment epithelium (RPE), which rapidly clears shed POS. Daily phagocytosis of aging POS is essential for the function and longevity of photoreceptor neurons. Failure of this process causes accumulation of photoreceptor cell debris that compromises the normal vision (Nandrot et al., 2004; Young and Bok, 1969).

4.1.3.4 Synaptic pruning in the developing mammalian CNS

Maturation of neuronal circuits requires selective elimination of excessive synaptic connections generated during early development (reviewed by Chung and Barres, 2012; Wilton et al., 2019). The disruption of synaptic remodeling has been suggested to play a role in neurodevelopmental disorders such as autism and schizophrenia (reviewed by Salter and Stevens, 2017; Wilton et al., 2019). Synaptic pruning often involves glial engulfment of synaptic material (Figure 4.1(C)). Microglia and astrocytes, tissue-resident phagocytes of the vertebrate CNS, play important roles in removing redundant synapses (reviewed by Riccomagno and Kolodkin, 2015; Wilton et al., 2019). The dorsolateral geniculate nucleus (dLGN) of the thalamus and the hippocampus are two regions of the developing mammalian brain where synaptic pruning has been extensively studied.

During early postnatal stages, the axons of retinal ganglion cells (RGCs) extend into the mouse dLGN and form excessive synaptic connections with relay neurons. Overlapping RGC inputs from both eyes undergo a process of remodeling called eye-specific segregation, resulting in the separation of ipsilateral and contralateral inputs into distinct non-overlapping domains in the mature dLGN (Katz and Shatz, 1996). Defective synaptic pruning of RGC inputs to the relay neurons in the dLGN leads to incomplete eye-specific segregation (Huberman, 2007; Jaubert-Miazza et al., 2005). Microglia participate in the pruning of excess RGC synaptic inputs during peak retinogeniculate pruning at around postnatal day (P) 5 in mouse (Lehrman et al., 2018; Li et al., 2020; Schafer et al., 2012; Scott-Hewitt et al., 2020; Stevens et al., 2007). This microglia-mediated engulfment of presynaptic terminals is regulated by RGC activity such that microglia preferentially engulf inputs from the "weaker" eye (Schafer et al., 2012). Astrocytes also actively engulf excessive synapses in the dLGN during the same developmental period (Chung et al., 2013). Disrupting microglia-mediated or astrocyte-mediated phagocytosis results in sustained deficits in synaptic connectivity (Chung et al., 2013; Schafer et al., 2012).

Synaptic pruning continues in the dLGN from eye opening to later developmental stages (P8–P30 in mouse). Initially, each dLGN neuron is innervated by multiple RGC axons. Between P11 and P16, spontaneous retinal activity drives bulk elimination of excess connections while strengthening the remaining synapses. Later, visual experience is required for synaptic plasticity

(Hooks and Chen, 2006). Microglia are involved in eliminating excessive synapses during both the early and later stages (Vainchtein et al., 2018).

Synaptic elimination in the hippocampus happens around P8–P18 as neural circuits mature (Filipello et al., 2018; Paolicelli et al., 2011; Scott-Hewitt et al., 2020; Weinhard et al., 2018) and in the adult during memory formation (Attardo et al., 2015). Again, microglia are involved in the elimination of excessive synapses in this brain region during development (Filipello et al., 2018; Paolicelli et al., 2011; Scott-Hewitt et al., 2020; Weinhard et al., 2018). Disruptions in microglia function result in delayed maturation of hippocampal synaptic circuits (Paolicelli et al., 2011). In the adult hippocampus, astrocytes phagocytose synapses to maintain proper hippocampal synaptic connectivity and plasticity (Lee et al., 2021).

4.2 Induction of Phagocytosis in Neuronal Remodeling

Phagocytosis of neurons during remodeling results from both neuronal-intrinsic and neuronal-extrinsic mechanisms. Intrinsically, molecular events that occur globally in the cell or locally in specific neurites or compartments lead to changes in cell surface properties, which ultimately induce engulfment by phagocytes. The molecular pathways leading to these changes are diverse and context-specific. For instance, caspase-mediated self-destruction underlies both neuronal PCD and at least some cases of neurite pruning; transcriptional control mediated by ecdysone receptor (EcR) is essential for large-scale axon and dendrite pruning during *Drosophila* metamorphosis; neuronal activity is an important regulator of synaptic pruning in mammals. Many cell-intrinsic pathways have been extensively discussed in previous reviews (Boulanger and Dura, 2015; Faust et al., 2021; Fricker et al., 2018; Riccomagno and Kolodkin, 2015; Yu and Schuldiner, 2014) or in other chapters of this book, and thus are not discussed here.

Extracellularly, phagocytosis is induced by the so-called "eat-me" signals that are exposed on the surface of neurons. "Eat-me" signals tag the neurons and neuronal compartments destined for phagocytosis so that they are distinguishable from other healthy neurons or healthy parts of neurons. Several membrane-anchored "eat-me" signals, including phosphatidylserine (PS), Calreticulin (Calr), Pretaporter (Prtp), and *Drosophila* calcium-binding protein 1 (DmCaBP1), have been identified from earlier work on the clearance of apoptotic cells (Gardai et al., 2005; Kuraishi et al., 2009; Okada et al., 2012; Ravichandran, 2010). Among these, PS is the best studied and its involvement in the clearance of neuronal materials is well-documented across species. In the last couple of decades, much has been learned regarding the roles of PS in phagocytosis of neuronal materials, recognition of PS by phagocytic receptors, and the signaling downstream of phagocytic receptor activation.

4.2.1 Phosphatidylserine (PS) as a major "eat-me" signal

PS is a negatively charged phospholipid that is normally confined to the cytoplasmic leaflet of the plasma membrane in healthy cells (reviewed by Leventis and Grinstein, 2010). However, during apoptosis, PS is externalized to the exoplasmic leaflet of dying cells and is recognized by phagocytes (Segawa and Nagata, 2015). Recent studies show that PS also functions as a potent "eat-me" signal exposed on neurons during developmental remodeling of the nervous system (Figure 4.1), clearance after neurite injury, and in neurological disease conditions. Below, we focus on the role of PS as an "eat-me" signal in the nervous system.

4.2.2 PS exposure marks degenerating neurites and synapses during nervous system remodeling

Given that PS is an "eat-me" signal for apoptotic cells (Mapes et al., 2012; Segawa and Nagata, 2015), PS is expected to be exposed globally on the surface of dying neurons. Interestingly, during neuronal remodeling, PS also specifically tags the compartments of neurons (axons or dendrites) that are destined to be phagocytosed. Compartmentalized PS exposure on degenerating axons was first shown using a PS sensor based on Annexin V in axotomy-treated mouse dorsal root ganglia (DRG) explants (Sievers et al., 2003). This finding was later corroborated by experiments using another PS sensor MFG-E8^{D89E}, a mutant version of milk fat globule-EGF factor 8 (MFG-E8, also called lactadherin) that cannot interact with integrin receptors, to label mouse DRG explants treated by vincristine or axotomy (Shacham-Silverberg et al., 2018). The first *in vivo* evidence that PS is specifically exposed on degenerative parts of neurons came from a study with injured rat sciatic nerves (Kim et al., 2010). PS exposure on injured, but not intact, nerves was shown with a polarity-sensitive annexin-based biosensor (pSIVA) that fluoresces only when binding to PS on membranes. Sapar et al. provided further *in vivo* evidence in *Drosophila* indicating that PS is an "eat-me" signal on neurites in intact live animals. Using genetically encoded PS binding proteins, Annexin V and the Lactadherin C1C2 domain, local PS exposure was found on dendrites undergoing injury-induced (or Wallerian) degeneration (Sapar et al., 2018) and dendrites of neurons deficient in NAD$^+$ biosynthesis, which molecularly resembles Wallerian degeneration (Ji et al., 2022). Long-term time-lapse live imaging revealed that PS exposure occurs prior to dendrite fragmentation and phagocytic engulfment of neuronal debris, supporting the role of PS as an "eat-me" signal (Ji et al., 2022; Sapar et al., 2018).

PS is also exposed on degenerating neurites during developmental remodeling. In an *in vitro* model for axon pruning, cultured mouse DRG explants under nerve growth factor (NGF) deprivation exposed PS on sub-axonal segments during degeneration (Kim et al., 2010; Shacham-Silverberg et al., 2018). The *in vivo* evidence came from experiments examining dendrite pruning during *Drosophila* metamorphosis, in which PS was exposed specifically on pruned dendrites that were severed from the cell body of C4da neurons (Sapar et al., 2018).

Besides neurites that have been detached from the cell body, PS exposure is also observed on locally restricted neuronal compartments that are degenerative. For example, in freshly dissected mouse retina, PS externalization was found to be restricted to POS tips with discrete boundaries using pSIVA (Ruggiero et al., 2012). At the synaptic level, PS exposure was detected at synapses in mouse dLGN and hippocampus with the fluorescent probe PSVue during the periods when microglial-mediated developmental pruning takes place (Li et al., 2020; Scott-Hewitt et al., 2020). In these contexts, PS-flagged pre-synaptic material was engulfed by microglia (Li et al., 2020; Scott-Hewitt et al., 2020), suggesting that local PS exposure instructs engulfment of synapses. Consistent with this idea, in brains of juvenile mice, PS was found preferentially exposed on inhibitory post-synapses, which are frequently engulfed by microglia (Park et al., 2021).

In all the above examples, PS exposure marks the compartments destined to be engulfed. The fact that PS can be exposed transiently on a restricted portion of the plasma membrane suggests that PS exposure can be regulated locally within the neuron.

4.2.3 Exposed PS dominantly triggers phagocytosis of neurons or neuronal processes

The PS asymmetry in the plasma membrane is established and maintained by transmembrane aminophospholipid flippases encoded by the P4-ATPase family. Several members in the P4-ATPase family have been demonstrated to be PS-specific flippases that unidirectionally transport PS from the outer leaflet of the plasma membrane to the inner leaflet (reviewed by Bevers and Williamson, 2016; Leventis and Grinstein, 2010). The PS-specific flippases involved in nervous system remodeling include mammalian ATP8A1/2, their

Drosophila homolog ATP8A, and their *C. elegans* homolog TAT-1 (Darland-Ransom et al., 2008; Sapar et al., 2018; Zhu et al., 2012). These PS-flippases require a chaperone protein called CDC50A for proper subcellular localization and function (Takatsu et al., 2011; Tanaka et al., 2011; van der Velden et al., 2010). PS asymmetry on the plasma membrane can be disrupted by the activity of lipid scramblases, enzymes that bi-directionally translocate PS between the two leaflets of biomembranes (reviewed by Bevers and Williamson, 2016; Leventis and Grinstein, 2010). One of the scramblases, Xk-related protein 8 (Xkr8), is activated by caspase-mediated cleavage and is responsible for PS exposure on apoptotic cells (Suzuki et al., 2013). Members of TMEM16 family are Ca^{2+}-activated scramblases in non-apoptotic cells (Falzone et al., 2018). For example, TMEM16F activation by Ca^{2+} induces PS exposure on platelets during blood clotting (Fujii et al., 2015; Suzuki et al., 2010).

The loss of PS flippases induces ectopic PS exposure on otherwise normal cells, offering an opportunity for investigating the consequence of non-apoptotic PS exposure. *TAT-1* LOF in living neurons caused PS exposure, and these cells were removed by neighboring phagocytes in *C. elegans* (Darland-Ransom et al., 2008), demonstrating an example of phagoptosis. Studies in *Drosophila* larval PNS further demonstrated the sufficiency of PS exposure in inducing neurite degeneration of sensory neurons. LOF of *CDC50A* or *ATP8A* in C4da neurons resulted in low levels of ectopic PS exposure at distal terminal dendrites, which were phagocytosed by surrounding epidermal cells (Sapar et al., 2018). This PS-induced neurite loss was exacerbated by combining *CDC50* knockout (KO) with the overexpression (OE) of a hypersensitive mutant of TMEM16F that is known to elevate PS exposure (Segawa et al., 2011). These results suggest that PS exposure is sufficient to induce neuronal membrane loss and that distal dendrites are more sensitive to disruptions of the PS asymmetry than proximal dendrites and the cell body.

The approaches of inducing ectopic PS exposure with flippase KO and scramblase OE also helped to reveal the role of PS-mediated phagocytosis in promoting dendrite fragmentation during Wallerian degeneration. PS exposure and fragmentation of injured dendrites is strongly blocked if the neuron overexpresses a chimeric protein called Wallerian degeneration slow (Wld[S]) (Ji et al., 2022; Sapar et al., 2018). Reintroducing PS exposure by knocking out *CDC50* or overexpressing TMEM16F in Wld[S]-expressing neurons restored fragmentation of injured dendrites (Ji et al., 2022). Considering that *CDC50* KO and TMEM16F OE cause milder PS exposure than that induced by injury (Sapar et al., 2018), PS-mediated phagocytosis should be sufficient to drive dendrite fragmentation after injury.

Dysregulation of PS asymmetry shows conserved effects in mammals. Mice with *wabbler-lethal* (*wl*) mutations develop progressive ataxia due to axonal degeneration in both the CNS and the PNS. The disease-causing *wl* mutations are in *ATP8A2*, the gene encoding the ATP8A2 flippase. Although spontaneous PS exposure on axons has not been demonstrated in *wl* mutant mice, the neurodegeneration phenotype discovered in *wl* mutant mice suggests that PS exposure due to flippase LOF can cause axonal degeneration in mammals (Zhu et al., 2012). In the context of synaptic pruning in mice, neuronal-specific deletion of *CDC50A* led to PS exposure on neuronal outer membranes, which caused specific loss of inhibitory post-synapses and audiogenic seizures (Park et al., 2021). These results collectively suggest that LOF of PS flippases induces axonal or synaptic degeneration in mammalian brains.

Interestingly, PS exposure induced by flippase LOF and scramblase GOF can cause distinct degeneration patterns in the fly CNS. In *Drosophila* OR22a olfactory receptor neurons (ORNs), *CDC50* KO led to a progressive age-dependent axon degeneration, suggesting that a low level of PS externalization can have a cumulative effect in causing axon loss over time. Overexpression of TMEM16F in OR22a neurons, in contrast, led to a rapid, neuronal activity-dependent axon loss (Sapar et al., 2018), consistent with TMEM16F being a Ca^{2+}-activated scramblase.

The above studies involving ectopic PS exposure in multiple species show that PS is a conserved neuronal "eat-me" signal that can dominantly induce dendrite and axon loss in both PNS and CNS due to attacks by phagocytes. These findings provide a potential mechanistic base for understanding neurodegeneration associated with aging and disease conditions.

4.2.4 PS exposure is required for phagocytosis of neurites or synapses in some contexts

The requirement of PS exposure in phagocytosis of neurons has been studied by masking PS signals using PS binding proteins. Blocking exposed PS using PS antibody or Annexin V reduced phagocytosis of POS by RPE in culture (Ruggiero et al., 2012). Direct masking of PS using MFG-E8[D89E] reduced engulfment of axonal debris in NGF-deprived neuronal culture (Shacham-Silverberg et al., 2018). Masking of PS using Annexin V also partially prevented synapse elimination in hippocampal neuron and microglia co-cultures (Scott-Hewitt et al., 2020). Corroborating this *in vitro* evidence, a more recent *in vivo* study showed that Annexin V injection in juvenile brains was sufficient to increase the number of inhibitory post-synapses and to prevent the loss of inhibitory post-synapses in *CDC50* conditional knockout (cKO) mice, presumably by masking the exposed PS (Park et al., 2021).

The above data are consistent with the idea that PS contributes to phagocytosis during neuronal remodeling. A more recent study on the degeneration of *Nmnat* KO neurons provides evidence for the requirement of PS exposure in phagocytosis of neurites (Ji et al., 2022). The *Drosophila Nmnat* gene encodes the nicotinamide mononucleotide adenylyltransferase required for NAD$^+$ production; *Nmnat* KO in C4da neurons resulted in spontaneous dendrite degeneration. This NAD$^+$ loss-induced neurodegeneration was previously thought to result from neuronal self-destruction (Zhai et al., 2006). Surprisingly, the dendrite degeneration of *Nmnat* KO neurons was completely rescued by either overexpressing ATP8A in neurons or suppressing epidermal phagocytosis, suggesting that PS-induced phagocytosis drives the degeneration of *Nmnat* KO neurons in *vivo* (Ji et al., 2022). These results also suggest that the maintenance of PS asymmetry on the plasma membrane requires sufficient levels of NAD$^+$ in the cell, a conclusion also supported by the observation that NAD$^+$ supplementation inhibited PS exposure on degenerating axons of cultured DRG neurons (Shacham-Silverberg et al., 2018).

Given that multiple "eat-me" signals can contribute to phagocytosis of apoptotic cells, it remains unclear whether PS exposure is required for phagocytosis in all developmental remodeling contexts.

4.3 Engulfment Receptors Mediating Phagocytosis during Neuronal Morphogenesis

Phagocytes rely on transmembrane engulfment receptors on their surface to detect and engulf neuronal material (Figure 4.2). Given the importance of PS exposure in phagocytosis, animals have evolved complex systems to recognize PS exposed on the surface of engulfment targets. While some of these systems are conserved from worms to flies and to humans, many others are new inventions of the evolution that are found only in vertebrates. Many engulfment receptors involved in neuronal morphogenesis have been shown to mediate PS recognition: some of them interact with PS directly while others recognize PS through bridging molecules. Here, we review the roles of these engulfment receptors in neuronal remodeling (see Table 4.1 for a summary) and the molecular pathways they activate to drive phagocytosis. We elaborate more on the Draper pathway in *Drosophila* and the complement system in mammals, as their mechanisms are better characterized, while summarizing work related to other receptors.

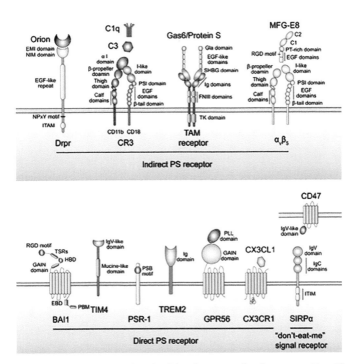

Figure 4.2   Engulfment receptors involved in phagocytosis of neurons. Engulfment receptors on phagocytes can recognize targets through a variety of mechanisms. These mechanisms include indirect recognition of neuronal PS through soluble bridging molecules, direct interactions with neuronal PS, and PS-independent ligand–receptor interactions. Recognition of neuronal PS by the indirect PS receptors Drpr, CR3, TAM receptors, and integrin $\alpha_v\beta_5$ requires specific PS-binding bridging molecules, Orion, C1q/C3, Gas6/Protein S, and MFG-E8, respectively. Direct PS receptors include BAI1, TIM4, PSR-1, TREM2, and GPR56. Drpr can also bind to PS directly *in vitro* and may do so *in vivo* when overexpressed. In addition to PS receptors, the chemokine receptor CX3CR1 is involved in synaptic pruning by interacting with its ligand CX3CL1. Lastly, the receptor SIPRα prevents phagocytosis of synapses by interacting with its ligand, the "don't-eat-me" signal CD47, on neuronal membranes. Domain/motif abbreviations: EGF, epidermal growth factor; ITAM, immunoreceptor tyrosine-based activation motif; PSI, plexin/semaphorin/integrin; Gla, gamma-carboxyglutamic acid-rich; SHBG, sex hormone binding globulin; Ig, immunoglobulin; FNIII, fibronectin type III; TK, tyrosine kinase; RGD, arginine-glycine-aspartate; PT, proline/threonine; TSR, thrombospondin type 1 repeat; HBD, hormone-binding domain; GAIN, GPCR autoproteolysis-inducing; EBD, ELMO-binding domain; PBM, PDZ domain-binding motif; IgV, immunoglobulin variable; PSB, PS-binding; PLL, pentraxin/laminin/neurexin/sex-hormone-binding-globulin-like; IgC, immunoglobulin constant; ITIM, immunoreceptor tyrosine-based inhibitory motif. Protein domain structures are based on (Behrens et al., 2022; Boulanger et al., 2021; Druart and Le Magueresse, 2019; Hanayama et al., 2002; Lamers et al., 2021; Lemke and Rothlin, 2008; Miyanishi et al., 2007; Park et al., 2020; Salzman et al., 2016; Ulland and Colonna, 2018; Weng et al., 2019; Wojdasiewicz et al., 2014; Wu et al., 2009; Yang et al., 2015; Ziegenfuss et al., 2008).

Table 4.1 Models of phagocytosis in the developing nervous system and the corresponding engulfment pathways

Morphogenesis type	Species	Phagocyte	"eat-me" signal	Bridging molecule	Engulfment receptor
Elimination of dead neurons	Fly	Cortex glia (Etchegaray et al., 2016; Kurant et al., 2008; McLaughlin et al., 2019; Nakano et al., 2019), astrocyte-like glia (Hilu-Dadia et al., 2018), and ensheathing glia (Hilu-Dadia et al., 2018)	PS? (Segawa and Nagata, 2015)		Drpr (Freeman et al., 2003; Tung et al., 2013)
	Zebrafish	Microglia (Mazaheri et al., 2014)			BAI1, and TIM4 (Mazaheri et al., 2014)
	Mammal	Microglia in CNS (Dalmau et al., 2003; Sierra et al., 2013; Sierra et al., 2010)		Gas6, and Pros1 (Fourgeaud et al., 2016; Grommes et al., 2008)	Mer, and Axl (Fourgeaud et al., 2016; Ji et al., 2013)
	Mammal	Satellite glial cell precursors in DRG (Wu et al., 2009)			Jedi-1, and MEGF10 (Scheib et al., 2012; Wu et al., 2009)
Developmental phagocytosis of live neuronal precursors	Worm		PS? (Darland-Ransom et al., 2008)		PSR-1, and CED-1 (Darland-Ransom et al., 2008; Hoeppner et al., 2001; Reddien et al., 2001)
	Mammal	Microglia (Cunningham et al., 2013; Marin-Teva et al., 2004; Wakselman et al., 2008)			CR3 subunit CD11b (Wakselman et al., 2008)
Pruning of mushroom body γ-neuron axons	Fly	Astrocyte-like glia (Awasaki and Ito, 2004; Awasaki et al., 2006; Hakim et al., 2014; Tasdemir-Yilmaz and Freeman, 2014; Watts et al., 2004)		Orion? (Boulanger et al., 2021)	Drpr (Awasaki et al., 2006; Hakim et al., 2014; Hoopfer et al., 2006; Tasdemir-Yilmaz and Freeman, 2014)

Process	Organism	Phagocyte (cell type)	Signal	Bridging molecule	Receptor
Pruning of da neuron dendrites	Fly	Epidermal cells (Han et al., 2014)	PS (Han et al., 2014; Ji et al., 2022; Sapar et al., 2018)	Orion (Ji, bioRxiv 2022)	Drpr (Han et al., 2014; Williams et al., 2006)
Elimination of axons at NMJ	Mammal	Schwann cells (Song et al., 2008)			
Growth of axons at NMJ	Fly	Glia, and muscles (Fuentes-Medel et al., 2009)			Drpr (Fuentes-Medel et al., 2009)
Elimination of AFP neuron sensory microvilli	Worm	AMsh glia (Raiders et al., 2021)	PS? (Raiders et al., 2021)		PSR-1, and PAT-2 (Raiders et al., 2021)
Phagocytosis of POS in retina	Mammal	RPE (Nandrot et al., 2004; Young and Bok 1969)	PS (Ruggiero et al., 2012)	MFG-E8 (Nandrot et al., 2007) Gas6, and Protein S (Burstyn-Cohen et al., 2012)	$\alpha_v\beta_5$ (Nandrot et al., 2007; Nandrot et al., 2004) Mer (D'Cruz et al., 2000; Duncan et al., 2003; Prasad et al., 2006; Vollrath et al., 2001)
Synaptic pruning in dLGN	Mammal	Microglia (Lehrman et al., 2018; Li et al., 2020; Schafer et al., 2012; Scott-Hewitt et al., 2020; Stevens et al., 2007; Vainchtein et al., 2018), and astrocytes (Chung et al., 2013)	PS (Li et al., 2020; Scott-Hewitt et al., 2020)	C1q (and C3?) (Stevens et al., 2007)	CR3 (Schafer et al., 2012) MEGF10 (Chung et al., 2013), Mer (Chung et al., 2013), and GPR56 (Li et al., 2020)
Synaptic pruning in hippocampus	Mammal	Microglia (Filipello et al., 2018; Paolicelli et al., 2011; Scott-Hewitt et al., 2020; Weinhard et al., 2018, and astrocytes (Lee et al., 2021)	PS (Li et al., 2020)		MEGF10 (Lee et al., 2021), TREM2 (Filipello et al., 2018; Scott-Hewitt et al., 2020), GPR56 (Li et al., 2020), and CX3CR1 (Paolicelli et al., 2011)

4.3.1 Draper (Drpr), an important engulfment receptor in phagocytosis of neurons in *Drosophila*

C. elegans CED-1, *Drosophila* Drpr, and mammalian MEGF10 and Jedi-1 represent a conserved MEGF family of engulfment receptors that are important in the recognition and removal of apoptotic cells (Wu et al., 2009). The founding member CED-1 was identified for its role in the engulfment of cell corpses in the worm (Hedgecock et al., 1983; Zhou et al., 2001b), and later CED-1 was also found to be required for phagocytosis of *TAT-1*-deficient neurons (Darland-Ransom et al., 2008) and the debris of injured axons (Chiu et al., 2018). Drpr (Freeman et al., 2003) is involved in many contexts of phagocytosis in and outside the nervous system in *Drosophila*. Jedi-1 and MEGF10 also function as engulfment receptors in the clearance of apoptotic neurons in developing DRG (Scheib et al., 2012; Wu et al., 2009). In addition, MEGF10 is partially required for astrocyte-mediated synapse elimination in the developing dLGN (Chung et al., 2013) and the adult hippocampus (Lee et al., 2021). Numerous studies on this family have contributed to the understanding of phagocytosis of neurons and the pathways involved. Here, we provide more details of *Drosophila* Drpr as its roles in the nervous system are best understood (Figure 4.3).

4.3.1.1 The involvement of Drpr in phagocytosis during neuronal remodeling

During embryonic development, Drpr is expressed in *Drosophila* glia to promote the clearance of apoptotic neurons (Freeman et al., 2003; Tung et al., 2013). Later in metamorphosis, astrocyte-like glia acquire phagocytic activity, and Drpr is localized on the membrane of astrocyte-like glia infiltrating MB axon bundles (Awasaki and Ito, 2004; Tasdemir-Yilmaz and Freeman, 2014). *drpr* mutations and knockdown of *drpr* in all glia strongly suppressed debris clearance of pruned MB axons (Awasaki et al., 2006; Hoopfer et al., 2006). Similarly, astrocyte-specific knockdown of *drpr* also produced clearance defects (Hakim et al., 2014).

The involvement of Drpr in the clearance of degenerating axons has also been demonstrated in axon injury models. After surgical removal of adult ORNs, ensheathing glia in the antenna lobe extend membrane processes to the injured axons and engulf axonal debris (Doherty et al., 2009; MacDonald et al., 2006). Drpr expression in the ensheathing glia is upregulated upon axonal injury (Doherty et al., 2009; MacDonald et al., 2006; Macdonald et al., 2013). In *drpr* mutants or when glial *drpr* expression is knocked down, glia fail to respond morphologically to axon injury, and severed axons are not cleared from the CNS (Doherty et al., 2009; MacDonald et al., 2006).

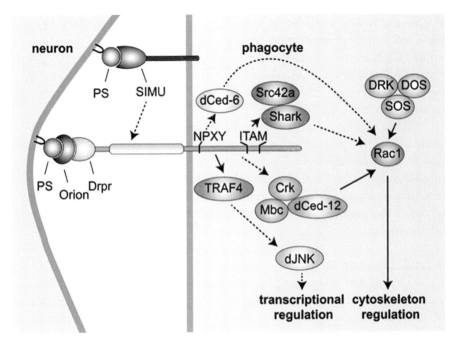

Figure 4.3 **Drpr-mediated phagocytosis in the nervous system of** *Drosophila***.** Drpr is an engulfment receptor expressed by phagocytes in *Drosophila*. *In vivo*, Drpr recognizes PS exposed on neurites through the PS-binding bridging molecule Orion. A tethering receptor SIMU acts upstream of Drpr in the phagocytosis of apoptotic neurons in embryos. Drpr can interact directly with PS *in vitro* and may do so *in vivo* when both the levels of PS exposure and Drpr expression are high. Downstream of Drpr activation, the adaptor protein dCed-6 and the kinases Src42a and Shark bind to the intracellular tail of Drpr and promote activation of the small GTPase Rac1, which regulates the subsequent cytoskeleton rearrangement. Rac1 can be activated by two GEF complexes, Crk/Mbc/dCed-12 and DRK/DOS/SOS, in *Drosophila* phagocytes. In another pathway downstream of Drpr, TRAF4 binds to Drpr and activates the dJNK pathway to regulate transcription.

Similarly, Drpr is required for the clearance of axons of gustatory receptor neurons in the ventral nerve cord (VNC) after axotomy (Purice et al., 2017).

The role of Drpr in dendrite clearance has been mainly investigated in the PNS, where C4da neurons serve as excellent models of dendrite pruning (Williams and Truman, 2005a) and dendrite injury (Tao and Rolls, 2011). When *drpr* is knocked down in epidermal cells, the resident phagocytes that engulf degenerating dendrites, the clearance of pruned C4da dendrites is strongly delayed at the pupal stage (Han et al., 2014). In the larva, Drpr-mediated phagocytosis promotes the fragmentation of injured C4da dendrites (Ji et al., 2022) and is required for the clearance of dendrite fragments (Han et al., 2014).

Drpr has also been reported to be involved in other scenarios of neuronal degeneration. Drpr is required for the clearance of destabilized boutons at growing NMJs at the larval stage (Fuentes-Medel et al., 2009). In aged flies, reduced Drpr activity in nearby glia results in delayed clearance of injured ORN axons (Purice et al., 2016). Furthermore, glial clearance of neurotoxic Aβ peptides in a *Drosophila* Alzheimer's disease (AD) model is Drpr-dependent, suggesting that Drpr can be protective in neurogenerative disease models (Ray et al., 2017).

Taken together, studies conducted in both the CNS and the PNS demonstrated that Drpr plays an important role in a variety of neuronal degeneration contexts. Interestingly, Drpr seems to be absolutely required for clearing injured neurites but is only partially required for clearing neurite debris resulting from developmental pruning. This suggests that other engulfment receptors and pathways likely work in parallel with Drpr during developmental pruning.

4.3.1.2 Ligands for Drpr

Since Drpr and its homologs play important roles in phagocytosis in the nervous system, whether Drpr recognizes PS exposed on neuronal membranes became an interesting question. Recent studies reveal the requirement of Drpr in PS-induced phagocytosis. In the *Drosophila* PNS, PS-exposing dendrites of *CDC50* KO and TEME16F OE C4da neurons shed membranes in a Drpr-dependent manner (Sapar et al., 2018), suggesting that Drpr is involved in PS recognition. However, whether PS is a direct ligand of Drpr *in vivo* had been elusive.

On the one hand, the Drpr extracellular EMI and NIM domains have been shown to bind to PS *in vitro* (Tung et al., 2013). Consistent with this finding, PS exposed on lipid bilayer-coated beads is sufficient to induce engulfment of the beads by Drpr-transfected *Drosophila* S2 cells (Williamson and Vale, 2018). In this system, PS is sufficient to locally trigger Drpr phosphorylation at the intracellular ITAM motif and to activate downstream engulfment signaling (Williamson and Vale, 2018). On the other hand, evidence suggests that Drpr may need bridging molecules (or opsonins) to interact with PS. Drpr has been reported to work along with a tethering receptor called six-microns-under (SIMU) in clearing apoptotic neurons during embryogenesis (Kurant et al., 2008). SIMU can bind to PS with its extracellular domains (Shklyar et al., 2013) and appears to function upstream of Drpr (Kurant et al., 2008). In addition, CED-1, the *C. elegans* homolog of Drpr, requires a secreted bridging molecule TTR-52 to recognize PS during phagocytosis of apoptotic cells (Wang et al., 2010).

Two recent studies provided new insights into the mechanisms of Drpr-mediated PS sensing. In a forward genetic screen for factors involved in MB axon remodeling, a secreted protein called Orion was identified to be required for astrocyte infiltration and clearance of axonal debris (Boulanger et al., 2021). Orion was further analyzed in the larval PNS, where distributions of Orion-GFP fusion proteins can be examined in live animals (Ji et al., 2023). *In vivo* assays showed that Orion binds to both PS and Drpr and is required for Drpr-mediated phagocytosis of C4da neurons (Ji et al., 2023). Furthermore, a membrane-tethered version of Orion triggers PS-independent but Drpr-dependent phagocytosis of healthy dendrites when it is expressed in neurons, while its expression in epidermal cells suppresses engulfment of injured dendrites. These results provide strong evidence that Drpr normally requires Orion as a PS-binding bridging molecule to sense PS on neurons (Figure 4.3). The same study also shows that Drpr overexpression in epidermal cells can bypass the requirement of Orion in engulfing injured dendrites, presumably through direct Drpr–PS interaction (Figure 4.3). However, whether endogenous Drpr directly senses PS exposure under physiological conditions *in vivo* is unknown.

Drpr has also been reported to recognize Prtp and DmCaBP1 during the clearance of apoptotic cells in *Drosophila* embryos (Kuraishi et al., 2009; Okada et al., 2012). Prtp and DmCaBP1 are ER proteins that are exposed on the cell surface upon apoptosis, but these ligands are not involved in axonal pruning during metamorphosis (Kuraishi et al., 2009; Okada et al., 2012). Whether they function in other contexts of neuronal remodeling remains to be determined.

4.3.1.3 Upstream regulation of Drpr

Besides being activated by PS on the target cell surface, Drpr expression in phagocytes can be regulated by various degeneration cues and developmental signals. In the larval CNS, dying neurons signal to phagocytic cortex glia via releasing a toll receptor ligand, Spätzle5. This cue activates a Toll-6 transcriptional pathway, which upregulates the expression of the Drpr in glia (McLaughlin et al., 2019). During metamorphosis, Drpr transcription in glia is upregulated. Expression of a dominant-negative mutant of ecdysone receptor (EcR-DN) in glia suppresses this upregulation (Awasaki et al., 2006; Hakim et al., 2014), suggesting that Drpr expression is regulated by hormonal signaling at the time of large-scale remodeling. In contrast, upregulation of Drpr expression in glia in response to axonal injury is mediated through c-Jun N-terminal kinase (dJNK) signaling (Losada-Perez et al., 2021; Macdonald et al., 2013).

4.3.1.4 Signaling downstream of Drpr

Drpr and its homologs are large single-pass transmembrane proteins with many extracellular EGF-repeats and a short intracellular domain containing tyrosine (Tyr) phosphorylation sites (Scheib et al., 2012; Zhou et al., 2001b; Ziegenfuss et al., 2008). They share some common downstream effectors to trigger phagocytosis of neuronal debris.

The initial molecular insights into the signaling downstream of these engulfment receptors came from studies of *cell death abnormal* (*ced*) mutants in *C. elegans*. Two partially redundant pathways activate engulfment of cell corpses during development and in the germline (reviewed by Reddien and Horvitz, 2004). In one pathway, the CED-6 adaptor protein transduces signals from CED-1, through possible binding between the phosphotyrosine-binding-domain protein (PTB) in CED-6 and the conserved NPXY (Asn-Pro-any amino acid-Tyr) motif in the intracellular region of CED-1, to promote removal of cell corpses (Kavanaugh et al., 1995; Liu and Hengartner, 1999; Su et al., 2000). CED-1 and CED-6 act upstream of the small GTPase CED-10 (Rac1 in mammals) to regulate cytoskeleton changes in phagocytes (Kinchen et al., 2005). The second pathway involves CED-2 (CrkII in mammals), CED-5 (DOCK180 in humans and Myoblast City (Mbc) in *Drosophila*), and CED-12 (ELMO in mammals). CED-2, CED-5, and CED-12 appear to form a ternary guanine nucleotide exchange factor (GEF) complex in response to upstream engulfment signals and activate CED-10 to promote cytoskeletal reorganization and corpse engulfment (Brugnera et al., 2002; Gumienny et al., 2001; Reddien and Horvitz, 2000; Wu and Horvitz, 1998; Wu et al., 2001; Zhou et al., 2001a). Both pathways contribute to the removal of necrotic neurons in *C. elegans* (Yang et al., 2015).

dCed-6, the *Drosophila* homolog of CED-6, is involved in Drpr signaling during phagocytosis in the nervous system (Figure 4.3). Glia-specific knockdown of *dCed-6* by RNAi partially suppresses glial engulfment of MB axons during metamorphosis (Awasaki et al., 2006). A combination of *dCed-6* RNAi and heterozygous *drpr* mutation in the pupa resulted in significantly reduced glial action compared with *dCed-6* RNAi alone or heterozygous *drpr* mutation alone, suggesting that *drpr* and *dCed-6* interact genetically in the glial engulfment of the MB axons (Awasaki et al., 2006). During NMJ development, RNAi knockdown of *dCed-6* in muscles or glia phenocopies *drpr* RNAi knockdown in these tissues (Fuentes-Medel et al., 2009). In the adult brain, dCed-6 is expressed in ensheathing glia but not in astrocyte-like glia, indicating that it may play a role in clearance of injured ORN axons (Doherty et al., 2009).

Srk family proteins that share similar domains with components of the CED-2/CED-5/CED12 pathway are also involved in Drpr signal transduction (Figure 4.3). Studies on clearance of injured ORN axons reveal that Drpr activation initiates signals through its immunoreceptor tyrosine-based activation motif (ITAM) domain to recruit downstream effectors, the Src family kinase

Src42a and Syk-related Tyr kinase Shark (containing dual SH2 domains) (Ziegenfuss et al., 2008). The involvement of Shark in glial phagocytosis has been shown in the clearance of neuronal cell corpses in embryos and injured ORN axons in adult flies, and engulfment of apoptotic cell corpses by Drpr-transfected S2 cells *in vitro* (Doherty et al., 2009; Williamson and Vale, 2018; Ziegenfuss et al., 2008). Mammalian Drpr homologs, Jedi-1 and MEGF10, recruit Shark homolog, Syk, through their ITAM domains as well, suggesting that this engulfment pathway is conserved (Scheib et al., 2012).

Consistent with the CED-1-mediated engulfment pathway, the small GTPase Rac1 that regulates the actin cytoskeleton appears to be an important downstream effector of Drpr (Figure 4.3). Glia-specific knockdown of *rac1* potently suppressed clearance of axonal debris after ORN injury, phenocopying *drpr*-null mutants (Ziegenfuss et al., 2012). Rac1 activation requires two redundant sets of GEF complexes, the Crk/Mbc/dCed-12 complex and a complex composed of downstream of receptor kinase (DRK) (Grb2 in mammals)/ daughter of sevenless (DOS) (Gab2 in mammals)/son of sevenless (SOS) (mSOS in mammals) (Lu et al., 2014; Ziegenfuss et al., 2012). Rac1 activity promotes the activation of glia after axon injury and internalization of axonal debris by glia (Lu et al., 2014; Ziegenfuss et al., 2012). Cytoskeleton changes that are potentially downstream of Rac1 have been studied in the *Drosophila* PNS. The association of actin-rich epidermal membranes with degenerating dendrites was reduced when *drpr* was knocked down in the epidermis, confirming that Drpr activation results in actin polymerization surrounding the engulfment target (Han et al., 2014).

The recent identification of tissue necrosis factor receptor associated factor 4 (TRAF4) as a Drpr binding partner links Drpr to the JNK pathway (Figure 4.3). TRAF4 acts downstream of Drpr to activate the JNK pathway, resulting in changes of gene expression in glia after ORN axon injury (Lu et al., 2017). JNK signaling is also important for neuronal remodeling in multiple contexts, including glial phagocytosis of apoptotic neurons downstream of Drpr during *Drosophila* metamorphosis (Hilu-Dadia et al., 2018), glia-mediated functional regeneration of the CNS after crush injury in adult *Drosophila* (Losada-Perez et al., 2021), CED-1-mediated axon regrowth in *C. elegans* (Chiu et al., 2018), and astrocyte proliferation in mammals (Gadea et al., 2008).

4.3.2 CR3 and the complement system in mammalian synaptic pruning

In mammals, CR3 and the complement system are a better-characterized pathway in phagocytosis of neuronal material. As a part of the innate immune system, the classical complement pathway contributes to the recognition and phagocytosis of invading pathogens and stimulates other components of the immune system (reviewed by van Lookeren Campagne et al., 2007). A simplified complement pathway involves soluble proteins C1q, C4, C3, and complement receptor 3 (CR3, also named as Mac-1, integrin $\alpha_M\beta_2$, or CD11b/CD18) expressed by macrophages. C1q, the first component of the pathway, binds to the engulfment target and activates the complement cascade through a series of proteolytic events, ending in activation of C3. Activated C3 is recruited to the target and triggers phagocytosis by interacting with its receptor CR3 (reviewed by Presumey et al., 2017).

Intriguingly, components of the complement system are also found in the brain, and they are involved in neuronal death in the mouse hippocampus (Wakselman et al., 2008) and activity-dependent synapse elimination by microglia in the developing mouse visual system (Stevens et al., 2007). Complement-dependent phagocytosis of synapses is also dysregulated in developmental disorders, such as schizophrenia (Sekar et al., 2016), and neurodegenerative disorders, such as glaucoma (Howell et al., 2011; Stevens et al., 2007), aging-related cognitive decline (Stephan et al., 2013), Alzheimer's disease (Hong et al., 2016), and frontotemporal dementia (Lui et al., 2016). Here, we review the molecular mechanisms of complement-dependent phagocytosis in the development of healthy dLGN.

4.3.2.1 CR3 as an engulfment receptor required for synaptic pruning in the developing dLGN

In the developing dLGN, the complement receptor CR3 is exclusively expressed in microglia, which phagocytose "weak" RGC inputs during the peak synaptic pruning period (Schafer et al., 2012). CR3 is highly expressed at P5 and its expression decreases over time (Schafer et al., 2012). CR3 on cultured microglia mediates the removal of desialylated neurites of co-cultured neurons (Linnartz et al., 2012). Consistent with these *in vitro* results, microglia in brain slices of CR3 KO mice had decreased capacity to engulf RGC inputs (Schafer et al., 2012), suggesting that phagocytosis by microglia is mediated by CR3. Furthermore, CR3 KO resulted in sustained deficits in eye-specific segregation and excessive immature synapses in the adult dLGN (Schafer et al., 2012), suggesting that CR3-mediated engulfment is important for synaptic pruning.

4.3.2.2 Components of the complement system upstream of CR3

CR3 is a receptor for activated C3 (Figure 4.2) (reviewed by Vorup-Jensen and Jensen, 2018). Before CR3's role was identified in synaptic pruning, C3 had been shown to tag subsets of synapses and to be required for synapse elimination in the developing brain (Stevens et al., 2007). C3 is enriched in synaptic regions of the postnatal dLGN but is downregulated when pruning is largely completed (Schafer et al., 2012; Stephan et al., 2013; Stevens et al., 2007). C3 KO mice displayed defects in eye-specific segregation and synapse elimination, which was phenocopied by CR3 KO mice (Schafer et al., 2012; Stevens et al., 2007). Together, these results suggest that C3/CR3 signaling is required for synaptic pruning.

Being required for C3 activation, C4 is also involved in synaptic refinement in the developing brain. In *C4*-deficient mice, C3 immunostaining in the dLGN was greatly reduced and fewer synaptic inputs were tagged by C3 (Sekar et al., 2016). Furthermore, similar to C3/CR3 KOs, mice lacking C4 had deficits in eye-segregation (Sekar et al., 2016).

As the initiator of the complement cascade, C1q has a similar distribution to C3 on synapses in the developing retina and brain (Stevens et al., 2007). Interestingly, C1q predominantly binds to presynaptic membranes of the synaptosomes isolated from the adult cerebral cortex tissue (Gyorffy et al., 2018). *In vitro*, C1q binds to desialylated neurons (Linnartz et al., 2012), suggesting that C1q recognizes neurons with altered glycocalyx. C1q KO resulted in significant defects in eye-specific segregation in the dLGN, consistent with C1q being upstream of C3 and CR3 (Stevens et al., 2007). Due to their ability to tag synapses during developmental pruning, C1q and C3 function like bridging molecules for CR3 (Figure 4.2).

4.3.2.3 PS exposure specifies the synapses to be eliminated by complement-mediated phagocytosis

What is unique about the synapses tagged by C1q and C3? Recent studies revealed that PS exposure on neuronal membranes acts upstream of the complement cascade in synapse elimination. Cell culture studies suggest that C1q can recognize PS directly (Paidassi et al., 2008) or indirectly (Martin et al., 2012) to facilitate phagocytic removal of apoptotic cells. Consistent with these results, C1q co-localizes with the PS marker Annexin V *ex vivo* on isolated synaptosomes (Gyorffy et al., 2018). Furthermore, in the developing dLGN, C1q and PSVue co-localize at a subset of retinogeniculate presynaptic inputs, and the loss of C1q resulted in an increase in PS-positive presynaptic inputs due to reduced microglial engulfment (Scott-Hewitt et al., 2020). These findings support a model in which locally exposed PS interacts with complement factors (and perhaps other proteins) to promote microglial engulfment during the critical periods of synaptic refinement.

So far, the complement signaling has been mainly studied in the visual system. Given that the loss of C1q, C3, or CR3 greatly interfered with eye-specific segregation but did not completely prevent it (Schafer et al., 2012; Stevens et al., 2007), other engulfment receptors are likely involved in this process as well.

4.3.3 Other engulfment receptors requiring PS-binding bridging molecules for phagocytosis of neurons

Besides CR3 and MEGF receptors, TAM receptors and integrins are also known to mediate PS-induced phagocytosis through extracellular bridging molecules. Their roles in the nervous system are mostly characterized in mammals.

4.3.3.1 Tyro3, Axl, and Mer (TAM) receptors

TAM receptors (Figure 4.2) are receptor tyrosine kinases that play important roles in several scenarios of phagocytosis in the nervous system, including synaptic pruning (Chung et al., 2013; Park et al., 2021), engulfment of retinal POS (Duncan et al., 2003), and clearance of apoptotic neurons (Fourgeaud et al., 2016). TAM receptors do not bind to PS directly but instead recognize PS via the bridging molecules Growth arrest-specific-6 (Gas6) and Protein S (Dransfield et al., 2015; Stitt et al., 1995; Zagorska et al., 2014). Gas6 and Protein S bridge TAM receptors on phagocytes to PS exposed on phagocytic targets (Dransfield et al., 2015; Lemke, 2017; Lew et al., 2014; Zagorska et al., 2014). Gas6 binds to and activates all three TAMs, whereas Protein S binds to and activates only Tyro3 and Mer (Lew et al., 2014). Although TAM receptors have also been extensively studied in the immune system (reviewed by Lemke, 2013), here, we focus only on the role of TAM receptors and their bridging molecules in the context of the developing nervous system.

The requirement of Mer in the phagocytosis of distal POS in the retina was demonstrated by two rodent models. In a retinal degeneration rat model called Royal College of Surgeons (RCS), photoreceptors are lost due to an LOF deletion within the rat *Mertk* gene (which encodes Mer) (D'Cruz et al., 2000). Gene transfer of *Mertk* to the RPEs in RCS rat retina resulted in correction of the RPE phagocytosis defect and preservation of photoreceptors (Vollrath et al., 2001). Similarly, in mice deficient of *Mertk*, photoreceptors undergo progressive degeneration due to the lack of phagocytosis of POS by RPEs (Duncan et al., 2003). Consistent with these findings, Mer and Tyro3 were found to be expressed in RPE cells in the mouse retina (Prasad et al., 2006). Later, the bridging molecules of Mer, Gas6, and Protein S were found to act redundantly in mediating phagocytosis of retinal POS (Burstyn-Cohen et al., 2012).

In the mouse brain, Mer is expressed by both astrocytes and microglia (Cahoy et al., 2008; Chung et al., 2013; Gautier et al., 2012; Grommes et al., 2008; Ji et al., 2013). In the developing dLGN, Mer is required for synaptic elimination mediated by phagocytic astrocytes but is dispensable for the phagocytic function of microglia (Chung et al., 2013). Evidence suggests that Mer mediates engulfment of PS-exposing synapses: deleting microglial *Mertk* saved the loss of inhibitory post-synapses and seizure phenotype in *CDC50A* cKO mice and increased the number of PS-exposing inhibitory post-synapses in the wild-type juvenile brains (Park et al., 2021).

The signaling downstream of TAM receptors has been mostly studied using *in vitro* assays in the context of phagocytosis of apoptotic cells (reviewed by Lemke, 2013, 2019). In brief, the activation of the TAM kinase activity is necessary for phagocytosis (Zagorska et al., 2014). Mer also works with the integrin pathway to regulate CrkII/DOCK180/Rac1 modules in controlling rearrangements of the actin cytoskeleton in phagocytes (Wu et al., 2005).

4.3.3.2 Integrin receptors

Integrin receptors (Figure 4.2) are another major player in the phagocytosis of retinal POS in mammals. In rodent and human retinas, the integrin receptor $\alpha_v\beta_5$ localizes specifically to the apical surface of RPE cells (Anderson et al., 1995; Finnemann et al., 1997) and is required for diurnal bursts of RPE phagocytosis of POS (Nandrot et al., 2007; Nandrot et al., 2004). $\alpha_v\beta_5$ has been shown to recognize PS indirectly through the bridging molecule MFG-E8 (Akakura et al., 2004). A discoidin-like domain at the carboxyl terminus of MFG-E8 recognizes PS exposed on apoptotic cells (Hanayama et al., 2002). In the retina, extracellular MFG-E8 promotes phagocytosis of shed POS by ligating $\alpha_v\beta_5$ on RPE cells (Nandrot et al., 2007). These results suggest that the phagocytosis of POS by RPEs is mediated by PS-MFG-E8-$\alpha_v\beta_5$ signaling. Intracellularly, the engagement of $\alpha_v\beta_5$ activates focal adhesion kinase, at the same time recruiting CrkII-Dock180 complex to activate Rac1, the common effector involved in phagocytosis (Akakura et al., 2004; Albert et al., 2000; Finnemann, 2003; Wu et al., 2005).

4.3.4 Direct PS receptors involved in phagocytosis of neurons

Several engulfment receptors, including brain-specific angiogenesis inhibitor 1 (BAI1), T-cell immunoglobulin- and mucin-domain-containing 4 (TIM4), triggering receptor expressed on myeloid cells 2 (TREM2), adhesion G protein-coupled receptor G1 (ADGRG1), and PSR-1 are known to directly interact with PS (Figure 4.2). With the exception of PSR-1, which is conserved from worms to humans, all of the above are microglial surface receptors that exist only in vertebrates. Compared to indirect PS receptors discussed above, relatively less is known about the roles of these receptors in the nervous system. Here, we summarize the main findings pointing to their involvement in phagocytosis of neurons.

BAI1 is a seven-transmembrane protein belonging to the adhesion-type G-protein-coupled receptor family (Park et al., 2007). TIM4 is a type I transmembrane protein (Miyanishi et al., 2007). Both BAI1 and TIM4 can directly bind to PS on apoptotic cells (Kobayashi et al., 2007; Miyanishi et al., 2007; Park et al., 2007; Sokolowski et al., 2011). Microglia lacking BAI1 and TIM-4 display clearance defects in removing dying neurons in the embryonic zebrafish brain (Mazaheri et al., 2014).

TREM2 is known for its association with AD (reviewed by Colonna and Wang, 2016). It can bind to PS directly (Wang et al., 2015) and is found to regulate microglial function in response to PS exposed on apoptotic cells *in vitro* (Shirotani et al., 2019). Recent studies revealed that TREM2 is essential for microglia-mediated synaptic refinement during brain development in mice (Filipello et al., 2018; Scott-Hewitt et al., 2020).

ADGRG1 (also called GPR56) is another adhesion G protein-coupled receptor expressed by microglia (Bennett et al., 2016; Singer et al., 2013). A recent study shows that one of its splicing isoforms is involved in microglia-mediated synaptic pruning in the mouse dLGN via direct PS binding (Li et al., 2020).

Lastly, PSR-1 is an engulfment receptor whose roles are not limited to the nervous system. In *C. elegans*, loss of RSP-1 (Yang et al., 2015) causes a mild delay in the clearance of apoptotic cells (Wang et al., 2003) and necrotic neuronal corpses (Yang et al., 2015). PSR-1 acts in the CED-2 phagocytosis pathway, in parallel with CED-1, to promote phagocytosis (Yang et al., 2015). A recent study revealed that the glial PSR-1 is required for the engulfment of sensory endings of the AFD neuron (Raiders et al., 2021), possibly by recognizing PS on the dendrites. In the same study, PAT-2, an α-integrin subunit implicated in apoptotic cell phagocytosis in *C. elegans* (Hsieh et al., 2012), was found to coordinate with PSR-1 to regulate glial engulfment of neuronal debris (Raiders et al., 2021).

4.3.5 Other immune molecules involved in phagocytosis of neurons

In addition to known PS receptors, several immune molecules that are not known to recognize PS have been shown to be involved in phagocytosis of neurons. CX3CR1, the receptor for the chemokine CX3CL1 (fractalkine) (Figure 4.2), is expressed by microglia in the mammalian brain (Harrison et al., 1998; Jung et al., 2000). Paolicelli et al. first identified a role for CX3CR1 in synaptic pruning in the mouse hippocampus (Paolicelli et al., 2011). CX3CR1 was also found to be involved in dendritic spine elimination and formation in the motor cortex (Parkhurst et al., 2013), reduced functional connectivity in the hippocampus (Zhan et al., 2014), and activity-dependent synaptic pruning in barrel cortex (Gunner et al., 2019). Even though CXCR1 has not been reported as a PS receptor, the sequence and functional similarity between CX3CL1 and the *Drosophila* chemokine-like Orion (Boulanger et al., 2021; Ji et al., 2023) points to a potential link between PS and CXC3L1-CXCR1 signaling.

Besides CX3CR1, some other immune molecules have also been described in the contexts of synaptic pruning. The major histocompatibility complex (MHC) class I proteins (Figure 4.2) are required for synaptic elimination in the mouse dLGN (Lee et al., 2014). Astrocyte-derived cytokine, IL-33, is also required for synaptic development in the thalamus and the spinal cord by signaling to microglia to promote synaptic engulfment (Vainchtein et al., 2018). To counteract the effect of "eat-me" signal, the so-called "don't-eat-me" signals have been proposed to protect synapses from being engulfed. The best studied "don't-eat-me" signal is the transmembrane immunoglobulin-related cell surface protein CD47 (Figure 4.2). The expression patterns of CD47 and its receptor, SIRPα, correlate with peak pruning in the dLGN. Supporting a role for CD47-SIRPα signaling in preventing excess microglial phagocytosis, *CD47* KO or *SIRPα* KO mice have fewer synapses and increased pruning in the dLGN (Lehrman et al., 2018). It remains unclear how CD47 as a "don't-eat-me" signal and PS as an "eat-me" signal coordinate in synaptic pruning.

4.4 Perspectives

The contribution of phagocytosis in sculpting the nervous system during morphogenesis has been increasingly appreciated. In the last two decades, the field of phagocytosis in the nervous system has made important advances. First, evidence suggests that phagocytosis not only clears neuronal corpses or degenerating neurites but also actively breaks and removes non-fragmenting neurites or synapses in many cases, refuting the conception that phagocytes merely passively clear neuronal debris after apoptosis or neurite fragmentation. Second, recent work deciphering the identity of the "eat-me" signal for degenerating neurites and weak synapses in diverse contexts has filled important gaps in understanding the trigger and specificity of phagocytosis.

Third, multiple engulfment receptors and pathways have been identified as being involved in sculpting neural circuits, providing a more complete picture of the major players in phagocytosis. Moreover, many studies took advantage of *in vivo* model systems to elucidate molecular mechanisms of phagocytosis in more physiologically relevant settings. These findings greatly expanded our understanding of how phagocytosis contributes to the morphogenesis of the nervous system.

However, several important questions in the field remain unanswered. Most crucially, since PS has been shown as an "eat-me" signal in most of the phagocytosis scenarios, including elimination of dying neurons, fragmented neurites, and intact neurites and synapses destined to be pruned, how does this same molecule trigger various degrees of phagocytosis in different scenarios? Interestingly, PS has been shown to play a role in axon fusion instead of triggering phagocytosis in *C. elegans* (Neumann et al., 2015). What properties of the PS exposed on neuronal surface instruct surround phagocytes to engulf the entire neuron, engulf a local branch, or leave the neuron alone? One possibility could be that the levels, the rates, and the regions of PS exposure on neuronal surfaces are distinct among different scenarios. The spatiotemporal pattern of PS exposure may dictate, to some extent, the bridging molecules or engulfment receptors recruited to trigger a specific behavior of phagocytes. In this model, PS exposure must be tightly regulated at a local scale for a controlled phagocytosis. How PS exposure is regulated, especially by the neuronal activity, is thus an important question to answer in coming years. The second possibility is that the exposed PS coordinates with other surface molecules, such as other "eat-me" signals or "don't-eat-me" signals, to generate a precise phagocytosis trigger. The involvement of the "don't-eat-me" signal CD47 in synaptic pruning (Lehrman et al., 2018) has provided some evidence for this possibility. The interesting cases of PS-exposing cells without being phagocytosed (Bevers and Williamson, 2016) could be good models to study the interplay between "eat-me" signals and "don't-eat-me" signals.

Yet another possibility is that the consequence of phagocytosis is determined by the status of the phagocytes. Some phagocyte types are known to be more potent in engulfing neuronal debris than others. For example, microglia are professional phagocytes, while other glial types are considered amateur phagocytes, because the latter normally fulfill other functions but turn into phagocytes when needed. So a cell could be programmed to execute a certain phagocytosis task in a given developmental window. Although cytoskeletal changes seem to be the convergent point of many phagocytosis behaviors, a lot is still unknown about how signaling is transduced in each type of phagocyte to regulate cytoskeletal changes. It would be interesting to investigate what factors determine the baseline potency of phagocytes and how cell signaling modulates this potency. Some phagocytes also maintain the homeostasis of the nervous system. For example, besides eliminating pruned synapses, microglia play an important role in regulating synapse growth and plasticity in the CNS (Wilton et al., 2019). How phagocytes balance their phagocytosis functions and other functions is an interesting question worth exploring.

Another interesting observation is that a number of engulfment receptors and pathways are involved in synaptic pruning in the mammalian CNS, including CR3, CX3CR1, Mer, TREM2, GPR56, and MEGF10. Why are so many receptors involved in synaptic pruning? One possibility is that they may function redundantly to back each other up. For instance, the complement system, Mer, and GPR56 all seem to be involved in synaptic elimination in the developing dLGN (Chung et al., 2013; Li et al., 2020; Schafer et al., 2012; Stevens et al., 2007). They may coordinate to ensure synaptic pruning happens at the right time and location. Alternatively, each engulfment receptor is only responsible for phagocytosis in certain brain regions and/ or at certain developmental stages. A piece of evidence is that complement system and CX3CR1 are involved in synaptic pruning in non-overlapping brain regions (Gunner et al., 2019; Paolicelli et al., 2011; Parkhurst et al., 2013; Schafer et al., 2012; Stevens et al., 2007). Thus, restricted expressions of receptors and PS bridging molecules may provide specificity in synaptic pruning. A systematic survey of these receptors in different brain regions and developmental stages could provide a more complete picture of the contribution of each pathway.

Finally, many of the players involved in phagocytosis in the developing nervous system are implicated in neurodevelopmental and neurodegenerative disorders (Chung et al., 2015; Colonna and Wang, 2016; Galloway et al., 2019; Neniskyte and Gross, 2017; Salter and Stevens, 2017; Sierra et al., 2014; Stephan et al., 2012). The fact that phagocytes actively engulf non-dying neurons and break neurites during development (Brown and Neher, 2014; Hakim et al., 2014; Han et al., 2014; Ji et al., 2022; Raiders et al., 2021) further implies possible contributions of active phagocytosis in pathogenesis. The research on how phagocytosis contributes to neuronal remodeling during development could thus help us to understand the causes of neurological disorders and to explore potential phagocytosis-dependent therapies.

Acknowledgements

We apologize for not being able to include all literature relevant to neuronal remodeling in this review due to the space limit. This work was supported by a Cornell start-up fund and NIH grants (R01NS099125, R21OD023824, and R21NS127052) awarded to C.H.

Conflict of Interest Statement

Nothing declared.

References

Akakura, S., Singh, S., Spataro, M., Akakura, R., Kim, J.I., Albert, M.L., and Birge, R.B. (2004). The opsonin MFG-E8 is a ligand for the alphavbeta5 integrin and triggers DOCK180-dependent Rac1 activation for the phagocytosis of apoptotic cells. Exp Cell Res **292**, 403–416.
Albert, M.L., Kim, J.I., and Birge, R.B. (2000). alphavbeta5 integrin recruits the CrkII-Dock180-rac1 complex for phagocytosis of apoptotic cells. Nat Cell Biol **2**, 899–905.
Anderson, D.H., Johnson, L.V., and Hageman, G.S. (1995). Vitronectin receptor expression and distribution at the photoreceptor-retinal pigment epithelial interface. J Comp Neurol **360**, 1–16.
Attardo, A., Fitzgerald, J.E., and Schnitzer, M.J. (2015). Impermanence of dendritic spines in live adult CA1 hippocampus. Nature **523**, 592–596.
Awasaki, T., and Ito, K. (2004). Engulfing action of glial cells is required for programmed axon pruning during Drosophila metamorphosis. Curr Biol **14**, 668–677.
Awasaki, T., Tatsumi, R., Takahashi, K., Arai, K., Nakanishi, Y., Ueda, R., and Ito, K. (2006). Essential role of the apoptotic cell engulfment genes draper and ced-6 in programmed axon pruning during Drosophila metamorphosis. Neuron **50**, 855–867.
Baek, M., Enriquez, J., and Mann, R.S. (2013). Dual role for Hox genes and Hox co-factors in conferring leg motoneuron survival and identity in Drosophila. Development **140**, 2027–2038.
Behrens, L.M., van den Berg, T.K., and van Egmond, M. (2022). Targeting the CD47-SIRPalpha Innate Immune Checkpoint to Potentiate Antibody Therapy in Cancer by Neutrophils. Cancers (Basel) **14**.
Bennett, M.L., Bennett, F.C., Liddelow, S.A., Ajami, B., Zamanian, J.L., Fernhoff, N.B., Mulinyawe, S.B., Bohlen, C.J., Adil, A., Tucker, A., *et al.* (2016). New tools for studying microglia in the mouse and human CNS. Proc Natl Acad Sci U S A **113**, E1738–1746.
Bevers, E.M., and Williamson, P.L. (2016). Getting to the Outer Leaflet: Physiology of Phosphatidylserine Exposure at the Plasma Membrane. Physiol Rev **96**, 605–645.

Bishop, D.L., Misgeld, T., Walsh, M.K., Gan, W.B., and Lichtman, J.W. (2004). Axon branch removal at developing synapses by axosome shedding. Neuron **44**, 651–661.

Boulanger, A., and Dura, J.M. (2015). Nuclear receptors and Drosophila neuronal remodeling. Biochim Biophys Acta **1849**, 187–195.

Boulanger, A., Thinat, C., Zuchner, S., Fradkin, L.G., Lortat-Jacob, H., and Dura, J.M. (2021). Axonal chemokine-like Orion induces astrocyte infiltration and engulfment during mushroom body neuronal remodeling. Nat Commun **12**, 1849.

Brown, G.C., and Neher, J.J. (2012). Eaten alive! Cell death by primary phagocytosis: 'phagoptosis'. Trends Biochem Sci **37**, 325–332.

Brown, G.C., and Neher, J.J. (2014). Microglial phagocytosis of live neurons. Nat Rev Neurosci **15**, 209–216.

Brugnera, E., Haney, L., Grimsley, C., Lu, M., Walk, S.F., Tosello-Trampont, A.C., Macara, I.G., Madhani, H., Fink, G.R., and Ravichandran, K.S. (2002). Unconventional Rac-GEF activity is mediated through the Dock180-ELMO complex. Nat Cell Biol **4**, 574–582.

Burstyn-Cohen, T., Lew, E.D., Traves, P.G., Burrola, P.G., Hash, J.C., and Lemke, G. (2012). Genetic dissection of TAM receptor-ligand interaction in retinal pigment epithelial cell phagocytosis. Neuron **76**, 1123–1132.

Buss, R.R., Sun, W., and Oppenheim, R.W. (2006). Adaptive roles of programmed cell death during nervous system development. Annu Rev Neurosci **29**, 1–35.

Cahoy, J.D., Emery, B., Kaushal, A., Foo, L.C., Zamanian, J.L., Christopherson, K.S., Xing, Y., Lubischer, J.L., Krieg, P.A., Krupenko, S.A., et al. (2008). A transcriptome database for astrocytes, neurons, and oligodendrocytes: a new resource for understanding brain development and function. J Neurosci **28**, 264–278.

Cecconi, F., Alvarez-Bolado, G., Meyer, B.I., Roth, K.A., and Gruss, P. (1998). Apaf1 (CED-4 homolog) regulates programmed cell death in mammalian development. Cell **94**, 727–737.

Chiu, H., Zou, Y., Suzuki, N., Hsieh, Y.W., Chuang, C.F., Wu, Y.C., and Chang, C. (2018). Engulfing cells promote neuronal regeneration and remove neuronal debris through distinct biochemical functions of CED-1. Nat Commun **9**, 4842.

Choi, Y.J., Lee, G., and Park, J.H. (2006). Programmed cell death mechanisms of identifiable peptidergic neurons in Drosophila melanogaster. Development **133**, 2223–2232.

Chung, W.S., and Barres, B.A. (2012). The role of glial cells in synapse elimination. Curr Opin Neurobiol **22**, 438–445.

Chung, W.S., Clarke, L.E., Wang, G.X., Stafford, B.K., Sher, A., Chakraborty, C., Joung, J., Foo, L.C., Thompson, A., Chen, C., *et al.* (2013). Astrocytes mediate synapse elimination through MEGF10 and MERTK pathways. Nature **504**, 394–400.

Chung, W.S., Welsh, C.A., Barres, B.A., and Stevens, B. (2015). Do glia drive synaptic and cognitive impairment in disease? Nat Neurosci **18**, 1539–1545.

Clarke, P.G. (1992). Neuron death in the developing avian isthmo-optic nucleus, and its relation to the establishment of functional circuitry. J Neurobiol **23**, 1140–1158.

Colman, H., Nabekura, J., and Lichtman, J.W. (1997). Alterations in synaptic strength preceding axon withdrawal. Science **275**, 356–361.

Colonna, M., and Wang, Y. (2016). TREM2 variants: new keys to decipher Alzheimer disease pathogenesis. Nat Rev Neurosci **17**, 201–207.

Corty, M.M., and Freeman, M.R. (2013). Cell biology in neuroscience: Architects in neural circuit design: glia control neuron numbers and connectivity. J Cell Biol **203**, 395–405.

Cunningham, C.L., Martinez-Cerdeno, V., and Noctor, S.C. (2013). Microglia regulate the number of neural precursor cells in the developing cerebral cortex. J Neurosci **33**, 4216–4233.

D'Cruz, P.M., Yasumura, D., Weir, J., Matthes, M.T., Abderrahim, H., LaVail, M.M., and Vollrath, D. (2000). Mutation of the receptor tyrosine kinase gene Mertk in the retinal dystrophic RCS rat. Hum Mol Genet **9**, 645–651.

Dalmau, I., Vela, J.M., Gonzalez, B., Finsen, B., and Castellano, B. (2003). Dynamics of microglia in the developing rat brain. J Comp Neurol **458**, 144–157.

Darland-Ransom, M., Wang, X., Sun, C.L., Mapes, J., Gengyo-Ando, K., Mitani, S., and Xue, D. (2008). Role of C. elegans TAT-1 protein in maintaining plasma membrane phosphatidylserine asymmetry. Science **320**, 528–531.

de Belle, J.S., and Heisenberg, M. (1994). Associative odor learning in Drosophila abolished by chemical ablation of mushroom bodies. Science **263**, 692–695.

Doherty, J., Logan, M.A., Tasdemir, O.E., and Freeman, M.R. (2009). Ensheathing glia function as phagocytes in the adult Drosophila brain. J Neurosci **29**, 4768–4781.

Dransfield, I., Zagorska, A., Lew, E.D., Michail, K., and Lemke, G. (2015). Mer receptor tyrosine kinase mediates both tethering and phagocytosis of apoptotic cells. Cell Death Dis **6**, e1646.

Druart, M., and Le Magueresse, C. (2019). Emerging Roles of Complement in Psychiatric Disorders. Front Psychiatry **10**, 573.

Duncan, J.L., LaVail, M.M., Yasumura, D., Matthes, M.T., Yang, H., Trautmann, N., Chappelow, A.V., Feng, W., Earp, H.S., Matsushima, G.K., *et al.* (2003). An RCS-like retinal dystrophy phenotype in mer knockout mice. Invest Ophthalmol Vis Sci **44**, 826–838.

Etchegaray, J.I., Elguero, E.J., Tran, J.A., Sinatra, V., Feany, M.B., and McCall, K. (2016). Defective Phagocytic Corpse Processing Results in Neurodegeneration and Can Be Rescued by TORC1 Activation. J Neurosci **36**, 3170–3183.

Falzone, M.E., Malvezzi, M., Lee, B.C., and Accardi, A. (2018). Known structures and unknown mechanisms of TMEM16 scramblases and channels. J Gen Physiol **150**, 933–947.

Faust, T.E., Gunner, G., and Schafer, D.P. (2021). Mechanisms governing activity-dependent synaptic pruning in the developing mammalian CNS. Nat Rev Neurosci **22**, 657–673.

Filipello, F., Morini, R., Corradini, I., Zerbi, V., Canzi, A., Michalski, B., Erreni, M., Markicevic, M., Starvaggi-Cucuzza, C., Otero, K., *et al.* (2018). The Microglial Innate Immune Receptor TREM2 Is Required for Synapse Elimination and Normal Brain Connectivity. Immunity **48**, 979–991 e978.

Finnemann, S.C. (2003). Focal adhesion kinase signaling promotes phagocytosis of integrin-bound photoreceptors. EMBO J **22**, 4143–4154.

Finnemann, S.C., Bonilha, V.L., Marmorstein, A.D., and Rodriguez-Boulan, E. (1997). Phagocytosis of rod outer segments by retinal pigment epithelial cells requires alpha(v)beta5 integrin for binding but not for internalization. Proc Natl Acad Sci U S A **94**, 12932–12937.

Forger, N.G. (2009). Control of cell number in the sexually dimorphic brain and spinal cord. J Neuroendocrinol **21**, 393–399.

Fourgeaud, L., Traves, P.G., Tufail, Y., Leal-Bailey, H., Lew, E.D., Burrola, P.G., Callaway, P., Zagorska, A., Rothlin, C.V., Nimmerjahn, A., *et al.* (2016). TAM receptors regulate multiple features of microglial physiology. Nature **532**, 240–244.

Freeman, M.R., Delrow, J., Kim, J., Johnson, E., and Doe, C.Q. (2003). Unwrapping glial biology: Gcm target genes regulating glial development, diversification, and function. Neuron **38**, 567–580.

Fricker, M., Tolkovsky, A.M., Borutaite, V., Coleman, M., and Brown, G.C. (2018). Neuronal Cell Death. Physiol Rev **98**, 813–880.

Fuentes-Medel, Y., Logan, M.A., Ashley, J., Ataman, B., Budnik, V., and Freeman, M.R. (2009). Glia and muscle sculpt neuromuscular arbors by engulfing destabilized synaptic boutons and shed presynaptic debris. PLoS Biol **7**, e1000184.

Fujii, T., Sakata, A., Nishimura, S., Eto, K., and Nagata, S. (2015). TMEM16F is required for phosphatidylserine exposure and microparticle release in activated mouse platelets. Proc Natl Acad Sci U S A **112**, 12800–12805.

Gadea, A., Schinelli, S., and Gallo, V. (2008). Endothelin-1 regulates astrocyte proliferation and reactive gliosis via a JNK/c-Jun signaling pathway. J Neurosci **28**, 2394–2408.

Galloway, D.A., Phillips, A.E.M., Owen, D.R.J., and Moore, C.S. (2019). Phagocytosis in the Brain: Homeostasis and Disease. Front Immunol **10**, 790.

Gardai, S.J., McPhillips, K.A., Frasch, S.C., Janssen, W.J., Starefeldt, A., Murphy-Ullrich, J.E., Bratton, D.L., Oldenborg, P.A., Michalak, M., and Henson, P.M. (2005). Cell-surface calreticulin initiates clearance of viable or apoptotic cells through trans-activation of LRP on the phagocyte. Cell **123**, 321–334.

Gautier, E.L., Shay, T., Miller, J., Greter, M., Jakubzick, C., Ivanov, S., Helft, J., Chow, A., Elpek, K.G., Gordonov, S., *et al.* (2012). Gene-expression profiles and transcriptional regulatory pathways that underlie the identity and diversity of mouse tissue macrophages. Nat Immunol **13**, 1118–1128.

Grommes, C., Lee, C.Y., Wilkinson, B.L., Jiang, Q., Koenigsknecht-Talboo, J.L., Varnum, B., and Landreth, G.E. (2008). Regulation of microglial phagocytosis and inflammatory gene expression by Gas6 acting on the Axl/Mer family of tyrosine kinases. J Neuroimmune Pharmacol **3**, 130–140.

Gumienny, T.L., Brugnera, E., Tosello-Trampont, A.C., Kinchen, J.M., Haney, L.B., Nishiwaki, K., Walk, S.F., Nemergut, M.E., Macara, I.G., Francis, R., *et al.* (2001). CED-12/ELMO, a novel member of the CrkII/Dock180/Rac pathway, is required for phagocytosis and cell migration. Cell **107**, 27–41.

Gunner, G., Cheadle, L., Johnson, K.M., Ayata, P., Badimon, A., Mondo, E., Nagy, M.A., Liu, L., Bemiller, S.M., Kim, K.W., *et al.* (2019). Sensory lesioning induces microglial synapse elimination via ADAM10 and fractalkine signaling. Nat Neurosci **22**, 1075–1088.

Gyorffy, B.A., Kun, J., Torok, G., Bulyaki, E., Borhegyi, Z., Gulyassy, P., Kis, V., Szocsics, P., Micsonai, A., Matko, J., *et al.* (2018). Local apoptotic-like mechanisms underlie complement-mediated synaptic pruning. Proc Natl Acad Sci U S A **115**, 6303–6308.

Hakim, Y., Yaniv, S.P., and Schuldiner, O. (2014). Astrocytes play a key role in Drosophila mushroom body axon pruning. PLoS One **9**, e86178.

Han, C., Song, Y., Xiao, H., Wang, D., Franc, N.C., Jan, L.Y., and Jan, Y.N. (2014). Epidermal cells are the primary phagocytes in the fragmentation and clearance of degenerating dendrites in Drosophila. Neuron **81**, 544–560.

Hanayama, R., Tanaka, M., Miwa, K., Shinohara, A., Iwamatsu, A., and Nagata, S. (2002). Identification of a factor that links apoptotic cells to phagocytes. Nature **417**, 182–187.

Harrison, J.K., Jiang, Y., Chen, S., Xia, Y., Maciejewski, D., McNamara, R.K., Streit, W.J., Salafranca, M.N., Adhikari, S., Thompson, D.A., *et al.* (1998). Role for neuronally derived fractalkine in mediating interactions between neurons and CX3CR1-expressing microglia. Proc Natl Acad Sci U S A **95**, 10896–10901.

Hedgecock, E.M., Sulston, J.E., and Thomson, J.N. (1983). Mutations affecting programmed cell deaths in the nematode Caenorhabditis elegans. Science **220**, 1277–1279.

Heisenberg, M., Borst, A., Wagner, S., and Byers, D. (1985). Drosophila mushroom body mutants are deficient in olfactory learning. J Neurogenet **2**, 1–30.

Hilu-Dadia, R., Hakim-Mishnaevski, K., Levy-Adam, F., and Kurant, E. (2018). Draper-mediated JNK signaling is required for glial phagocytosis of apoptotic neurons during Drosophila metamorphosis. Glia **66**, 1520–1532.

Hoeppner, D.J., Hengartner, M.O., and Schnabel, R. (2001). Engulfment genes cooperate with ced-3 to promote cell death in Caenorhabditis elegans. Nature **412**, 202–206.

Hong, S., Beja-Glasser, V.F., Nfonoyim, B.M., Frouin, A., Li, S., Ramakrishnan, S., Merry, K.M., Shi, Q., Rosenthal, A., Barres, B.A., *et al.* (2016). Complement and microglia mediate early synapse loss in Alzheimer mouse models. Science **352**, 712–716.

Hooks, B.M., and Chen, C. (2006). Distinct roles for spontaneous and visual activity in remodeling of the retinogeniculate synapse. Neuron **52**, 281–291.

Hoopfer, E.D., McLaughlin, T., Watts, R.J., Schuldiner, O., O'Leary, D.D., and Luo, L. (2006). Wlds protection distinguishes axon degeneration following injury from naturally occurring developmental pruning. Neuron **50**, 883–895.

Howell, G.R., Macalinao, D.G., Sousa, G.L., Walden, M., Soto, I., Kneeland, S.C., Barbay, J.M., King, B.L., Marchant, J.K., Hibbs, M., *et al.* (2011). Molecular clustering identifies complement and endothelin induction as early events in a mouse model of glaucoma. J Clin Invest **121**, 1429–1444.

Hsieh, H.H., Hsu, T.Y., Jiang, H.S., and Wu, Y.C. (2012). Integrin alpha PAT-2/CDC-42 signaling is required for muscle-mediated clearance of apoptotic cells in Caenorhabditis elegans. PLoS Genet **8**, e1002663.

Huberman, A.D. (2007). Mechanisms of eye-specific visual circuit development. Curr Opin Neurobiol **17**, 73–80.

Jaubert-Miazza, L., Green, E., Lo, F.S., Bui, K., Mills, J., and Guido, W. (2005). Structural and functional composition of the developing retinogeniculate pathway in the mouse. Vis Neurosci **22**, 661–676.

Ji, H., Sapar, M.L., Sarkar, A., Wang, B., and Han, C. (2022). Phagocytosis and self-destruction break down dendrites of Drosophila sensory neurons at distinct steps of Wallerian degeneration. Proc Natl Acad Sci U S A **119**.

Ji, H., Wang, B., Shen, Y., Labib, D., Lei, J., Chen, X., Sapar, M., Boulanger, A., Dura, J. M., & Han, C. (2023). The Drosophila chemokine-like Orion bridges phosphatidylserine and Draper in phagocytosis of neurons. Proc Natl Acad Sci U S A, **120(24)**.

Ji, R., Tian, S., Lu, H.J., Lu, Q., Zheng, Y., Wang, X., Ding, J., Li, Q., and Lu, Q. (2013). TAM receptors affect adult brain neurogenesis by negative regulation of microglial cell activation. J Immunol **191**, 6165–6177.

Jiang, Y., and Reichert, H. (2012). Programmed cell death in type II neuroblast lineages is required for central complex development in the Drosophila brain. Neural Dev **7**, 3.

Jung, S., Aliberti, J., Graemmel, P., Sunshine, M.J., Kreutzberg, G.W., Sher, A., and Littman, D.R. (2000). Analysis of fractalkine receptor CX(3)CR1 function by targeted deletion and green fluorescent protein reporter gene insertion. Mol Cell Biol **20**, 4106–4114.

Katz, L.C., and Shatz, C.J. (1996). Synaptic activity and the construction of cortical circuits. Science **274**, 1133–1138.

Kavanaugh, W.M., Turck, C.W., and Williams, L.T. (1995). PTB domain binding to signaling proteins through a sequence motif containing phosphotyrosine. Science **268**, 1177–1179.

Kim, Y.E., Chen, J., Chan, J.R., and Langen, R. (2010). Engineering a polarity-sensitive biosensor for time-lapse imaging of apoptotic processes and degeneration. Nat Methods **7**, 67–73.

Kinchen, J.M., Cabello, J., Klingele, D., Wong, K., Feichtinger, R., Schnabel, H., Schnabel, R., and Hengartner, M.O. (2005). Two pathways converge at CED-10 to mediate actin rearrangement and corpse removal in C. elegans. Nature **434**, 93–99.

Kobayashi, N., Karisola, P., Pena-Cruz, V., Dorfman, D.M., Jinushi, M., Umetsu, S.E., Butte, M.J., Nagumo, H., Chernova, I., Zhu, B., *et al.*

(2007). TIM-1 and TIM-4 glycoproteins bind phosphatidylserine and mediate uptake of apoptotic cells. Immunity **27**, 927–940.

Kuo, C.T., Jan, L.Y., and Jan, Y.N. (2005). Dendrite-specific remodeling of Drosophila sensory neurons requires matrix metalloproteases, ubiquitin-proteasome, and ecdysone signaling. Proc Natl Acad Sci U S A **102**, 15230–15235.

Kuraishi, T., Nakagawa, Y., Nagaosa, K., Hashimoto, Y., Ishimoto, T., Moki, T., Fujita, Y., Nakayama, H., Dohmae, N., Shiratsuchi, A., *et al.* (2009). Pretaporter, a Drosophila protein serving as a ligand for Draper in the phagocytosis of apoptotic cells. EMBO J **28**, 3868–3878.

Kurant, E., Axelrod, S., Leaman, D., and Gaul, U. (2008). Six-microns-under acts upstream of Draper in the glial phagocytosis of apoptotic neurons. Cell **133**, 498–509.

Lamers, C., Pluss, C.J., and Ricklin, D. (2021). The Promiscuous Profile of Complement Receptor 3 in Ligand Binding, Immune Modulation, and Pathophysiology. Front Immunol **12**, 662164.

Lance-Jones, C. (1982). Motoneuron cell death in the developing lumbar spinal cord of the mouse. Brain Res **256**, 473–479.

LaVail, M.M. (1976). Rod outer segment disk shedding in rat retina: relationship to cyclic lighting. Science **194**, 1071–1074.

Lee, H., Brott, B.K., Kirkby, L.A., Adelson, J.D., Cheng, S., Feller, M.B., Datwani, A., and Shatz, C.J. (2014). Synapse elimination and learning rules co-regulated by MHC class I H2-Db. Nature **509**, 195–200.

Lee, H.H., Jan, L.Y., and Jan, Y.N. (2009). Drosophila IKK-related kinase Ik2 and Katanin p60-like 1 regulate dendrite pruning of sensory neuron during metamorphosis. Proc Natl Acad Sci U S A **106**, 6363–6368.

Lee, J.H., Kim, J.Y., Noh, S., Lee, H., Lee, S.Y., Mun, J.Y., Park, H., and Chung, W.S. (2021). Astrocytes phagocytose adult hippocampal synapses for circuit homeostasis. Nature **590**, 612–617.

Lee, T., Lee, A., and Luo, L. (1999). Development of the Drosophila mushroom bodies: sequential generation of three distinct types of neurons from a neuroblast. Development **126**, 4065–4076.

Lehrman, E.K., Wilton, D.K., Litvina, E.Y., Welsh, C.A., Chang, S.T., Frouin, A., Walker, A.J., Heller, M.D., Umemori, H., Chen, C., *et al.* (2018). CD47 Protects Synapses from Excess Microglia-Mediated Pruning during Development. Neuron **100**, 120–134 e126.

Lemke, G. (2013). Biology of the TAM receptors. Cold Spring Harb Perspect Biol **5**, a009076.

Lemke, G. (2017). Phosphatidylserine Is the Signal for TAM Receptors and Their Ligands. Trends Biochem Sci **42**, 738–748.

Lemke, G. (2019). How macrophages deal with death. Nat Rev Immunol **19**, 539–549.

Lemke, G., and Rothlin, C.V. (2008). Immunobiology of the TAM receptors. Nat Rev Immunol **8**, 327–336.

Leventis, P.A., and Grinstein, S. (2010). The distribution and function of phosphatidylserine in cellular membranes. Annu Rev Biophys **39**, 407–427.

Lew, E.D., Oh, J., Burrola, P.G., Lax, I., Zagorska, A., Traves, P.G., Schlessinger, J., and Lemke, G. (2014). Differential TAM receptor-ligand-phospholipid interactions delimit differential TAM bioactivities. Elife **3**.

Li, T., Chiou, B., Gilman, C.K., Luo, R., Koshi, T., Yu, D., Oak, H.C., Giera, S., Johnson-Venkatesh, E., Muthukumar, A.K., *et al.* (2020). A splicing isoform of GPR56 mediates microglial synaptic refinement via phosphatidylserine binding. EMBO J **39**, e104136.

Linnartz, B., Kopatz, J., Tenner, A.J., and Neumann, H. (2012). Sialic acid on the neuronal glycocalyx prevents complement C1 binding and complement receptor-3-mediated removal by microglia. J Neurosci **32**, 946–952.

Liu, Q.A., and Hengartner, M.O. (1999). Human CED-6 encodes a functional homologue of the Caenorhabditis elegans engulfment protein CED-6. Curr Biol **9**, 1347–1350.

Losada-Perez, M., Garcia-Guillen, N., and Casas-Tinto, S. (2021). A novel injury paradigm in the central nervous system of adult Drosophila: molecular, cellular and functional aspects. Dis Model Mech **14**.

Lu, T.Y., Doherty, J., and Freeman, M.R. (2014). DRK/DOS/SOS converge with Crk/Mbc/dCed-12 to activate Rac1 during glial engulfment of axonal debris. Proc Natl Acad Sci U S A **111**, 12544–12549.

Lu, T.Y., MacDonald, J.M., Neukomm, L.J., Sheehan, A.E., Bradshaw, R., Logan, M.A., and Freeman, M.R. (2017). Axon degeneration induces glial responses through Draper-TRAF4-JNK signalling. Nat Commun **8**, 14355.

Lui, H., Zhang, J., Makinson, S.R., Cahill, M.K., Kelley, K.W., Huang, H.Y., Shang, Y., Oldham, M.C., Martens, L.H., Gao, F., *et al.* (2016). Progranulin Deficiency Promotes Circuit-Specific Synaptic Pruning by Microglia via Complement Activation. Cell **165**, 921–935.

Luo, L., and O'Leary, D.D. (2005). Axon retraction and degeneration in development and disease. Annu Rev Neurosci **28**, 127–156.

MacDonald, J.M., Beach, M.G., Porpiglia, E., Sheehan, A.E., Watts, R.J., and Freeman, M.R. (2006). The Drosophila cell corpse engulfment receptor Draper mediates glial clearance of severed axons. Neuron **50**, 869–881.

Macdonald, J.M., Doherty, J., Hackett, R., and Freeman, M.R. (2013). The c-Jun kinase signaling cascade promotes glial engulfment activity through activation of draper and phagocytic function. Cell Death Differ **20**, 1140–1148.

Mapes, J., Chen, Y.Z., Kim, A., Mitani, S., Kang, B.H., and Xue, D. (2012). CED-1, CED-7, and TTR-52 regulate surface phosphatidylserine expression on apoptotic and phagocytic cells. Curr Biol **22**, 1267–1275.

Marin-Teva, J.L., Dusart, I., Colin, C., Gervais, A., van Rooijen, N., and Mallat, M. (2004). Microglia promote the death of developing Purkinje cells. Neuron **41**, 535–547.

Martin, M., Leffler, J., and Blom, A.M. (2012). Annexin A2 and A5 serve as new ligands for C1q on apoptotic cells. J Biol Chem **287**, 33733–33744.

Mazaheri, F., Breus, O., Durdu, S., Haas, P., Wittbrodt, J., Gilmour, D., and Peri, F. (2014). Distinct roles for BAI1 and TIM-4 in the engulfment of dying neurons by microglia. Nat Commun **5**, 4046.

McLaughlin, C.N., Perry-Richardson, J.J., Coutinho-Budd, J.C., and Broihier, H.T. (2019). Dying Neurons Utilize Innate Immune Signaling to Prime Glia for Phagocytosis during Development. Dev Cell **48**, 506–522 e506.

Miyanishi, M., Tada, K., Koike, M., Uchiyama, Y., Kitamura, T., and Nagata, S. (2007). Identification of Tim4 as a phosphatidylserine receptor. Nature **450**, 435–439.

Nakano, R., Iwamura, M., Obikawa, A., Togane, Y., Hara, Y., Fukuhara, T., Tomaru, M., Takano-Shimizu, T., and Tsujimura, H. (2019). Cortex glia clear dead young neurons via Drpr/dCed-6/Shark and Crk/Mbc/dCed-12 signaling pathways in the developing Drosophila optic lobe. Dev Biol **453**, 68–85.

Nandrot, E.F., Anand, M., Almeida, D., Atabai, K., Sheppard, D., and Finnemann, S.C. (2007). Essential role for MFG-E8 as ligand for alphavbeta5 integrin in diurnal retinal phagocytosis. Proc Natl Acad Sci U S A **104**, 12005–12010.

Nandrot, E.F., Kim, Y., Brodie, S.E., Huang, X., Sheppard, D., and Finnemann, S.C. (2004). Loss of synchronized retinal phagocytosis and age-related blindness in mice lacking alphavbeta5 integrin. J Exp Med **200**, 1539–1545.

Neniskyte, U., and Gross, C.T. (2017). Errant gardeners: glial-cell-dependent synaptic pruning and neurodevelopmental disorders. Nat Rev Neurosci **18**, 658–670.

Neumann, B., Coakley, S., Giordano-Santini, R., Linton, C., Lee, E.S., Nakagawa, A., Xue, D., and Hilliard, M.A. (2015). EFF-1-mediated regenerative axonal fusion requires components of the apoptotic pathway. Nature **517**, 219–222.

Nonomura, K., Yamaguchi, Y., Hamachi, M., Koike, M., Uchiyama, Y., Nakazato, K., Mochizuki, A., Sakaue-Sawano, A., Miyawaki, A., Yoshida, H., *et al.* (2013). Local apoptosis modulates early mammalian brain development through the elimination of morphogen-producing cells. Dev Cell **27**, 621–634.

O'Leary, D.D. (1992). Development of connectional diversity and specificity in the mammalian brain by the pruning of collateral projections. Curr Opin Neurobiol **2**, 70–77.

O'Leary, D.D., and Koester, S.E. (1993). Development of projection neuron types, axon pathways, and patterned connections of the mammalian cortex. Neuron **10**, 991–1006.

Offner, N., Duval, N., Jamrich, M., and Durand, B. (2005). The pro-apoptotic activity of a vertebrate Bar-like homeobox gene plays a key role in patterning the Xenopus neural plate by limiting the number of chordin- and shh-expressing cells. Development **132**, 1807–1818.

Okada, R., Nagaosa, K., Kuraishi, T., Nakayama, H., Yamamoto, N., Nakagawa, Y., Dohmae, N., Shiratsuchi, A., and Nakanishi, Y. (2012). Apoptosis-dependent externalization and involvement in apoptotic cell clearance of DmCaBP1, an endoplasmic reticulum protein of Drosophila. J Biol Chem **287**, 3138–3146.

Oppenheim, R.W. (1986). The absence of significant postnatal motoneuron death in the brachial and lumbar spinal cord of the rat. J Comp Neurol **246**, 281–286.

Oppenheim, R.W., Prevette, D., Houenou, L.J., Pincon-Raymond, M., Dimitriadou, V., Donevan, A., O'Donovan, M., Wenner, P., McKemy, D.D., and Allen, P.D. (1997). Neuromuscular development in the avian paralytic mutant crooked neck dwarf (cn/cn): further evidence for the role of neuromuscular activity in motoneuron survival. J Comp Neurol **381**, 353–372.

Paidassi, H., Tacnet-Delorme, P., Garlatti, V., Darnault, C., Ghebrehiwet, B., Gaboriaud, C., Arlaud, G.J., and Frachet, P. (2008). C1q binds phosphatidylserine and likely acts as a multiligand-bridging molecule in apoptotic cell recognition. J Immunol **180**, 2329–2338.

Paolicelli, R.C., Bolasco, G., Pagani, F., Maggi, L., Scianni, M., Panzanelli, P., Giustetto, M., Ferreira, T.A., Guiducci, E., Dumas, L., *et al.* (2011). Synaptic pruning by microglia is necessary for normal brain development. Science **333**, 1456–1458.

Park, D., Tosello-Trampont, A.C., Elliott, M.R., Lu, M., Haney, L.B., Ma, Z., Klibanov, A.L., Mandell, J.W., and Ravichandran, K.S. (2007). BAI1 is an engulfment receptor for apoptotic cells upstream of the ELMO/Dock180/Rac module. Nature **450**, 430–434.

Park, E.J., Myint, P.K., Ito, A., Appiah, M.G., Darkwah, S., Kawamoto, E., and Shimaoka, M. (2020). Integrin-Ligand Interactions in Inflammation, Cancer, and Metabolic Disease: Insights Into the Multifaceted Roles of an Emerging Ligand Irisin. Front Cell Dev Biol **8**, 588066.

Park, J., Choi, Y., Jung, E., Lee, S.H., Sohn, J.W., and Chung, W.S. (2021). Microglial MERTK eliminates phosphatidylserine-displaying inhibitory post-synapses. EMBO J **40**, e107121.

Parkhurst, C.N., Yang, G., Ninan, I., Savas, J.N., Yates, J.R., 3rd, Lafaille, J.J., Hempstead, B.L., Littman, D.R., and Gan, W.B. (2013). Microglia promote learning-dependent synapse formation through brain-derived neurotrophic factor. Cell **155**, 1596–1609.

Prasad, D., Rothlin, C.V., Burrola, P., Burstyn-Cohen, T., Lu, Q., Garcia de Frutos, P., and Lemke, G. (2006). TAM receptor function in the retinal pigment epithelium. Mol Cell Neurosci **33**, 96–108.

Presumey, J., Bialas, A.R., and Carroll, M.C. (2017). Complement System in Neural Synapse Elimination in Development and Disease. Adv Immunol **135**, 53–79.

Purice, M.D., Ray, A., Munzel, E.J., Pope, B.J., Park, D.J., Speese, S.D., and Logan, M.A. (2017). A novel Drosophila injury model reveals severed axons are cleared through a Draper/MMP-1 signaling cascade. Elife **6**.

Purice, M.D., Speese, S.D., and Logan, M.A. (2016). Delayed glial clearance of degenerating axons in aged Drosophila is due to reduced PI3K/Draper activity. Nat Commun **7**, 12871.

Raiders, S., Black, E.C., Bac, A., MacFarlane, S., Klein, M., Shaham, S., and Singhvi, A. (2021). Glia actively sculpt sensory neurons by controlled phagocytosis to tune animal behavior. Elife **10**.

Rasmussen, J.P., Sack, G.S., Martin, S.M., and Sagasti, A. (2015). Vertebrate epidermal cells are broad-specificity phagocytes that clear sensory axon debris. J Neurosci **35**, 559–570.

Ravichandran, K.S. (2010). Find-me and eat-me signals in apoptotic cell clearance: progress and conundrums. J Exp Med **207**, 1807–1817.

Ray, A., Speese, S.D., and Logan, M.A. (2017). Glial Draper Rescues Abeta Toxicity in a Drosophila Model of Alzheimer's Disease. J Neurosci **37**, 11881–11893.

Reddien, P.W., Cameron, S., and Horvitz, H.R. (2001). Phagocytosis promotes programmed cell death in C. elegans. Nature **412**, 198–202.

Reddien, P.W., and Horvitz, H.R. (2000). CED-2/CrkII and CED-10/Rac control phagocytosis and cell migration in Caenorhabditis elegans. Nat Cell Biol **2**, 131–136.

Reddien, P.W., and Horvitz, H.R. (2004). The engulfment process of programmed cell death in caenorhabditis elegans. Annu Rev Cell Dev Biol **20**, 193–221.

Riccomagno, M.M., and Kolodkin, A.L. (2015). Sculpting neural circuits by axon and dendrite pruning. Annu Rev Cell Dev Biol **31**, 779–805.

Rogulja-Ortmann, A., Luer, K., Seibert, J., Rickert, C., and Technau, G.M. (2007). Programmed cell death in the embryonic central nervous system of Drosophila melanogaster. Development **134**, 105–116.

Ruggiero, L., Connor, M.P., Chen, J., Langen, R., and Finnemann, S.C. (2012). Diurnal, localized exposure of phosphatidylserine by rod outer segment tips in wild-type but not Itgb5-/- or Mfge8-/- mouse retina. Proc Natl Acad Sci U S A **109**, 8145–8148.

Salter, M.W., and Stevens, B. (2017). Microglia emerge as central players in brain disease. Nat Med **23**, 1018–1027.

Salzman, G.S., Ackerman, S.D., Ding, C., Koide, A., Leon, K., Luo, R., Stoveken, H.M., Fernandez, C.G., Tall, G.G., Piao, X., *et al.* (2016). Structural Basis for Regulation of GPR56/ADGRG1 by Its Alternatively Spliced Extracellular Domains. Neuron **91**, 1292–1304.

Sapar, M.L., Ji, H., Wang, B., Poe, A.R., Dubey, K., Ren, X., Ni, J.Q., and Han, C. (2018). Phosphatidylserine Externalization Results from and Causes Neurite Degeneration in Drosophila. Cell Rep **24**, 2273–2286.

Schafer, D.P., Lehrman, E.K., Kautzman, A.G., Koyama, R., Mardinly, A.R., Yamasaki, R., Ransohoff, R.M., Greenberg, M.E., Barres, B.A., and Stevens, B. (2012). Microglia sculpt postnatal neural circuits in an activity and complement-dependent manner. Neuron **74**, 691–705.

Scheib, J.L., Sullivan, C.S., and Carter, B.D. (2012). Jedi-1 and MEGF10 signal engulfment of apoptotic neurons through the tyrosine kinase Syk. J Neurosci **32**, 13022–13031.

Scott-Hewitt, N., Perrucci, F., Morini, R., Erreni, M., Mahoney, M., Witkowska, A., Carey, A., Faggiani, E., Schuetz, L.T., Mason, S., *et al.* (2020). Local externalization of phosphatidylserine mediates developmental synaptic pruning by microglia. EMBO J **39**, e105380.

Segawa, K., and Nagata, S. (2015). An Apoptotic 'Eat Me' Signal: Phosphatidylserine Exposure. Trends Cell Biol **25**, 639–650.

Segawa, K., Suzuki, J., and Nagata, S. (2011). Constitutive exposure of phosphatidylserine on viable cells. Proc Natl Acad Sci U S A **108**, 19246–19251.

Sekar, A., Bialas, A.R., de Rivera, H., Davis, A., Hammond, T.R., Kamitaki, N., Tooley, K., Presumey, J., Baum, M., Van Doren, V., *et al.* (2016). Schizophrenia risk from complex variation of complement component 4. Nature **530**, 177–183.

Shacham-Silverberg, V., Sar Shalom, H., Goldner, R., Golan-Vaishenker, Y., Gurwicz, N., Gokhman, I., and Yaron, A. (2018). Phosphatidylserine is a marker for axonal debris engulfment but its exposure can be decoupled from degeneration. Cell Death Dis **9**, 1116.

Shimono, K., Fujimoto, A., Tsuyama, T., Yamamoto-Kochi, M., Sato, M., Hattori, Y., Sugimura, K., Usui, T., Kimura, K., and Uemura, T. (2009). Multidendritic sensory neurons in the adult Drosophila abdomen: origins, dendritic morphology, and segment- and age-dependent programmed cell death. Neural Dev **4**, 37.

Shirotani, K., Hori, Y., Yoshizaki, R., Higuchi, E., Colonna, M., Saito, T., Hashimoto, S., Saito, T., Saido, T.C., and Iwata, N. (2019). Aminophospholipids are signal-transducing TREM2 ligands on apoptotic cells. Sci Rep **9**, 7508.

Shklyar, B., Levy-Adam, F., Mishnaevski, K., and Kurant, E. (2013). Caspase activity is required for engulfment of apoptotic cells. Mol Cell Biol **33**, 3191–3201.

Sierra, A., Abiega, O., Shahraz, A., and Neumann, H. (2013). Janus-faced microglia: beneficial and detrimental consequences of microglial phagocytosis. Front Cell Neurosci **7**, 6.

Sierra, A., Encinas, J.M., Deudero, J.J., Chancey, J.H., Enikolopov, G., Overstreet-Wadiche, L.S., Tsirka, S.E., and Maletic-Savatic, M. (2010). Microglia shape adult hippocampal neurogenesis through apoptosis-coupled phagocytosis. Cell Stem Cell **7**, 483–495.

Sierra, A., Tremblay, M.E., and Wake, H. (2014). Never-resting microglia: physiological roles in the healthy brain and pathological implications. Front Cell Neurosci **8**, 240.

Sievers, C., Platt, N., Perry, V.H., Coleman, M.P., and Conforti, L. (2003). Neurites undergoing Wallerian degeneration show an apoptotic-like process with Annexin V positive staining and loss of mitochondrial membrane potential. Neurosci Res **46**, 161–169.

Singer, K., Luo, R., Jeong, S.J., and Piao, X. (2013). GPR56 and the developing cerebral cortex: cells, matrix, and neuronal migration. Mol Neurobiol **47**, 186–196.

Singhvi, A., Liu, B., Friedman, C.J., Fong, J., Lu, Y., Huang, X.Y., and Shaham, S. (2016). A Glial K/Cl Transporter Controls Neuronal Receptive Ending Shape by Chloride Inhibition of an rGC. Cell **165**, 936–948.

Smith, I.W., Mikesh, M., Lee, Y., and Thompson, W.J. (2013). Terminal Schwann cells participate in the competition underlying neuromuscular synapse elimination. J Neurosci **33**, 17724–17736.

Sokolowski, J.D., Nobles, S.L., Heffron, D.S., Park, D., Ravichandran, K.S., and Mandell, J.W. (2011). Brain-specific angiogenesis inhibitor-1 expression in astrocytes and neurons: implications for its dual function as an apoptotic engulfment receptor. Brain Behav Immun **25**, 915–921.

Song, J.W., Misgeld, T., Kang, H., Knecht, S., Lu, J., Cao, Y., Cotman, S.L., Bishop, D.L., and Lichtman, J.W. (2008). Lysosomal activity associated with developmental axon pruning. J Neurosci **28**, 8993–9001.

Stephan, A.H., Barres, B.A., and Stevens, B. (2012). The complement system: an unexpected role in synaptic pruning during development and disease. Annu Rev Neurosci **35**, 369–389.

Stephan, A.H., Madison, D.V., Mateos, J.M., Fraser, D.A., Lovelett, E.A., Coutellier, L., Kim, L., Tsai, H.H., Huang, E.J., Rowitch, D.H., *et al.* (2013). A dramatic increase of C1q protein in the CNS during normal aging. J Neurosci **33**, 13460–13474.

Stevens, B., Allen, N.J., Vazquez, L.E., Howell, G.R., Christopherson, K.S., Nouri, N., Micheva, K.D., Mehalow, A.K., Huberman, A.D., Stafford, B., *et al.* (2007). The classical complement cascade mediates CNS synapse elimination. Cell **131**, 1164–1178.

Stitt, T.N., Conn, G., Gore, M., Lai, C., Bruno, J., Radziejewski, C., Mattsson, K., Fisher, J., Gies, D.R., Jones, P.F., *et al.* (1995). The anticoagulation factor protein S and its relative, Gas6, are ligands for the Tyro 3/Axl family of receptor tyrosine kinases. Cell **80**, 661–670.

Su, H.P., Brugnera, E., Van Criekinge, W., Smits, E., Hengartner, M., Bogaert, T., and Ravichandran, K.S. (2000). Identification and characterization of a dimerization domain in CED-6, an adapter protein involved in engulfment of apoptotic cells. J Biol Chem **275**, 9542–9549.

Suzuki, J., Denning, D.P., Imanishi, E., Horvitz, H.R., and Nagata, S. (2013). Xk-related protein 8 and CED-8 promote phosphatidylserine exposure in apoptotic cells. Science **341**, 403–406.

Suzuki, J., Umeda, M., Sims, P.J., and Nagata, S. (2010). Calcium-dependent phospholipid scrambling by TMEM16F. Nature **468**, 834–838.

Takatsu, H., Baba, K., Shima, T., Umino, H., Kato, U., Umeda, M., Nakayama, K., and Shin, H.W. (2011). ATP9B, a P4-ATPase (a putative aminophospholipid translocase), localizes to the trans-Golgi network in a CDC50 protein-independent manner. J Biol Chem **286**, 38159–38167.

Tanaka, K., Fujimura-Kamada, K., and Yamamoto, T. (2011). Functions of phospholipid flippases. J Biochem **149**, 131–143.

Tao, J., and Rolls, M.M. (2011). Dendrites have a rapid program of injury-induced degeneration that is molecularly distinct from developmental pruning. J Neurosci **31**, 5398–5405.

Tasdemir-Yilmaz, O.E., and Freeman, M.R. (2014). Astrocytes engage unique molecular programs to engulf pruned neuronal debris from distinct subsets of neurons. Genes Dev **28**, 20–33.

Togane, Y., Ayukawa, R., Hara, Y., Akagawa, H., Iwabuchi, K., and Tsujimura, H. (2012). Spatio-temporal pattern of programmed cell death in the developing Drosophila optic lobe. Dev Growth Differ **54**, 503–518.

Tung, T.T., Nagaosa, K., Fujita, Y., Kita, A., Mori, H., Okada, R., Nonaka, S., and Nakanishi, Y. (2013). Phosphatidylserine recognition and induction of apoptotic cell clearance by Drosophila engulfment receptor Draper. J Biochem **153**, 483–491.

Ulland, T.K., and Colonna, M. (2018). TREM2 - a key player in microglial biology and Alzheimer disease. Nat Rev Neurol **14**, 667–675.

Vainchtein, I.D., Chin, G., Cho, F.S., Kelley, K.W., Miller, J.G., Chien, E.C., Liddelow, S.A., Nguyen, P.T., Nakao-Inoue, H., Dorman, L.C., *et al.* (2018). Astrocyte-derived interleukin-33 promotes microglial synapse engulfment and neural circuit development. Science **359**, 1269–1273.

van der Velden, L.M., Wichers, C.G., van Breevoort, A.E., Coleman, J.A., Molday, R.S., Berger, R., Klomp, L.W., and van de Graaf, S.F. (2010). Heteromeric interactions required for abundance and subcellular localization of human CDC50 proteins and class 1 P4-ATPases. J Biol Chem **285**, 40088–40096.

van Lookeren Campagne, M., Wiesmann, C., and Brown, E.J. (2007). Macrophage complement receptors and pathogen clearance. Cell Microbiol **9**, 2095–2102.

Vollrath, D., Feng, W., Duncan, J.L., Yasumura, D., D'Cruz, P.M., Chappelow, A., Matthes, M.T., Kay, M.A., and LaVail, M.M. (2001). Correction of the retinal dystrophy phenotype of the RCS rat by viral gene transfer of Mertk. Proc Natl Acad Sci U S A **98**, 12584–12589.

Vorup-Jensen, T., and Jensen, R.K. (2018). Structural Immunology of Complement Receptors 3 and 4. Front Immunol **9**, 2716.

Wakselman, S., Bechade, C., Roumier, A., Bernard, D., Triller, A., and Bessis, A. (2008). Developmental neuronal death in hippocampus requires the microglial CD11b integrin and DAP12 immunoreceptor. J Neurosci **28**, 8138–8143.

Walsh, M.K., and Lichtman, J.W. (2003). In vivo time-lapse imaging of synaptic takeover associated with naturally occurring synapse elimination. Neuron **37**, 67–73.

Wang, X., Li, W., Zhao, D., Liu, B., Shi, Y., Chen, B., Yang, H., Guo, P., Geng, X., Shang, Z., *et al.* (2010). Caenorhabditis elegans transthyretin-like protein TTR-52 mediates recognition of apoptotic cells by the CED-1 phagocyte receptor. Nat Cell Biol **12**, 655–664.

Wang, X., Wu, Y.C., Fadok, V.A., Lee, M.C., Gengyo-Ando, K., Cheng, L.C., Ledwich, D., Hsu, P.K., Chen, J.Y., Chou, B.K., *et al.* (2003). Cell corpse engulfment mediated by C. elegans phosphatidylserine receptor through CED-5 and CED-12. Science **302**, 1563–1566.

Wang, Y., Cella, M., Mallinson, K., Ulrich, J.D., Young, K.L., Robinette, M.L., Gilfillan, S., Krishnan, G.M., Sudhakar, S., Zinselmeyer, B.H., *et al.* (2015). TREM2 lipid sensing sustains the microglial response in an Alzheimer's disease model. Cell **160**, 1061–1071.

Watts, R.J., Hoopfer, E.D., and Luo, L. (2003). Axon pruning during Drosophila metamorphosis: evidence for local degeneration and requirement of the ubiquitin-proteasome system. Neuron **38**, 871–885.

Watts, R.J., Schuldiner, O., Perrino, J., Larsen, C., and Luo, L. (2004). Glia engulf degenerating axons during developmental axon pruning. Curr Biol **14**, 678–684.

Weinhard, L., di Bartolomei, G., Bolasco, G., Machado, P., Schieber, N.L., Neniskyte, U., Exiga, M., Vadisiute, A., Raggioli, A., Schertel, A., *et al.* (2018). Microglia remodel synapses by presynaptic trogocytosis and spine head filopodia induction. Nat Commun **9**, 1228.

Weng, Z., Situ, C., Lin, L., Wu, Z., Zhu, J., and Zhang, R. (2019). Structure of BAI1/ELMO2 complex reveals an action mechanism of adhesion GPCRs via ELMO family scaffolds. Nat Commun **10**, 51.

Williams, D.W., Kondo, S., Krzyzanowska, A., Hiromi, Y., and Truman, J.W. (2006). Local caspase activity directs engulfment of dendrites during pruning. Nat Neurosci **9**, 1234-1236.

Williams, D.W., and Truman, J.W. (2005a). Cellular mechanisms of dendrite pruning in Drosophila: insights from in vivo time-lapse of remodeling dendritic arborizing sensory neurons. Development **132**, 3631–3642.

Williams, D.W., and Truman, J.W. (2005b). Remodeling dendrites during insect metamorphosis. J Neurobiol **64**, 24–33.

Williamson, A.P., and Vale, R.D. (2018). Spatial control of Draper receptor signaling initiates apoptotic cell engulfment. J Cell Biol **217**, 3977–3992.

Wilton, D.K., Dissing-Olesen, L., and Stevens, B. (2019). Neuron-Glia Signaling in Synapse Elimination. Annu Rev Neurosci **42**, 107–127.

Winbush, A., and Weeks, J.C. (2011). Steroid-triggered, cell-autonomous death of a Drosophila motoneuron during metamorphosis. Neural Dev **6**, 15.

Wojdasiewicz, P., Poniatowski, L.A., Kotela, A., Deszczynski, J., Kotela, I., and Szukiewicz, D. (2014). The chemokine CX3CL1 (fractalkine) and its receptor CX3CR1: occurrence and potential role in osteoarthritis. Arch Immunol Ther Exp (Warsz) **62**, 395–403.

Wu, H.H., Bellmunt, E., Scheib, J.L., Venegas, V., Burkert, C., Reichardt, L.F., Zhou, Z., Farinas, I., and Carter, B.D. (2009). Glial precursors clear sensory neuron corpses during development via Jedi-1, an engulfment receptor. Nat Neurosci **12**, 1534–1541.

Wu, Y., Singh, S., Georgescu, M.M., and Birge, R.B. (2005). A role for Mer tyrosine kinase in alphavbeta5 integrin-mediated phagocytosis of apoptotic cells. J Cell Sci **118**, 539–553.

Wu, Y.C., and Horvitz, H.R. (1998). C. elegans phagocytosis and cell-migration protein CED-5 is similar to human DOCK180. Nature **392**, 501–504.

Wu, Y.C., Tsai, M.C., Cheng, L.C., Chou, C.J., and Weng, N.Y. (2001). C. elegans CED-12 acts in the conserved crkII/DOCK180/Rac pathway to control cell migration and cell corpse engulfment. Dev Cell **1**, 491–502.

Yang, H., Chen, Y.Z., Zhang, Y., Wang, X., Zhao, X., Godfroy, J.I., 3rd, Liang, Q., Zhang, M., Zhang, T., Yuan, Q., *et al.* (2015). A lysine-rich motif in the phosphatidylserine receptor PSR-1 mediates recognition and removal of apoptotic cells. Nat Commun **6**, 5717.

Young, R.W. (1967). The renewal of photoreceptor cell outer segments. J Cell Biol **33**, 61–72.

Young, R.W. (1971). The renewal of rod and cone outer segments in the rhesus monkey. J Cell Biol **49**, 303–318.

Young, R.W. (1977). The daily rhythm of shedding and degradation of cone outer segment membranes in the lizard retina. J Ultrastruct Res **61**, 172–185.

Young, R.W., and Bok, D. (1969). Participation of the retinal pigment epithelium in the rod outer segment renewal process. J Cell Biol **42**, 392–403.

Yu, F., and Schuldiner, O. (2014). Axon and dendrite pruning in Drosophila. Curr Opin Neurobiol **27**, 192–198.

Zagorska, A., Traves, P.G., Lew, E.D., Dransfield, I., and Lemke, G. (2014). Diversification of TAM receptor tyrosine kinase function. Nat Immunol **15**, 920–928.

Zhai, R.G., Cao, Y., Hiesinger, P.R., Zhou, Y., Mehta, S.Q., Schulze, K.L., Verstreken, P., and Bellen, H.J. (2006). Drosophila NMNAT maintains neural integrity independent of its NAD synthesis activity. PLoS Biol **4**, e416.

Zhan, Y., Paolicelli, R.C., Sforazzini, F., Weinhard, L., Bolasco, G., Pagani, F., Vyssotski, A.L., Bifone, A., Gozzi, A., Ragozzino, D., *et al.* (2014). Deficient neuron-microglia signaling results in impaired functional brain connectivity and social behavior. Nat Neurosci **17**, 400–406.

Zhou, Z., Caron, E., Hartwieg, E., Hall, A., and Horvitz, H.R. (2001a). The C. elegans PH domain protein CED-12 regulates cytoskeletal reorganization via a Rho/Rac GTPase signaling pathway. Dev Cell **1**, 477–489.

Zhou, Z., Hartwieg, E., and Horvitz, H.R. (2001b). CED-1 is a transmembrane receptor that mediates cell corpse engulfment in C. elegans. Cell **104**, 43–56.

Zhu, X., Libby, R.T., de Vries, W.N., Smith, R.S., Wright, D.L., Bronson, R.T., Seburn, K.L., and John, S.W. (2012). Mutations in a P-type ATPase gene cause axonal degeneration. PLoS Genet **8**, e1002853.

Ziegenfuss, J.S., Biswas, R., Avery, M.A., Hong, K., Sheehan, A.E., Yeung, Y.G., Stanley, E.R., and Freeman, M.R. (2008). Draper-dependent glial phagocytic activity is mediated by Src and Syk family kinase signalling. Nature **453**, 935–939.

Ziegenfuss, J.S., Doherty, J., and Freeman, M.R. (2012). Distinct molecular pathways mediate glial activation and engulfment of axonal debris after axotomy. Nat Neurosci **15**, 979–987.

5

Molecular Underpinnings of Developmental Axon Degeneration

Yu Yong[1], Kanchana Gamage[1], Sarah Hunter-Chang[1,2],
Ekaterina Stepanova[1,2], Sushanth Kumar[1,2], O. Yipkin Calhan[1,2],
Sarah Kucenas[1,2], and Christopher D. Deppmann[1,2]

[1]Department of Biology, University of Virginia, USA
[2]Program in Fundamental Neuroscience, University of Virginia, USA
Email: deppmann@virginia.edu

Abstract

During nervous system development, an overabundance of neurons, axons, and synapses is selectively eliminated to establish functional circuits. Axons compete for trophic cues, with winners stabilizing and losers degenerating. This chapter explores molecular pathways involved in axon degeneration, focusing on progressive axon stabilization pathways (e.g., PI3K-AKT, MAPK/ERK, calpastatin, etc.) and regressive pro-degenerative pathways (e.g., death receptors, JNK, DLK, calcium, calpain, etc.). Additionally, distinct axonal death pathways include soma-derived pro- and anti-degenerative cues. A more comprehensive understanding of the molecular mechanisms behind axon degeneration, the transitions between early and late degeneration phases, and the role of cell death pathways will provide invaluable insights into not only the development of the nervous system but also related diseases.

5.1 Introduction

During development of the nervous system, neurons are initially overproduced and then selectively eliminated to sculpt circuits (Burek & Oppenheim 1996). This process is mediated by the access to limited supply of trophic factors, molecules required for neuronal survival, which are produced by innervation targets (Levi-Montalcini 1987). Neurons then compete for these survival cues, and winners induce death in their neighbors via paracrine signaling to leave behind appropriately wired systems (Deppmann et al. 2008; Luo & O'Leary 2005).

Elimination of axons is a common feature in nervous system development, trauma, and neurodegenerative diseases. During nervous system development, an overabundance of neurons is born and many more axon branches are created than are ultimately required. At later stages of development, these excess neurons and axon branches are removed, leaving what is remaining to participate in the functional circuit. It is believed that the pathways involved in this process of developmental degeneration may also play a role in certain pathological conditions, where excessive pruning/degeneration occurs. As such, both pathological and developmental degeneration share morphological characteristics including beading and blebbing of axonal membranes as well as fragmentation and breakdown of the cytoskeleton (Martin et al. 1988; Raff et al. 2002; Wang et al. 2012). Consistent with this idea, neurodegenerative diseases such as Alzheimer's, Parkinson's, amyotrophic lateral sclerosis, and multiple sclerosis (MS) display axon loss morphologically indistinguishable from developmental degeneration (Coleman & Perry 2002; Luo & O'Leary 2005). Preservation of axonal structure has become an important therapeutic target for these disorders (Coleman & Perry 2002; De Vos et al. 2008; Luo & O'Leary 2005; Wang et al. 2012). While there are several excellent reviews on axon degeneration in pathologies like injury (Neukomm & Freeman 2014; Vargas & Barres 2007; Yong et al. 2021), there has been less emphasis of late on the emerging themes in developmental axon degeneration, which will be focused on herein. This chapter primarily focuses on developmental degeneration in vertebrate systems, but there are several excellent reviews on the seminal work performed in invertebrates (Furusawa & Emoto 2021; Lu & Mizumoto 2019; Williams & Truman 2005).

5.2 Models of Developmental Degeneration

There are two main categories of developmental axonal regressive events: retraction-like pruning and degeneration-like pruning (Riccomagno & Kolodkin 2015). Retraction occurs when axons draw back without shedding axonal material and can be observed during axon remodeling of the hippocampal infrapyramidal tract (IPT) (Bagri et al. 2003; Riccomagno et al. 2012). While retraction is a developmental regressive event, it is not generally considered a degenerative event. In contrast, developmental pruning eliminates circuitry by breakdown and elimination of the axonal material. It has hallmarks similar to non-developmental degeneration (e.g., injury-induced

Wallerian degeneration (WD)) including membrane blebbing/beading, formation of spheroids, loss of cytoskeletal integrity, and engulfment of debris by phagocytes (Nazareth et al. 2021; Van Broeckhoven et al. 2021; Yong et al. 2021). Pruning occurs in virtually all vertebrate neuron types; however, the molecular mechanism underlying stabilization versus degeneration is not as well characterized in the central nervous system (CNS) as it is in the peripheral nervous system (PNS). In the PNS, the decision to stabilize or degenerate is dictated by a competition for limiting amounts of target derived trophic factors like the neurotrophin family of ligands (Deppmann et al. 2008; Martin et al. 1992; Wang et al. 2012). Those that receive sufficient quantities of these trophic cues persist and those that do not, degenerate. Significantly, the mechanisms regulating degeneration induced by local and global triggers (such as trophic withdrawal on distal axons versus mass culture) are overlapping but distinct from caspase-dependent cell death pathways (Cusack et al. 2013; Geden et al. 2019). This may be important when an axon collateral is being degenerated while sparing the rest of the axonal arbor and/or entire neuron (Geden & Deshmukh 2016; Riccomagno & Kolodkin 2015).

Although all of the necessary components for developmental degeneration can be found within the axon, it is important to consider how non-neuronal cells influence degeneration. Such cells include ensheathing glia and phagocytic responders. Because of these roles for non-neuronal cells, a comprehensive understanding of degeneration requires its study in an *in vivo* context. In mammals like mice and rats, investigators have examined pruning in response to axonal interactions with repulsive cues like myelin, which is produced by non-neuronal Schwann cells and oligodendrocytes. Such an interaction occurs between septal neurons and the white matter of the corpus callosum (Park et al. 2010). Branch elimination is studied *in vivo* using whole mount organ staining and retrograde injection into final innervation targets (Glebova & Ginty 2004; Singh et al. 2008). While these approaches are advantageous because they are a reasonable approximation of general mammalian physiology (i.e., humans), conclusions drawn from them about axon degeneration are all based on inference because we can only examine developmental snap shots. Additionally, while genetic manipulations are both possible and common, mammals' slower gestation and maturation times, gamete inaccessibility, and smaller litter sizes can make the process of establishing a new transgenic line slow, difficult, and costly.

To overcome the disadvantages of mammalian *in vivo* studies, there are several other model systems well suited to study degeneration. Models such as zebrafish (*Danio rerio*), fruit flies (*Drosophila melanogaster*), and roundworms (*Caenorhabditis elegans*) are transparent, which allows for real-time imaging of axon degeneration *in vivo*. These live imaging studies frequently require cell labeling with an endogenously produced fluorescent marker to visualize processes of interest, which is made possible by the insertion of a transgene. Conveniently, transgenic zebrafish, fruit flies, and *C. elegans* are all easily generated through established methods such as injecting transgene-carrying plasmids into a fertilized egg. Such methods are used in tandem with live imaging to study developmental degeneration signaling pathways in *C. elegans* and in *Drosophila* (Lu & Mizumoto 2019; Williams & Truman 2005).

In vitro models have also been useful to interrogate the molecular pathways underlying developmental axon degeneration. By and large, sympathetic or sensory neurons from mice or rats are used to examine degeneration pathways. This is due to their relative ease of isolation and culture. These neurons are also exquisitely dependent on neurotrophic factors for both soma and axon survival (Levi-Montalcini 1965; Martin et al. 1992). When sympathetic or sensory neurons are grown in culture and deprived of nerve growth factor (NGF), the axons degenerate at (18–24 h later) and the cell bodies apoptose shortly thereafter (Deckwerth & Johnson 1993). This timing is typical of a global deprivation paradigm whereby both the cell body and axons lack access to trophic factor. While this is a convenient method to study axon degeneration, it is a bit different from the *in vivo* situation, where trophic factors responsible for promoting cell body and axon survival are derived from target tissues, setting up a scenario whereby axon collaterals from the same neuron might be receiving different amounts of target-derived trophic factor. Compartmentalized culture systems like Campenot chambers and microfluidic devices have been very useful toward modeling local trophic deprivation paradigms (Yong et al. 2020c). For example, a three chambered device where cell bodies are in the middle and axon branches can project into one of two chambers have been instrumental in uncovering the notion that branches may compete with each other (Singh et al. 2008). Another model of local trophic deprivation comes from two chambered Campenot chambers and microfluidic devices. In this paradigm, cell bodies are established in NGF and allowed to project to the other side of the device, which also contains a trophic factor. Once axons have projected, trophic factor is withdrawn from the axonal, but not cell body, side of the chamber. In this scenario, the cell body survives, but axons degenerate within 36–48 h (Cusack et al. 2013; MacInnis & Campenot 2005; Yong et al. 2019). It is important to note that the timing of degeneration appears to be sensitive to the volume of media that axons are bathed in, suggesting the role of autocrine/paracrine degenerative factors, which will be discussed more in the next section. Interestingly, the mechanism by which this degeneration occurs in local trophic deprivation appears to be distinct from the mechanism triggered in response to global deprivation. This axonal deprivation also triggers long-distance regressive signaling, which we have previously reviewed (Pathak et al. 2021).

5.3 Stages of Axon Degeneration

Axon degeneration is an evolutionary conserved process that can be activated by different stimuli, including trophic factor deprivation, mechanical damage, oxidative stress, and toxic drug incubation. After a degenerative trigger, axons undergo three distinct stages of degeneration: latent, transition, and catastrophic.

1. The latent phase varies in length of time depending on the trigger (typically 18–20 h after global trophic withdrawal in MFDs). In developmental degeneration, several factors are known to influence the length of this latency phase including transcription, anterograde transport of degenerative factors, activation of death receptors, and activation of caspases (Deckwerth & Johnson 1993; Deshmukh & Johnson 1997; Gamage et al. 2017a; Maor-Nof et al. 2016; Simon et al. 2016; Singh et al. 2008; Yong et al. 2019). In WD scenarios, there is a very short latent phase (roughly an hour after enucleation in MFDs) (Yong et al. 2020a). The molecular pathways regulating the duration of the latent phase in injury contexts is less well characterized; however, it does not appear to rely on de novo synthesis or death receptor activation (Yong et al. 2020a).

2. We have previously defined the onset of the transition phase with the formation of spheroids (Yong et al. 2019). These structures were first observed in spinal cord, distal to a site of injury by Ramon y Cajal, who indicated that "the voluminous balls along the nerves were the seat of destructive process," as they appeared earlier than nerve fragmentation (Ramón y Cajal 1928). Similar to injury in the CNS, crushed peripheral nerve fibers swell, causing a beaded spherical morphology (Gershenbaum & Roisen 1978). Axonal spheroids are also observed in the aging brain (Bridge et al. 2009), traumatic brain injury (TBI) (Newell et al. 1999), and many neurodegenerative diseases including Alzheimer's disease (AD) (Stokin et al. 2005), Parkinson's disease (PD) (Galvin et al. 1999), and amyotrophic lateral sclerosis (ALS) (Carpenter 1968). We recently found that spheroids arise at the transition between latency and catastrophic degeneration in both trophic

withdrawal and injury (Yong et al. 2019, 2020a). The function of axonal spheroids in degeneration has been largely overlooked. However, we have suggested that the rupture of growing spheroids corresponds to the release of a pro-degenerative molecule that helps a field of susceptible axons coordinately enter catastrophic degeneration. This transition phase lasts 20–40 min (Yong et al. 2019).

3.   The final stage of degeneration is a rapid and near synchronous "catastrophic"/execution phase, in which the cytoskeleton disintegrates (Beirowski et al. 2005; Rosenberg et al. 2012; Wang et al. 2012). In the catastrophic phase, molecules related to cytoskeleton breakdown, such as calpain, drive the final stage of axon disintegration (Ma et al. 2013; Salvadores et al. 2017). The degradation of calpastatin and activation of calpain are implicated in the common downstream pathways shared by both developmental degeneration and WD (Yang et al. 2013). Importantly, re-supplementation of NGF in previously trophically deprived axons in the early latent phase, but not in the late catastrophic phase, is able to reverse the degeneration progress in a manner dependent on *de novo* synthesis, suggesting the existence of "point of no return" in axon and neuronal death (Deckwerth & Johnson 1993).

5.4   Role of Cell Death Pathways in Developmental Axon Degeneration

Neuronal axons can be 1000 times larger in surface area and volume than their cell bodies (Friede 1963), giving rise to demanding axonal transport needs that make them susceptible to rupture and "supply chain issues." The intense metabolic demands of these transport processes combined with those of neuronal ion pumps result in extreme sensitivity to decreases in ATP availability and, subsequently, vulnerability to degeneration (Fricker et al. 2018). Axons typically degenerate before the neuronal soma must choose how it will die, a phenomenon sometimes termed "dying back" for its retrograde progression (Conforti et al. 2014; Raff et al. 2002). The interplay between axonal and neuronal death programs is complex and frequently involves multiple exchanges between the two compartments of the neuron.

A classic model for developmental pruning is trophic withdrawal. In sympathetic and some sensory neurons, this is accomplished by removing NGF either from the entire neuron or locally on axons using compartmentalized culture approaches. The mechanism by which NGF-TrkA signaling prevents apoptosis and degeneration is through activation of the pro-survival

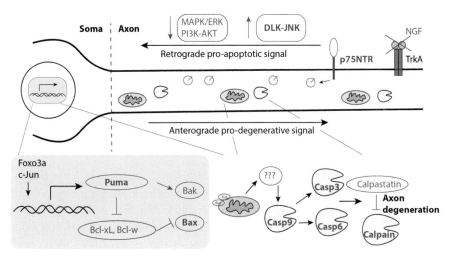

Figure 5.1 Developmental axon degeneration pathways. When neurons are deprived of NGF, the retrograde pro-apoptotic pathway initiated from p75NTR is activated, with decreased ERK and AKT signaling and increased DLK/JNK activity. The upregulation of transcriptional factors leads to increased expression of the pro-death BH3-only gene, Puma and inhibition of Bcl-2 family genes (Bcl-xL, Bcl-w) in the cell body. Puma induces anterograde pro-degenerative signaling by activating Bax. APAF-1 is dispensable for trophic withdrawal induced pruning so that the mechanism by which Bax transloaction induces caspase activation remains unclear. Activation of downstream caspase cascade leads to degredation of calpastatin and catastrophic axon degeneration.

PI3K-AKT (phosphoinositide 3-kinase-AKT/protein kinase B) and MAPK/ERK (mitogen-activated protein kinase/extracellular signal-regulated kinase) pathways.

The molecular pathways underlying local axon degeneration in development are well documented (Figure 5.1). Loss of these trophic signaling pathways initiates a retrograde activation of prodegenerative JNK and DLK signaling (Ghosh et al. 2011). Tessier-Lavigne and colleagues as well as Yaron and colleagues observed that locally depriving distal axons of NGF increased somal expression of the pro-apoptotic protein Puma (Maor-Nof et al. 2016; Simon et al. 2016). Puma overcomes the inhibition by pro-survival factors Bcl-xL and Bcl-w and initiates axon degeneration, indicating an important role for the cell body in developmental axon degeneration (Courchesne et al. 2011; Maor-Nof et al. 2016; Pease-Raissi et al. 2017; Pease & Segal 2014; Simon et al. 2016, 2021). Puma activation then triggers a change in anterograde trafficking of an as-yet unknown degeneration-inducing protein along the axon, which could be prevented by transection from the soma. Curiously, this is the opposite of a speculative, anterogradely trafficked anti-degeneration cue hypothesized to be lost during WD (Lubińska 1982). The Coleman group has definitively shown that the NAD+ producing enzyme, and NMNAT2 is likely to be this anterograde survival cue (Coleman & Freeman 2010; Coleman & Höke 2020; Gilley et al. 2013; Milde et al. 2013). This suggests at least two distinct pathways for axonal death: one for delivery of a soma-derived pro-degenerative cue, and one for transection-like deaths that could also involve a soma-derived anti-degenerative cue. However, it is likely that there are more trafficked degeneration regulators to be elucidated (Pathak et al. 2021).

It is important to note that there are differences in trophic withdrawal-induced cell death versus axon degeneration pathways. While Bax is involved in both axon degeneration and cell death, Apaf-1 appears to be dispensable for axonal pruning induced by local NGF deprivation (Geden et al. 2019). Apaf-1 is a crucial component of the apoptosome, along with Caspase 9 and cytochrome C, which raises questions about how Caspase-9 is activated during local deprivation in the absence of Apaf-1. This also casts doubt on whether the release of cytochrome C into the axoplasm is necessary to initiate the activation of Caspase 9 and the downstream effector caspases 3 and 6 following local trophic deprivation (Cusack et al. 2013; Simon et al. 2012). Interestingly, aging can also play a role in neuronal susceptibility to trophic withdrawal. Sympathetic neurons aged 28 days *in vitro* do not degenerate in response to global trophic withdrawal but are still susceptible to degeneration triggered by local withdrawal (Cusack et al. 2013). Deshmukh and colleagues have proposed that the expression of XIAP may limit axon-selective degeneration and may be the mechanism underlying the age-related difference in susceptibility to global versus local trophic deprivation (Cusack et al. 2013).

Much of the work surrounding axon degeneration has centered around components of the apoptotic machinery. More recent evidence suggests that engagement of necroptotic signaling proteins may also play a role in mediating axon demise following injury and other pathological triggers. Necroptosis is a form of regulated necrosis traditionally orchestrated by the receptor interacting protein kinases 1 and 3 (RIPK1 and RIPK3) and the pseudokinase MLKL (Degterev et al. 2005, 2008; Linkermann & Green 2014). Pharmacologic inhibition of RIPK1 or genetic knockdown of either RIPK3 or MLKL offered protection against injury-induced degeneration in both CNS and PNS axons (Arrázola et al. 2019; Ko et al. 2020). Given the frequent overlap in axonal death mechanisms across contexts, whether or not necroptosis also occurs in developmental degeneration merits further consideration.

SARMoptosis, a type of non-caspase-dependent cell death, has primarily been associated with injury-induced degeneration and cell death after viral infection (DiAntonio 2019; Leak & Dixon 2023; Panneerselvam & Ding 2015; Sankar et al. 2023). Surprisingly, loss of *SARM1* appears to accelerate the spread of axon degeneration in response to trophic deprivation (Gamage et al. 2017b), which contrasts with the dramatic protection observed in injured *Sarm1$^{-/-}$* axons (Henninger et al. 2016; Osterloh et al. 2012).

5.5 Role of Death Receptors in Developmental Axon Degeneration

Death receptors (DRs) are members of the tumor necrosis factor receptor (TNFR) superfamily (TNFRSF) whose cytoplasmic tail contains a conserved death domain (DD). In spite of their name, DRs can trigger either cell death or survival. During development, DRs and their ligands regulate neuronal expansion, growth, differentiation, and regional pattern formation, processes critical for brain development (Twohig et al. 2011). In neurodegenerative diseases, DR expression and signaling mediate neuronal death, axon degeneration, excitotoxicity, and inflammation (Haase et al. 2008). Adapter proteins, along with other binding partners, are recruited by means of DD-interaction to transduce DR signals. For example, Fas, DR4, and DR5 primarily bind Fas-associated DD (FADD), while tumor necrosis factor receptor 1 (TNFR1), DR3, and DR6 primarily bind TNFR-associated DD (TRADD) to promote downstream signaling events (Mc Guire et al. 2011; Walczak 2013).

Previous studies describe that developmental axon pruning involves the death receptor p75 neurotrophin receptor (p75NTR) and one of its ligands, brain-derived neurotrophic factor (BDNF) (Park et al. 2010; Singh et al. 2008). Developmental cell death and axonal loss appear to be driven by competition between antagonistic trophic and "punishment" signaling pathways, which promote axon stability or degeneration, respectively (Deppmann et al. 2008; Singh et al. 2008). Interestingly, the punishment pathways appear to rely on autocrine/paracrine mechanisms allowing "strong" axons to expedite the elimination of weaker neighbors. The highly related TNFRSF members, p75NTR, TNFR1α, and DR6 are implicated in this extrinsic degeneration program in the peripheral nervous system (PNS) (Olsen et al. 2014; Park et al. 2010; Singh et al. 2008; Vilar et al. 2009; Wheeler et al. 2014). For example, mice deficient in p75NTR or its ligand, BDNF, display hyperinnervation of sympathetic target organs suggesting that p75NTR and BDNF are essential for axonal pruning *in vitro* and *in vivo* (Lee et al. 1994; Singh et al. 2008). Similarly, DR6 promotes axon degeneration in developmental paradigms (Olsen et al. 2014).

Axon degeneration induced by death receptors is also impacted by trophic signaling. When trophic signaling (e.g. NGF-TrkA) is high, TNFR family members are unable to induce degeneration. The molecular basis of this cross-talk remains unknown. Lack of NGF-TrkA signaling permits the prodegenerative cues originating from death receptors, including TNFR1a, p75NTR, and DR6, which have been implicated in developmental axon degeneration in the PNS (Barker et al. 2001; Olsen et al. 2014; Park et al. 2010; Wheeler et al. 2014). p75NTR and DR6 will be explored further below.

p75NTR:

p75NTR is widely expressed in the developing nervous system, including sympathetic, sensory, and motor neurons, as well as glial cells. The expression of p75NTR is diminished in adulthood but can be upregulated or re-expressed in response to injury or degenerative insult (Ibáñez & Simi 2012; Zeng et al. 2011). Similar to other DRs, the extracellular structure of p75NTR is highlighted by conserved cysteine-rich domains (CRDs), responsible for binding to all the neurotrophins (NGF, BDNF, NT-3, and NT-4/5) and their pro-forms with similar affinities (Chao 1994; Teng et al. 2010). Unlike other death receptors, p75NTR does not signal through the recruitment of adaptor proteins by its DD. Depending on the ligand and co-receptor, p75NTR can initiate pro-survival and pro-apoptotic signals and regulate cell cycle entry, axonal elongation, and synaptic transmission (Dechant & Barde 2002; Meeker & Williams 2015; Yamashita et al. 2005).

In the presence of NGF, p75NTR interacts with the TrkA receptor to promote sympathetic neuron survival through activation of phosphoinositide 3-kinase (PI3K)-AKT, Ras-mitogen-activated protein kinase (MAPK), and nuclear factor kappa light chain enhancer of activated B-cells (NF-κB) pathways (Gentry et al. 2004). However, when sympathetic neurons are maintained with low quantities of NGF or KCl, BDNF can activate the p75NTR and c-Jun N-terminal kinase (JNK) pathway to cause neuronal apoptosis (Bamji et al. 1998). During developmental sympathetic axon competition, BDNF secreted from active axons drives the activation of p75NTR on "losing" axons to cause degeneration (Singh et al. 2008). Moreover, p75NTR also modulates neural connectivity in the intact mature nervous system. Specifically, myelin triggers local axon degeneration by p75NTR-dependent sequestration of Rho guanine nucleotide dissociation inhibitor (Rho-GDI) and downstream activation of Rho and caspase-6 (Park et al. 2010). Importantly, p75NTR forms disulfide-linked dimers through the highly conserved Cys^{257}

in its transmembrane domain in both the liganded and unliganded condition. This suggests that the p75NTR is activated via conformational change rather than oligomerization. Upon neurotrophin binding, the close association between dimeric p75NTR DDs is transiently disrupted by a conformational change to allow binding of the caspase recruitment domain of RIP2 kinase for activation of the NF-kB pathway, competing with the binding of Rho-GDI for Rho activation (Lin et al. 2015; Tanaka et al. 2016; Vilar et al. 2009). Additionally, proteolysis of p75NTR in axons by the metalloprotease TNFα-converting enzyme (also known as a disintegrin and metalloprotease (ADAM)17) and γ-secretase are required for generation of the intracellular domain of p75NTR for retrograde degenerative signaling in response to trophic deprivation or oxidative stress (Kraemer et al. 2014; Pathak et al. 2018). Recent studies demonstrate that p75NTR mediates retrograde pro-apoptotic signaling in response to trophic deprivation or BDNF binding to p75NTR (Pathak et al. 2018). Whether and how p75NTR and other death receptors interact with retrograde and anterograde pro-degenerative signals in response to local NGF deprivation require further investigation.

It is widely appreciated that p75NTR is important for axon degeneration in sympathetic and basal forebrain cholinergic neurons (BFCNs) in response to trophic withdrawal; however, it has long been unclear what phase of axon degeneration p75NTR participates in (Park et al. 2010; Singh & Miller 2005; Singh et al. 2008). We recently reported that p75NTR acts during the latent phase of axon degeneration but not during the catastrophic phase (Yong et al. 2019, 2021). We also found that p75NTR is upstream of prodegenerative transcription, Rho and caspase activity, all of which are required to promote spheroid formation, thereby gating entry into the catastrophic phase of degeneration. It is possible that this pathway governs the length of the latency window. In the context of injury, p75NTR does not seem to impact the kinetics of degeneration; however, it is an integral protein for Schwann cell response to injury (Boerboom et al. 2017; Song et al. 2006; Yong et al. 2020a).

DR6:

DR6 is a single-pass transmembrane receptor that possesses four extracellular TNFR-like CRDs, a transmembrane domain, and a cytoplasmic DD related to those of all known DRs (Pan et al. 1998). DR6 is expressed in most human tissues, and abundant transcripts are detected in heart, brain, placenta, pancreas, thymus, lymph node, and several non-lymphoid cancer cell lines (Pan et al. 1998). Studies show that DR6 associates with TRADD but not FADD to couple to downstream caspases and activation of NF-κB and JNK (Kasof et al. 2001; Pan et al. 1998).

DR6 did not receive much attention in the field of degeneration until the identification of amyloid precursor protein (APP) as a potential ligand for DR6 in axonal pruning. It was reported that trophic factor deprivation could trigger β-secretase (BACE)-dependent shedding of surface APP, which binds DR6 and activates caspase 6 to promote axon degeneration (Nikolaev et al. 2009). However, further genetic and biochemical analyses revealed that the *n*-terminal portion of APP is not a *bona fide* ligand of DR6 (Kuester et al. 2011; Olsen et al. 2014). However, it has been suggested that DR6 and APP may act as co-receptors (Xu et al. 2015).

We previously described a role for DR6 in mediating degeneration in response to both trophic withdrawal and injury (Yong et al. 2019, 2020a). Interestingly, we found that DR6 is not required for the formation of spheroids. Instead, it is important for responding to the prodegenerative factors released by ruptured axons, placing its participation at the beginning of the catastrophic phase of degeneration (Yong et al. 2019). DR6 has also been shown to mediate spinal cord axonal degeneration induced by prion peptide (Wang et al. 2015). It is important to note that DR6 is not universally required for axon degeneration. For example, DR6 is not required for axonal degeneration in injured retinal ganglion cells (Fernandes et al. 2018; Vohra et al. 2010).

Interestingly, in addition to the cell autonomous function of DR6 in axon degeneration, a recent study has revealed a non-cell autonomous function of DR6 in Schwann cell proliferation (Colombo et al. 2018). As a novel substrate for ADAM10 and γ-secretase, neuronal DR6 was found to be cleaved and act *in trans* on Schwann cells to mediate their proliferation and myelination during development, independently of its cytoplasmic DD (Colombo et al. 2018).

Cultured sympathetic neurons deprived of NGF experience significant axon degeneration, with about 50% of neurites disintegrating within approximately 18 h (Deckwerth & Johnson 1993). However, this process can be delayed to roughly 24 h in the absence of *p75NTR* or *DR6* (Gamage et al. 2017b). By 36 h of trophic withdrawal in sensory neurons, *DR6$^{-/-}$ axons* displayed a very modest protection compared to wild-type controls (Olsen et al. 2014).

5.6 Calcium Signaling in Axon Degeneration

It is widely appreciated that axoplasmic calcium concentrations increase as axons degenerate (Wang et al. 2012; Yong et al. 2019). Such calcium transients act as temporal and spatial cues that trigger pruning and can be compartmentalized to branches targeted for destruction (Adalbert et al. 2012; Kanamori et al. 2013; Vargas et al. 2015). Even within such a compartment, however, calcium is not evenly distributed. Axonal spheroids concentrate up to 10 times more calcium compared to surrounding axonal regions (Barsukova et al. 2012). These spheroids can then rupture, expelling calcium into the surrounding areas *in vitro* (Yong et al. 2019), the effects of which are unknown. The calcium that remains within the axon continues to increase, eventually activating the protease calpain and another set of destructive machinery, the ubiquitin proteasome system, which culminates in breakdown of the axon (Yang et al. 2013; Watts et al. 2003). During the latency phase, there are robust axoplasmic calcium transients, but calpain-induced degeneration is prevented. According to Tessier-Lavigne and colleagues, this is due to the gradual degradation of the calpain inhibitor, Calpastatin, following injury or trophic withdrawal. This degradation can be reversed in the absence of Sarm1 or Caspase-3, respectively, indicating an important mechanism for controlling the transition from latent to catastrophic degeneration (Yang et al., 2013).

Where does rising axoplasmic calcium come from? It has been observed that chelating extracellular calcium delays fragmentation in response to trophic deprivation (Johnstone et al. 2019; Vargas et al. 2015). This extracellular calcium passes through membrane channels in a variety of degenerative contexts; blocking calcium-specific channels or their subunits such as voltage-gated calcium channels (VGCCs) and sodium-calcium exchanger (NCX) can delay axonal degeneration in response to injury or oxidative stress (Barsukova et al. 2012; Dombert et al. 2017; LoPachin & Lehning 1997; Ribas et al. 2017; Tabata et al. 2018; Tedeschi et al. 2016). This suggests that calcium influx from the extracellular space via calcium channels and NCX reversal contribute to axon degeneration. However, the subtypes of calcium channels involved in the degeneration process may be dependent on neuronal types and the degenerative trigger. It is also possible that extracellular calcium enters non-selectively across the axonal plasma membrane via nanoscale ruptures, as observed in a multiple sclerosis model of axon degeneration (Witte et al. 2019).

Intracellular stores within the endoplasmic reticulum (ER) and mitochondria also contribute to the axonal calcium rise observed in degeneration. Preventing calcium release through pharmacological depletion of ER calcium stores, blockage of ryanodine and IP_3 receptors, disruption of the mitochondrial permeability transition pore (mPTP), or inhibiting store-operated calcium entry (SOCE) inhibit cytoskeletal degradation and secondary axonal degeneration (Orem et al. 2017, 2020; Staal et al. 2010; Tian et al. 2020; Villegas et al. 2014). As such, both extracellular calcium and intracellular stores contribute to axon degeneration in various degenerative etiologies, though their exact mechanisms may vary depending on developmental context.

5.7 Contrasting Developmental Degeneration with Wallerian Degeneration

One of the best studied models of degeneration is injury-induced or WD. Similar to developmental degeneration, WD is characterized by break up of endoplasmic reticulum (ER), swelling, and local accumulation of mitochondria and fragmentation of neurofilaments (Vial 1958; Webster 1962). WD also has three stages of degeneration; however, in contrast to developmental degeneration, WD has a very short lag phase preceded by a rapid burst of calcium influx immediately after injury. The difference in latent phase duration between developmental pruning and injury paradigms suggests distinct pathways.

One of the most surprising differences between trophic withdrawal and injury is the role of Caspases. As outlined in Section 5.4, Caspases-3, -6, and -9, as well as Bax translocation have been implicated in trophic deprivation-mediated pruning (Cusack et al. 2013; Schoenmann et al. 2010; Simon et al. 2012). Notably, Deshmukh and colleagues make a compelling argument that degeneration induced by trophic degeneration of the entire neuron versus local axon trophic deprivation use distinct mechanisms, with global trophic deprivation more closely resembling conventional apoptotic pathways (Geden & Deshmukh 2016). In contrast, Caspase 3 and Bax are not essential for injury-induced degeneration (Simon et al. 2012; Whitmore et al. 2003).

In the past, we and others have found that pharmacologically inhibiting transcription blocks axon degeneration after trophic withdrawal (Deckwerth & Johnson 1993; Maor-Nof et al. 2016; Simon et al. 2016; Yong et al. 2019). However, this is not the case for injury-induced degeneration where axons lose their connection to the cell body and thus lose their ability to receive new transcripts. Collectively, these findings suggest that during the latent phase of trophic withdrawal-induced degeneration, *de novo* synthesis and caspase activation are required, whereas Wallerian degeneration (WD) does not require these processes.

It is known that injury-induced degeneration is regulated by the levels of nicotinamide adenine dinucleotide (NAD+) (Figure 5.2). Wallerian degeneration-slow (Wld^S) mutant mice contain an in-frame fusion protein composed of full-length nicotinamide mononucleotide adenylyltransferase 1 (NMNAT1) and N-terminal 70 amino acids of E4-type ubiquitin ligase

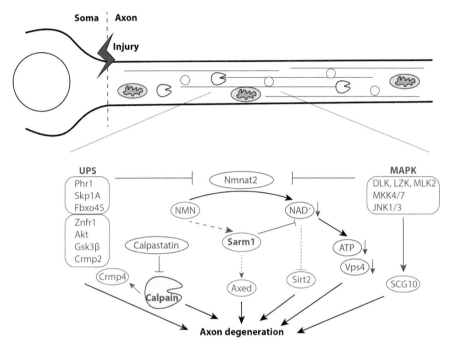

Figure 5.2 Wallerian degeneration pathways. In response to injury, activation of MAPK signaling cascade and UPS lead to NMNAT2 degradation, increase of NMN/NAD$^+$ ratio, and subsequent Sarm1 activation. Energy depletion along the axons and the cytoskeleton breakdown mediated by calpain, Axed, Sirt2, SCG10, and CRMP2/4 promote catastrophic axon degeneration.

(Ube4b) (Coleman & Freeman 2010; Conforti et al. 2000; Mack et al. 2001). This allows for increased biosynthesis of NAD$^+$, which prevents injured axons from degenerating. Likewise, axonal protection after injury can be provided by overexpressing the NMNAT enzyme (Magni et al. 2004). Three NMNAT mammalian isoforms have different subcellular localizations: Nmnat1 is localized to the nucleus; Nmnat2 is found in the cytoplasm and trafficked anterogradely in the axoplasm; and Nmnat3 is mostly localized to mitochondria, allowing compartmentalization of NAD$^+$ metabolic pools for diverse cellular activities (Di Stefano & Conforti 2013). When NAD+ catabolism is inhibited through loss of the NADase, Sterile alpha, and TIR motif containing 1 (Sarm1), injury-induced axon degeneration is also inhibited (Gerdts et al. 2013, 2015; Osterloh et al. 2012).

Do NAD+ levels also influence degeneration induced by trophic withdrawal? Neurons cultured from mice harboring *Wld^s* or overexpressing of

NMNAT display delayed degeneration in response to trophic withdrawal; however, the phenotype does not appear as dramatic as observed in injury indicating parallel and perhaps redundant pathways that are present in developmentally degenerating but not WD axons (Vohra et al. 2010; Gamage et al. 2017b). Interestingly, neurons lacking *Sarm1* remain susceptible to degeneration induced by trophic withdrawal (Gamage et al. 2017b; Osterloh et al. 2012). These findings suggest that the rate of NAD+ depletion determines the length of the latent phase in injured axons, but this does not apply to trophic deprivation.

Because of the morphological similarity between all forms of axon degeneration, it is tempting to speculate that disparate triggers funnel toward a common catastrophic degeneration pathway. Regardless of the degenerative trigger, the latent and catastrophic phases appear to be demarcated by the appearance of spheroids (Yong et al. 2021). Therefore, the regulators of latency in trophic deprivation or Wallerian degeneration are also upstream regulators of spheroid formation and rupture, within their respective contexts (Yong et al. 2019, 2020a).

Axon degeneration induced by trophic withdrawal and WD converge on the Calpain/calpastatin axis described above to enter the catastrophic phase of degeneration (Yang et al. 2013). We have previously found that spheroid formation and rupture are upstream of calpain activation after trophic deprivation (Yong et al. 2019). Whether and how spheroid formation and rupture leads to activation of degradation of calpastatin and activation of Calpain remains to be determined.

5.8 Conclusions and Future Directions

Developmental degeneration is an essential process in sculpting an efficient and functional nervous system. This type of pruning has long been studied apart from pathological degenerative triggers like Alzheimer's disease or injury. We now appreciate that although axonal degeneration can have many different triggers, the catastrophic phase of degeneration may be mediated by pathways common to different etiologies. While degeneration is described in many different developmental and pathological contexts, it remains to be seen whether these different "flavors" of degeneration are more like trophic withdrawal or more like injury (WD). Because many neurodegenerative disorders display impaired retrograde trafficking, which would mimic trophic withdrawal, it stands to reason that disorders like ALS or Parkinson's would be more similar to developmental degeneration. On the other hand, chemotherapeutic neuropathy, which is often the result of damaged neuronal cytoskeleton, may be similar to WD. Determining whether different etiologies of degeneration can be binned between developmental or WD types will be a profitable avenue of future investigation.

Beyond understanding the differences in molecular mechanisms between different etiologies of degeneration, there remain several open questions:

1. Because we now appreciate that degeneration occurs in different phases, it will be important to place previously identified molecular players in this degeneration timeline. This will be critical as we seek to understand how transitions from latent to catastrophic phases occur.

2. Determining how cell death pathways, particularly non-apoptotic pathways, are repurposed to promote axon degeneration.

3. Understanding the functionally antagonistic relationship between trophic signaling and regressive signaling.

4. Examining the role of phagocytosis in mediating degeneration.

A better mechanistic appreciation of degeneration will not only inform a general logic for neural development but will also help us rationalize anti-degeneration therapies.

References

Adalbert R, Morreale G, Paizs M, Conforti L, Walker SA, et al. 2012. Intra-axonal calcium changes after axotomy in wild-type and slow Wallerian degeneration axons. *Neuroscience.* **225**:44–54

Arrázola MS, Saquel C, Catalán RJ, Barrientos SA, Hernandez DE, et al. 2019. Axonal degeneration is mediated by necroptosis activation. *J. Neurosci.* **39(20)**:3832–44

Bagri A, Cheng H-J, Yaron A, Pleasure SJ, Tessier-Lavigne M. 2003. Stereotyped pruning of long hippocampal axon branches triggered by retraction inducers of the semaphorin family. *Cell.* **113(3)**:285–99

Bamji SX, Majdan M, Pozniak CD, Belliveau DJ, Aloyz R, et al. 1998. The p75 neurotrophin receptor mediates neuronal apoptosis and is essential for naturally occurring sympathetic neuron death. *J. Cell Biol.* **140(4)**:911–23

Barker V, Middleton G, Davey F, Davies AM. 2001. TNFalpha contributes to the death of NGF-dependent neurons during development. *Nat. Neurosci.* **4(12)**:1194–98

Barsukova AG, Forte M, Bourdette D. 2012. Focal increases of axoplasmic Ca2+, aggregation of sodium-calcium exchanger, N-type Ca2+ channel, and actin define the sites of spheroids in axons undergoing oxidative stress. *J. Neurosci.* **32(35)**:12028–37

Beirowski B, Adalbert R, Wagner D, Grumme DS, Addicks K, et al. 2005. The progressive nature of Wallerian degeneration in wild-type and slow Wallerian degeneration (WldS) nerves. *BMC Neurosci.* **6**:6

Boerboom A, Dion V, Chariot A, Franzen R. 2017. Molecular mechanisms involved in schwann cell plasticity. *Front. Mol. Neurosci.* **10**:38

Bridge KE, Berg N, Adalbert R, Babetto E, Dias T, et al. 2009. Late onset distal axonal swelling in YFP-H transgenic mice. *Neurobiol. Aging.* **30(2)**:309–21

Burek MJ, Oppenheim RW. 1996. Programmed cell death in the developing nervous system. *Brain Pathol.* **6(4)**:427–46

Carpenter S. 1968. Proximal axonal enlargement in motor neuron disease. *Neurology.* 18(9):841–51

Chao MV. 1994. The p75 neurotrophin receptor. *J. Neurobiol.* 25(11):1373–85

Coleman MP, Freeman MR. 2010. Wallerian degeneration, wld(s), and nmnat. *Annu. Rev. Neurosci.* **33**:245–67

Coleman MP, Höke A. 2020. Programmed axon degeneration: from mouse to mechanism to medicine. *Nat. Rev. Neurosci.* **21(4)**:183–96

Coleman MP, Perry VH. 2002. Axon pathology in neurological disease: a neglected therapeutic target. *Trends Neurosci.* **25(10)**:532–37

Colombo A, Hsia H-E, Wang M, Kuhn P-H, Brill MS, et al. 2018. Non-cell-autonomous function of DR6 in Schwann cell proliferation. *EMBO J.* **37(7)**:

Conforti L, Gilley J, Coleman MP. 2014. Wallerian degeneration: an emerging axon death pathway linking injury and disease. *Nat. Rev. Neurosci.* **15(6)**:394–409

Conforti L, Tarlton A, Mack TG, Mi W, Buckmaster EA, et al. 2000. A Ufd2/D4Cole1e chimeric protein and overexpression of Rbp7 in the slow Wallerian degeneration (WldS) mouse. *Proc Natl Acad Sci USA.* **97(21)**:11377–82

Courchesne SL, Karch C, Pazyra-Murphy MF, Segal RA. 2011. Sensory neuropathy attributable to loss of Bcl-w. *J. Neurosci.* **31(5)**:1624–34

Cusack CL, Swahari V, Hampton Henley W, Michael Ramsey J, Deshmukh M. 2013. Distinct pathways mediate axon degeneration during apoptosis and axon-specific pruning. *Nat. Commun.* **4**:1876

Dechant G, Barde Y-A. 2002. The neurotrophin receptor p75(NTR): novel functions and implications for diseases of the nervous system. *Nat. Neurosci.* **5(11)**:1131–36

Deckwerth TL, Johnson EM. 1993. Temporal analysis of events associated with programmed cell death (apoptosis) of sympathetic neurons deprived of nerve growth factor. *J. Cell Biol.* **123(5)**:1207–22

Degterev A, Hitomi J, Germscheid M, Ch'en IL, Korkina O, et al. 2008. Identification of RIP1 kinase as a specific cellular target of necrostatins. *Nat. Chem. Biol.* **4(5)**:313–21

Degterev A, Huang Z, Boyce M, Li Y, Jagtap P, et al. 2005. Chemical inhibitor of nonapoptotic cell death with therapeutic potential for ischemic brain injury. *Nat. Chem. Biol.* **1(2)**:112–19

Deppmann CD, Mihalas S, Sharma N, Lonze BE, Niebur E, Ginty DD. 2008. A model for neuronal competition during development. *Science.* **320**(5874):369–73

Deshmukh M, Johnson EM. 1997. Programmed cell death in neurons: focus on the pathway of nerve growth factor deprivation-induced death of sympathetic neurons. *Mol. Pharmacol.* **51(6)**:897–906

De Vos KJ, Grierson AJ, Ackerley S, Miller CCJ. 2008. Role of axonal transport in neurodegenerative diseases. *Annu. Rev. Neurosci.* **31**:151–73

DiAntonio A. 2019. Axon degeneration: mechanistic insights lead to therapeutic opportunities for the prevention and treatment of peripheral neuropathy. *Pain.* **160** Suppl 1(Suppl 1):S17–22

Di Stefano M, Conforti L. 2013. Diversification of NAD biological role: the importance of location. *FEBS J.* **280(19)**:4711–28

Dombert B, Balk S, Lüningschrör P, Moradi M, Sivadasan R, et al. 2017. BDNF/trkB Induction of Calcium Transients through Cav2.2 Calcium Channels in Motoneurons Corresponds to F-actin Assembly and Growth Cone Formation on β2-Chain Laminin (221). *Front. Mol. Neurosci.* **10**:346

Fernandes KA, Mitchell KL, Patel A, Marola OJ, Shrager P, et al. 2018. Role of SARM1 and DR6 in retinal ganglion cell axonal and somal degeneration following axonal injury. *Exp. Eye Res.* **171**:54–61

Fricker M, Tolkovsky AM, Borutaite V, Coleman M, Brown GC. 2018. Neuronal Cell Death. *Physiol. Rev.* **98(2)**:813–80

Friede RL. 1963. The relationship of body size, nerve cell size, axon length, and glial density in the cerebellum. *Proc Natl Acad Sci USA.* **49**:187–93

Furusawa K, Emoto K. 2021. Spatiotemporal regulation of developmental neurite pruning: Molecular and cellular insights from Drosophila models. *Neurosci. Res.* **167**:54–63

Galvin JE, Uryu K, Lee VM, Trojanowski JQ. 1999. Axon pathology in Parkinson's disease and Lewy body dementia hippocampus contains alpha-, beta-, and gamma-synuclein. *Proc Natl Acad Sci USA.* **96(23)**:13450–55

Gamage KK, Cheng I, Park RE, Karim MS, Edamura K, et al. 2017a. Death receptor 6 promotes wallerian degeneration in peripheral axons. *Curr. Biol.* **27(8)**:1250

Gamage KK, Cheng I, Park RE, Karim MS, Edamura K, et al. 2017b. Death receptor 6 promotes wallerian degeneration in peripheral axons. *Curr. Biol.* **27(6)**:890–96

Geden MJ, Deshmukh M. 2016. Axon degeneration: context defines distinct pathways. *Curr. Opin. Neurobiol.* **39**:108–15

Geden MJ, Romero SE, Deshmukh M. 2019. Apoptosis versus axon pruning: Molecular intersection of two distinct pathways for axon degeneration. *Neurosci. Res.* **139**:3–8

Gentry JJ, Barker PA, Carter BD. 2004. The p75 neurotrophin receptor: multiple interactors and numerous functions. In *NGF and Related Molecules in Health and Disease*, Vol. **146**, pp. 25–39. Elsevier

Gerdts J, Brace EJ, Sasaki Y, DiAntonio A, Milbrandt J. 2015. SARM1 activation triggers axon degeneration locally via NAD$^+$ destruction. *Science.* **348(6233)**:453–57

Gerdts J, Summers DW, Sasaki Y, DiAntonio A, Milbrandt J. 2013. Sarm1-mediated axon degeneration requires both SAM and TIR interactions. *J. Neurosci.* **33(33)**:13569–80

Gershenbaum MR, Roisen FJ. 1978. A scanning electron microscopic study of peripheral nerve degeneration and regeneration. *Neuroscience.* **3(12)**:1241–50

Ghosh AS, Wang B, Pozniak CD, Chen M, Watts RJ, Lewcock JW. 2011. DLK induces developmental neuronal degeneration via selective regulation of proapoptotic JNK activity. *J. Cell Biol.* **194(5)**:751–64

Gilley J, Adalbert R, Yu G, Coleman MP. 2013. Rescue of peripheral and CNS axon defects in mice lacking NMNAT2. *J. Neurosci.* **33(33)**:13410–24

Glebova NO, Ginty DD. 2004. Heterogeneous requirement of NGF for sympathetic target innervation in vivo. *J. Neurosci.* **24(3)**:743–51

Haase G, Pettmann B, Raoul C, Henderson CE. 2008. Signaling by death receptors in the nervous system. *Curr. Opin. Neurobiol.* **18(3)**:284–91

Henninger N, Bouley J, Sikoglu EM, An J, Moore CM, et al. 2016. Attenuated traumatic axonal injury and improved functional outcome after traumatic brain injury in mice lacking Sarm1. *Brain.* **139**(Pt 4):1094–1105

Ibáñez CF, Simi A. 2012. p75 neurotrophin receptor signaling in nervous system injury and degeneration: paradox and opportunity. *Trends Neurosci.* **35(7)**:431–40

Johnstone AD, de Léon A, Unsain N, Gibon J, Barker PA. 2019. Developmental Axon Degeneration Requires TRPV1-Dependent Ca2+ Influx. *eNeuro.* **6**(1):

Kanamori T, Kanai MI, Dairyo Y, Yasunaga K, Morikawa RK, Emoto K. 2013. Compartmentalized calcium transients trigger dendrite pruning in Drosophila sensory neurons. *Science.* **340(6139)**:1475–78

Kasof GM, Lu JJ, Liu D, Speer B, Mongan KN, et al. 2001. Tumor necrosis factor-alpha induces the expression of DR6, a member of the TNF receptor family, through activation of NF-kappaB. *Oncogene.* **20(55)**:7965–75

Ko KW, Milbrandt J, DiAntonio A. 2020. SARM1 acts downstream of neuroinflammatory and necroptotic signaling to induce axon degeneration. *J. Cell Biol.* **219(8)**:

Kraemer BR, Snow JP, Vollbrecht P, Pathak A, Valentine WM, et al. 2014. A role for the p75 neurotrophin receptor in axonal degeneration and apoptosis induced by oxidative stress. *J. Biol. Chem.* **289(31)**:21205–16

Kuester M, Kemmerzehl S, Dahms SO, Roeser D, Than ME. 2011. The crystal structure of death receptor 6 (DR6): a potential receptor of the amyloid precursor protein (APP). *J. Mol. Biol.* **409(2)**:189–201

Leak L, Dixon SJ. 2023. Surveying the landscape of emerging and understudied cell death mechanisms. *Biochim. Biophys. Acta Mol. Cell Res.* **1870(3)**:119432

Lee KF, Davies AM, Jaenisch R. 1994. p75-deficient embryonic dorsal root sensory and neonatal sympathetic neurons display a decreased sensitivity to NGF. *Development.* **120(4)**:1027–33

Levi-Montalcini R. 1965. Growth regulation of sympathetic nerve cells. *Arch. Ital. Biol.* **103(4)**:832–46

Levi-Montalcini R. 1987. The nerve growth factor 35 years later. *Science.* **237(4819)**:1154–62

Linkermann A, Green DR. 2014. Necroptosis. *N. Engl. J. Med.* **370(5)**:455–65

Lin Z, Tann JY, Goh ETH, Kelly C, Lim KB, et al. 2015. Structural basis of death domain signaling in the p75 neurotrophin receptor. *eLife.* **4**:e11692

LoPachin RM, Lehning EJ. 1997. Mechanism of calcium entry during axon injury and degeneration. *Toxicol. Appl. Pharmacol.* **143(2)**:233–44

Lubińska L. 1982. Patterns of Wallerian degeneration of myelinated fibres in short and long peripheral stumps and in isolated segments of rat phrenic nerve. Interpretation of the role of axoplasmic flow of the trophic factor. *Brain Res.* **233(2)**:227–40

Luo L, O'Leary DDM. 2005. Axon retraction and degeneration in development and disease. *Annu. Rev. Neurosci.* **28**:127–56

Lu M, Mizumoto K. 2019. Gradient-independent Wnt signaling instructs asymmetric neurite pruning in C. elegans. *eLife.* **8**:

MacInnis BL, Campenot RB. 2005. Regulation of Wallerian degeneration and nerve growth factor withdrawal-induced pruning of axons of sympathetic neurons by the proteasome and the MEK/Erk pathway. *Mol. Cell. Neurosci.* **28(3)**:430–39

Mack TG, Reiner M, Beirowski B, Mi W, Emanuelli M, et al. 2001. Wallerian degeneration of injured axons and synapses is delayed by a Ube4b/Nmnat chimeric gene. *Nat. Neurosci.* **4(12)**:1199–1206

Magni G, Amici A, Emanuelli M, Orsomando G, Raffaelli N, Ruggieri S. 2004. Enzymology of NAD+ homeostasis in man. *Cell. Mol. Life Sci.* **61(1)**:19–34

Maor-Nof M, Romi E, Sar Shalom H, Ulisse V, Raanan C, et al. 2016. Axonal Degeneration Is Regulated by a Transcriptional Program that Coordinates Expression of Pro- and Anti-degenerative Factors. *Neuron.* **92(5)**:991–1006

Martin DP, Ito A, Horigome K, Lampe PA, Johnson EM. 1992. Biochemical characterization of programmed cell death in NGF-deprived sympathetic neurons. *J. Neurobiol.* **23(9)**:1205–20

Martin DP, Schmidt RE, DiStefano PS, Lowry OH, Carter JG, Johnson EM. 1988. Inhibitors of protein synthesis and RNA synthesis prevent neuronal death caused by nerve growth factor deprivation. *J. Cell Biol.* **106(3)**:829–44

Ma M, Ferguson TA, Schoch KM, Li J, Qian Y, et al. 2013. Calpains mediate axonal cytoskeleton disintegration during Wallerian degeneration. *Neurobiol. Dis.* **56**:34–46

Mc Guire C, Beyaert R, van Loo G. 2011. Death receptor signalling in central nervous system inflammation and demyelination. *Trends Neurosci.* **34(12)**:619–28

Meeker RB, Williams KS. 2015. The p75 neurotrophin receptor: at the crossroad of neural repair and death. *Neural Regen. Res.* **10(5)**:721–25

Milde S, Gilley J, Coleman MP. 2013. Subcellular localization determines the stability and axon protective capacity of axon survival factor Nmnat2. *PLoS Biol.* **11(4)**:e1001539

Nazareth L, St John J, Murtaza M, Ekberg J. 2021. Phagocytosis by peripheral glia: importance for nervous system functions and implications in injury and disease. *Front. Cell Dev. Biol.* **9**:660259

Neukomm LJ, Freeman MR. 2014. Diverse cellular and molecular modes of axon degeneration. *Trends Cell Biol.* **24(9)**:515–23

Newell KL, Boyer P, Gomez-Tortosa E, Hobbs W, Hedley-Whyte ET, et al. 1999. Alpha-synuclein immunoreactivity is present in axonal swellings in neuroaxonal dystrophy and acute traumatic brain injury. *J. Neuropathol. Exp. Neurol.* **58(12)**:1263–68

Nikolaev A, McLaughlin T, O'Leary DDM, Tessier-Lavigne M. 2009. APP binds DR6 to trigger axon pruning and neuron death via distinct caspases. *Nature*. **457(7232)**:981–89

Olsen O, Kallop DY, McLaughlin T, Huntwork-Rodriguez S, Wu Z, et al. 2014. Genetic analysis reveals that amyloid precursor protein and death receptor 6 function in the same pathway to control axonal pruning independent of β-secretase. *J. Neurosci.* **34(19)**:6438–47

Orem BC, Partain SB, Stirling DP. 2020. Inhibiting store-operated calcium entry attenuates white matter secondary degeneration following SCI. *Neurobiol. Dis.* **136**:104718

Orem BC, Pelisch N, Williams J, Nally JM, Stirling DP. 2017. Intracellular calcium release through IP3R or RyR contributes to secondary axonal degeneration. *Neurobiol. Dis.* **106**:235–43

Osterloh JM, Yang J, Rooney TM, Fox AN, Adalbert R, et al. 2012. dSarm/Sarm1 is required for activation of an injury-induced axon death pathway. *Science*. **337(6093)**:481–84

Panneerselvam P, Ding JL. 2015. Beyond TLR signaling—the role of SARM in antiviral immune defense, apoptosis & development. *Int. Rev. Immunol.* **34(5)**:432–44

Pan G, Bauer JH, Haridas V, Wang S, Liu D, et al. 1998. Identification and functional characterization of DR6, a novel death domain-containing TNF receptor. *FEBS Lett.* **431(3)**:351–56

Park KJ, Grosso CA, Aubert I, Kaplan DR, Miller FD. 2010. p75NTR-dependent, myelin-mediated axonal degeneration regulates neural connectivity in the adult brain. *Nat. Neurosci.* **13(5)**:559–66

Pathak A, Clark S, Bronfman FC, Deppmann CD, Carter BD. 2021. Long-distance regressive signaling in neural development and disease. *Wiley Interdiscip. Rev. Dev. Biol.* **10(2)**:e382

Pathak A, Stanley EM, Hickman FE, Wallace N, Brewer B, et al. 2018. Retrograde Degenerative Signaling Mediated by the p75 Neurotrophin Receptor Requires p150Glued Deacetylation by Axonal HDAC1. *Dev. Cell.* **46(3)**:376-387.e7

Pease-Raissi SE, Pazyra-Murphy MF, Li Y, Wachter F, Fukuda Y, et al. 2017. Paclitaxel Reduces Axonal Bclw to Initiate IP3R1-Dependent Axon Degeneration. *Neuron*. **96(2)**:373-386.e6

Pease SE, Segal RA. 2014. Preserve and protect: maintaining axons within functional circuits. *Trends Neurosci.* **37(10)**:572–82

Raff MC, Whitmore AV, Finn JT. 2002. Axonal self-destruction and neurodegeneration. *Science*. **296(5569)**:868–71

Ramón y Cajal S. 1928. *Degeneration and Regeneration of the Nervous System*

Ribas VT, Koch JC, Michel U, Bähr M, Lingor P. 2017. Attenuation of axonal degeneration by calcium channel inhibitors improves retinal ganglion cell survival and regeneration after optic nerve crush. *Mol. Neurobiol.* **54(1)**:72–86

Riccomagno MM, Hurtado A, Wang H, Macopson JGJ, Griner EM, et al. 2012. The RacGAP β2-Chimaerin selectively mediates axonal pruning in the hippocampus. *Cell.* **149(7)**:1594–1606

Riccomagno MM, Kolodkin AL. 2015. Sculpting neural circuits by axon and dendrite pruning. *Annu. Rev. Cell Dev. Biol.* **31**:779–805

Rosenberg AF, Wolman MA, Franzini-Armstrong C, Granato M. 2012. *In vivo* nerve-macrophage interactions following peripheral nerve injury. *J. Neurosci.* **32(11)**:3898–3909

Salvadores N, Sanhueza M, Manque P, Court FA. 2017. Axonal Degeneration during Aging and Its Functional Role in Neurodegenerative Disorders. *Front. Neurosci.* **11**:451

Sankar S, Dhakshinamoorthy V, Rajakumar G. 2023. PARP in the neuropathogenesis of cytomegalovirus infection – Possible role and therapeutic perspective. *Microb. Pathog.* **176**:106018

Schoenmann Z, Assa-Kunik E, Tiomny S, Minis A, Haklai-Topper L, et al. 2010. Axonal degeneration is regulated by the apoptotic machinery or a NAD+-sensitive pathway in insects and mammals. *J. Neurosci.* **30(18)**:6375–86

Simon DJ, Belsky DM, Bowen ME, Ohn CYJ, O'Rourke MK, et al. 2021. An anterograde pathway for sensory axon degeneration gated by a cytoplasmic action of the transcriptional regulator P53. *Dev. Cell.* **56(7)**:976-984.e3

Simon DJ, Pitts J, Hertz NT, Yang J, Yamagishi Y, et al. 2016. Axon Degeneration Gated by Retrograde Activation of Somatic Pro-apoptotic Signaling. *Cell.* **164(5)**:1031–45

Simon DJ, Weimer RM, McLaughlin T, Kallop D, Stanger K, et al. 2012. A caspase cascade regulating developmental axon degeneration. *J. Neurosci.* **32(49)**:17540–53

Singh KK, Miller FD. 2005. Activity regulates positive and negative neurotrophin-derived signals to determine axon competition. *Neuron.* **45(6)**:837–45

Singh KK, Park KJ, Hong EJ, Kramer BM, Greenberg ME, et al. 2008. Developmental axon pruning mediated by BDNF-p75NTR-dependent axon degeneration. *Nat. Neurosci.* **11(6)**:649–58

Song X-Y, Zhou FH-H, Zhong J-H, Wu LLY, Zhou X-F. 2006. Knockout of p75(NTR) impairs re-myelination of injured sciatic nerve in mice. *J. Neurochem.* **96(3)**:833–42

Staal JA, Dickson TC, Gasperini R, Liu Y, Foa L, Vickers JC. 2010. Initial calcium release from intracellular stores followed by calcium dysregulation is linked to secondary axotomy following transient axonal stretch injury. *J. Neurochem.* **112(5)**:1147–55

Stokin GB, Lillo C, Falzone TL, Brusch RG, Rockenstein E, et al. 2005. Axonopathy and transport deficits early in the pathogenesis of Alzheimer's disease. *Science.* **307(5713)**:1282–88

Tabata Y, Imaizumi Y, Sugawara M, Andoh-Noda T, Banno S, et al. 2018. T-type Calcium Channels Determine the Vulnerability of Dopaminergic Neurons to Mitochondrial Stress in Familial Parkinson Disease. *Stem Cell Reports.* **11(5)**:1171–84

Tanaka K, Kelly CE, Goh KY, Lim KB, Ibáñez CF. 2016. Death Domain Signaling by Disulfide-Linked Dimers of the p75 Neurotrophin Receptor Mediates Neuronal Death in the CNS. *J. Neurosci.* **36(20)**:5587–95

Tedeschi A, Dupraz S, Laskowski CJ, Xue J, Ulas T, et al. 2016. The calcium channel subunit alpha2delta2 suppresses axon regeneration in the adult CNS. *Neuron.* **92(2)**:419–34

Teng KK, Felice S, Kim T, Hempstead BL. 2010. Understanding proneurotrophin actions: Recent advances and challenges. *Dev. Neurobiol.* **70(5)**:350–59

Tian N, Hanson KA, Canty AJ, Vickers JC, King AE. 2020. Microtubule-dependent processes precede pathological calcium influx in excitotoxin-induced axon degeneration. *J. Neurochem.* **152(5)**:542–55

Twohig JP, Cuff SM, Yong AA, Wang ECY. 2011. The role of tumor necrosis factor receptor superfamily members in mammalian brain development, function and homeostasis. *Rev. Neurosci.* **22(5)**:509–33

Van Broeckhoven J, Sommer D, Dooley D, Hendrix S, Franssen AJPM. 2021. Macrophage phagocytosis after spinal cord injury: when friends become foes. *Brain.* **144(10)**:2933–45

Vargas ME, Barres BA. 2007. Why is Wallerian degeneration in the CNS so slow? *Annu. Rev. Neurosci.* **30**:153–79

Vargas ME, Yamagishi Y, Tessier-Lavigne M, Sagasti A. 2015. Live Imaging of Calcium Dynamics during Axon Degeneration Reveals Two Functionally Distinct Phases of Calcium Influx. *J. Neurosci.* **35(45)**:15026–38

Vial JD. 1958. The Early Changes in the Axoplasm during Wallerian Degeneration. *J. Cell Biol.* **4(5)**:551–56

Vilar M, Charalampopoulos I, Kenchappa RS, Simi A, Karaca E, et al. 2009. Activation of the p75 neurotrophin receptor through conformational rearrangement of disulphide-linked receptor dimers. *Neuron.* **62(1)**:72–83

Villegas R, Martinez NW, Lillo J, Pihan P, Hernandez D, et al. 2014. Calcium release from intra-axonal endoplasmic reticulum leads to axon degeneration through mitochondrial dysfunction. *J. Neurosci.* **34(21)**:7179–89

Vohra BPS, Sasaki Y, Miller BR, Chang J, DiAntonio A, Milbrandt J. 2010. Amyloid precursor protein cleavage-dependent and -independent axonal degeneration programs share a common nicotinamide mononucleotide adenylyltransferase 1-sensitive pathway. *J. Neurosci.* **30(41)**:13729–38

Walczak H. 2013. Death receptor-ligand systems in cancer, cell death, and inflammation. *Cold Spring Harb. Perspect. Biol.* **5(5)**:a008698

Wang JT, Medress ZA, Barres BA. 2012. Axon degeneration: molecular mechanisms of a self-destruction pathway. *J. Cell Biol.* **196(1)**:7–18

Wang Y, Zhao D, Pan B, Song Z, Shah SZA, et al. 2015. Death Receptor 6 and Caspase-6 Regulate Prion Peptide-Induced Axonal Degeneration in Rat Spinal Neurons. *J. Mol. Neurosci.* **56(4)**:966–76

Watts RJ, Hoopfer ED, Luo L. 2003. Axon pruning during Drosophila metamorphosis: evidence for local degeneration and requirement of the ubiquitin-proteasome system. *Neuron.* **38(6)**:871–85

Webster HD. 1962. Transient, focal accumulation of axonal mitochondria during the early stages of wallerian degeneration. *J. Cell Biol.* **12**:361–83

Wheeler MA, Heffner DL, Kim S, Espy SM, Spano AJ, et al. 2014. TNF-α/TNFR1 signaling is required for the development and function of primary nociceptors. *Neuron.* **82(3)**:587–602

Whitmore AV, Lindsten T, Raff MC, Thompson CB. 2003. The proapoptotic proteins Bax and Bak are not involved in Wallerian degeneration. *Cell Death Differ.* **10(2)**:260–61

Williams DW, Truman JW. 2005. Cellular mechanisms of dendrite pruning in Drosophila: insights from in vivo time-lapse of remodeling dendritic arborizing sensory neurons. *Development.* **132(16)**:3631–42

Witte ME, Schumacher A-M, Mahler CF, Bewersdorf JP, Lehmitz J, et al. 2019. Calcium Influx through Plasma-Membrane Nanoruptures Drives Axon Degeneration in a Model of Multiple Sclerosis. *Neuron.* **101(4)**:615-624.e5

Xu K, Olsen O, Tzvetkova-Robev D, Tessier-Lavigne M, Nikolov DB. 2015. The crystal structure of DR6 in complex with the amyloid precursor protein provides insight into death receptor activation. *Genes Dev.* **29(8)**:785–90

Yamashita T, Fujitani M, Hata K, Mimura F, Yamagishi S. 2005. Diverse functions of the p75 neurotrophin receptor. *Anat. Sci. Int.* **80(1)**:37–41

Yang J, Weimer RM, Kallop D, Olsen O, Wu Z, et al. 2013. Regulation of axon degeneration after injury and in development by the endogenous calpain inhibitor calpastatin. *Neuron.* **80(5)**:1175–89

Yong Y, Gamage K, Cheng I, Barford K, Spano A, et al. 2019. p75NTR and DR6 Regulate Distinct Phases of Axon Degeneration Demarcated by Spheroid Rupture. *J. Neurosci.* **39(48)**:9503–20

Yong Y, Gamage K, Cushman C, Spano A, Deppmann C. 2020a. Regulation of degenerative spheroids after injury. *Sci. Rep.* **10(1)**:15472

Yong Y, Hughes C, Deppmann C. 2020b. A microfluidic culture platform to assess axon degeneration. *Methods Mol. Biol.* **2143**:83–96

Yong Y, Hunter-Chang S, Stepanova E, Deppmann C. 2021. Axonal spheroids in neurodegeneration. *Mol. Cell. Neurosci.* **117**:103679

Zeng F, Lu J-J, Zhou X-F, Wang Y-J. 2011. Roles of p75NTR in the pathogenesis of Alzheimer's disease: a novel therapeutic target. *Biochem. Pharmacol.* **82(10)**:1500–1509

6

Mechanisms of Pathological Axonal Degeneration

Ying Cao and Jing Yang

IDG/McGovern Institute for Brain Research, Center for Life Sciences,
School of Life Sciences, Peking University, China
Corresponding Email: jing.yang@pku.edu.cn

Abstract

Pathological axonal degeneration is one of the common features of neurode-generative diseases, which can occur independently from neuronal cell death. By interrupting the functional or structural connectivity of neurocircuits, such axonal pathology can directly contribute to the onset and progression of clinical symptoms in patients. Therefore, delay or prevention of axonal damage is indispensable for effectively treating neurodegenerative diseases. Notably, pathological axonal degeneration is often distinct from several known types of programmed cell death, for example, apoptosis, necroptosis, or pyroptosis. Instead, this destructive process is intrinsically linked to energy metabolism, particularly the co-enzyme nicotinamide adenine dinucleotide (NAD^+), within damaged axons. This book chapter reviews the history of the research field and highlights the landmark works elucidating the molecular mechanisms of pathological axonal degeneration. Also, critical questions that still await future investigations are discussed.

As one of the unique structures of neurons, axons act as the bridge between neurons and their innervating targets. By transducing action potentials, axonal connections form the foundation for neural development and functions. As a result, the structural and functional integrity of axons is essential for various neurophysiological processes, for example, sense, motility, memory, and cognition. Conversely, damage or destruction of axons causes the abnormality or breakdown of corresponding neural circuits, leading to

215

severe neuropathological defects such as numbness, pain, blindness, paralysis, ataxia, dementia, and even death.

Through decades of research, pathological loss of axons has been documented as a hallmark feature in almost all types of neurodegenerative diseases, including Alzheimer's disease, Parkinson's disease, Huntington's disease, amyotrophic lateral sclerosis (also known as Lou Gehrig's disease), multiple sclerosis, Guillain–Barré syndrome, Charcot–Marie–Tooth disease, glaucoma, traumatic neural injuries, and other types of central or peripheral neuropathy (Coleman, 2005; Coleman and Hoke, 2020; DiAntonio, 2019; Neukomm and Freeman, 2014; Wang et al., 2012). Further, it has become increasingly recognized that pathological axonal degeneration contributes to the onset and progression of clinical symptoms by directly interfering with normal neural functions. Therefore, molecular mechanisms underlying pathological axonal degeneration are integral to neurodegeneration, and preserving axonal structures inflicted by neurodegenerative insults should be indispensable for effective strategies to prevent, delay, or revert disease symptoms.

Research in the past decades has achieved some of the most important and exciting breakthroughs in unraveling pathological axonal degeneration. Such advances have opened up a new dimension to our understanding of this unique axonal pathology and neurodegenerative diseases in general. This book chapter aims to review the updated knowledge of pathological axonal degeneration, highlighting entry points that may eventually lead to conquering those currently incurable human diseases.

6.1 Overview of Pathological Axonal Degeneration

Pathological axonal degeneration is the programmed destruction of axons. Such axonal pathology can precede the demise of corresponding neuronal cells in neurodegenerative conditions, implicating the spatial and temporal separation of pathological axonal degeneration from neuronal cell death. In addition, pathological axonal degeneration may occur independently of neuronal death, that is, a neuron may survive after losing its axon. Therefore, although the loss of neurons and their axons are observed simultaneously in many neurodegenerative diseases, it is essential to distinguish pathological axonal degeneration as a self-standing process.

Pathological axonal degeneration in different disease scenarios shares similar morphological and functional features. This axonal pathology can be characterized in a simplified model by several temporally distinct but related

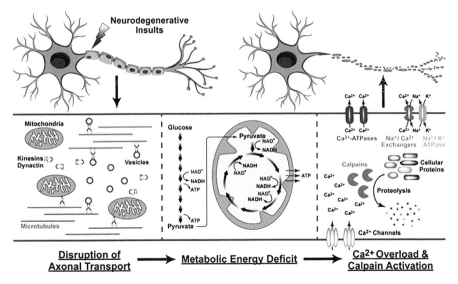

Figure 6.1 **An overview of pathological axonal degeneration.** Upon neurodegenerative insults, the concomitant or sequential occurrence of several key steps, including disruption of axonal transport, metabolic energy deficit, Ca^{2+} overload, and calpain activation, designates the process of pathological axonal degeneration.

steps (Figure 6.1). Disruption of axonal transport is often the first detectable sign of axonal damage. It has been well known that axonal transport moves a variety of cargoes, for example, mitochondria, vesicles, mRNAs, cytoskeletons, and other proteins, in both anterograde and retrograde directions within axons (De Vos et al., 2008; Maday et al., 2014; Millecamps and Julien, 2013). As a result, the disrupted axonal transport causes the focal accumulation of such cellular components, producing axonal swelling. Those swellings, ranging from several to tens of micrometers, may be randomly distributed distal to a site of neurodegenerative damage. The specialized motor proteins, that is, Kinesins and Dynactin, enact axonal transport (Goldstein and Yang, 2000; Maday et al., 2014; Schroer, 2004). Because all these motor proteins require ATP as the energy source to migrate on microtubule bundles, their malfunction can result from an inadequate energy supply in damaged axons.

Indeed, in concomitant to or following the disruption of axonal transport, the next step of pathological axonal degeneration is the profound defect of energy homeostasis. This metabolic event involves the pathological depletion of the co-enzyme nicotinamide adenine dinucleotide (NAD^+) and the vital energy source ATP. Importantly, this loss of axonal energy disables all essential biological processes such as axonal transport, protein synthesis or degradation, and transduction of action potentials. Such a systematic shutdown collectively results in the functional failure of axons even before any further structural destruction. This step of pathological axonal degeneration is sufficient to interfere with the normal function of neural circuits and likely correlate with the onset of disease symptoms.

The following step of pathological axonal degeneration is the massive Ca^{2+} overload. Intracellular Ca^{2+} levels in healthy axons are typically maintained within the range of submicromolar concentrations by the combinatorial action of Ca^{2+}-ATPases and Na^+/Ca^{2+} exchangers. Of importance, Ca^{2+}-ATPases depends on the energy input from ATP. Although Na^+/Ca^{2+} exchangers do not directly consume ATP, their function relies on the Na^+ gradient across the plasma membrane established by Na^+/K^+-ATPase that requires ATP as the energy source. Therefore, the metabolic energy deficit occurring in the previous step of pathological axonal degeneration leads to the inevitable buildup of Ca^{2+} influx via various Ca^{2+} channels. Such Ca^{2+} overload then triggers a specific group of Ca^{2+}-activated proteases, that is, calpains, which rapidly proteolyze axonal cytoskeletons and other cellular proteins (Goll et al., 2003; Liu et al., 2004). Also, blebbing and fragmentation of the plasma membrane of axons happen, morphologically resembling that observed in programmed cell death. This breakdown of structural integrity is the terminal, irreversible step of pathological axonal degeneration.

Notably, these steps of pathological axonal degeneration may proceed with drastically variable timelines under different neurodegenerative conditions, ranging from days to months or even years. Despite such temporal divergence, research has elucidated that pathological axonal degeneration shares specific molecular mechanisms (Coleman, 2005; Coleman and Hoke, 2020; DiAntonio, 2019). We will discuss several signaling pathways extensively investigated in this process of axonal pathology.

6.2 Apoptotic Pathway

As described above, pathological axonal degeneration shares certain aspects of morphological similarity to programmed cell death, for example, blebbing and fragmentation of the plasma membrane. Therefore, research efforts have been made to determine whether the signaling pathways involved in programmed cell death may also participate in such axonal pathology. The classic apoptotic pathway is one of the most prominent types of programmed cell death (Budihardjo et al., 1999; Elmore, 2007). In the intrinsic mechanism of apoptosis, releasing cytochrome c from mitochondria via BAX or BAK proteins is the primary trigger of cell death. The released cytochrome c binds to the apoptotic protease-activating factor 1 (APAF1) protein in the cytosol, forming a complex known as the apoptosome. This complex then recruits and activates caspase-9. The activated caspase-9 further cleaves to activate the effector caspases, that is, caspase-3, caspase-6, and caspase-7. These active caspases degrade many essential cellular proteins, thus destroying biological processes critical for cell survival. This intrinsic apoptotic mechanism can be initiated under various conditions, including loss of trophic signals, DNA damage, and other cellular stresses. In addition to such intrinsic signals, extrinsic stimuli also induce apoptotic cell death. In particular, the engagement of Fas ligand (FasL) or tumor necrosis factor-alpha (TNF-alpha) to their specific receptors, that is, Fas or tumor necrosis factor receptor 1 (TNFR1), respectively, leads to activation of the downstream caspase-8. The active caspase-8 then directly cleaves to activate the effector caspases, such as caspase-3, to induce apoptotic cell death. Alternatively, the active caspase-8 cleaves the BID protein into tBID. tBID then promotes the activation of BAX or BAK that causes the release of cytochrome c from mitochondria, thus establishing the crosstalk with the intrinsic mechanism. This combinatory action of the intrinsic and extrinsic mechanisms consists of the apoptotic pathway.

Apoptosis is broadly involved in neurodevelopment. In particular, studies have shown that axonal pruning, also known as developmental axonal degeneration, often depends on the apoptotic pathway (Geden and Deshmukh, 2016; Schuldiner and Yaron, 2015). Molecular mechanisms governing developmental axonal degeneration have been discussed in a previous chapter of this book. In contrast, evidence supporting the involvement of the apoptotic pathway in pathological axonal degeneration is relatively limited. For example, the activation of caspase-3 and caspase-6 was detected in the neuronal cells inflicted by Alzheimer's disease (Albrecht et al., 2009; Selznick et al., 1999). Although the overexpression of the anti-apoptotic BCL-2 protein could reduce the accumulation of amyloid plaques and neurofibrillary tangles in the mouse model of Alzheimer's disease (Rohn et al., 2008), the effect of such apoptosis inhibition on pathological axonal degeneration was unclear. Also, the caspase-9 activation was observed in the motor neurons damaged in amyotrophic lateral sclerosis (Inoue et al., 2003). The genetic deletion of BAX blocked the cell death of motor neurons in the mouse disease model induced by the overexpression of mutant human superoxide dismutase 1 (SOD1) protein but did not affect the loss of motor axons (Gould et al., 2006). Similarly, the BAX deletion preserved the survival of cerebellar granule neurons but not their axonal structures in the mouse model of prion disease (Chiesa et al.,

2005). Further, in the traumatic injury of optic nerves or the glaucoma condition, the genetic deletion of BAX or BAK effectively inhibited the death of retinal ganglion cells while failing to stop the pathological degeneration of optic axons (Libby et al., 2005; Whitmore et al., 2003). Therefore, a general theme has been proposed that neuronal cell death and pathological axonal degeneration are regulated separately, with the apoptotic pathway only controlling the demise of neuronal cells in many neurodegenerative conditions.

A few examples currently suggest the role of apoptosis in pathological axonal degeneration. For instance, the caspase-3 activation occurred in the dying dopaminergic neurons in Parkinson's disease (Hartmann et al., 2000). While the BAX deletion fully protected the dopaminergic neurons in the mouse disease models induced by 1-methyl-4-phenyl-1,2,3,6-tetrahydropyridine (MPTP) or 6-hydroxydopamine, this genetic blockage of apoptosis also partially mitigated the destruction of their axonal projections (Kim et al., 2011; Vila et al., 2001). In addition, there was the activation of caspase-3 and caspase-8 in the brain regions damaged by traumatic injuries (Clark et al., 1999; Zhang et al., 2003). The genetic deletion of caspase-8 was reported to lessen the death of cortical neurons and their axons in the mouse disease model (Krajewska et al., 2011). However, the involvement of the apoptotic pathway in this particular context might be indirect. At least in the in vitro cultured neurons, the caspase activation could not be detected in axons upon traumatic neural injuries, and the genetic deletion of BAX or caspases failed to prolong the survival of traumatically injured axons (Simon et al., 2012). It is plausible that while the apoptotic pathway has essential roles in neurodevelopment, its participation in pathological axonal degeneration is restricted.

6.3 Necroptotic Pathway

Necroptosis is another critical type of programmed cell death under pathological conditions (Christofferson and Yuan, 2010; Sun and Wang, 2014; Xu et al., 2021). The engagement of TNFR1 or Fas receptors represents a main trigger of the necroptotic pathway. Rather than inducing the downstream apoptotic signals described above, a kinase cascade involving RIPK1, RIPK3, and MLKL can initiate necroptotic cell death. Although RIPK1 also controls the caspase-8 activation, RIPK3 and MLKL are involved explicitly in necroptosis but not apoptosis. MLKL oligomerizes upon its phosphorylation by RIPK3 and then inserts into the plasma membrane to form the pore structure. This MLKL-mediated membrane permeabilization causes the rapid flux of intracellular and extracellular components such as proteins and ions.

Such destruction of the plasma membrane integrity leads to necrosis-like cell death.

Research efforts have begun to investigate the potential roles of necroptosis in neurodegenerative diseases. For instance, the phosphorylation of RIPK3 and MLKL was detected in the spinal cord tissues of patients with amyotrophic lateral sclerosis or multiple sclerosis (Ito et al., 2016; Ofengeim et al., 2015). The genetic deletion of RIPK3 delayed the disease symptoms, including the degeneration of motor axons, in the mouse models of amyotrophic lateral sclerosis induced by the mutant human SOD1 or the loss of Optineurin protein (Ito et al., 2016). Also, the RIPK3 deletion modestly protected the axonal structures inflicted by the cuprizone-induced demyelination in the mouse model of multiple sclerosis (Ofengeim et al., 2015). In addition, the RIPK3 deletion lessened the neuronal loss and the behavioral defects in the mouse models of traumatic brain injury or spinal cord injury (Fan et al., 2016; Liu et al., 2018), although the effect of such necroptosis inhibition on pathological axonal degeneration was not examined. Further, the genetic deletion of MLKL mitigated the axonal damage in the mouse experimental autoimmune encephalomyelitis that recapitulates the condition of multiple sclerosis (Zhang et al., 2019). However, recent studies have reported that the expression of MLKL protein appears undetectable in the central nervous system, and the MLKL deletion fails to exert any protection in the mouse model of SOD1-induced amyotrophic lateral sclerosis (Wang et al., 2020). Therefore, the definitive function of the necroptotic pathway in pathological axonal degeneration awaits clarification. While the genetic deletion or the pharmacological inhibition of RIPK1 has been reported to confer beneficial effects under various neurodegenerative conditions (Mifflin et al., 2020; Yuan et al., 2019), for example, Alzheimer's disease, Parkinson's disease, amyotrophic lateral sclerosis, multiple sclerosis, and traumatic neural injuries, it remains undetermined whether RIPK1 may directly instruct pathological axonal degeneration via the necroptotic pathway in such disease scenarios.

6.4 Pyroptotic Pathway and Other Cell Death Pathways

In addition to apoptosis and necroptosis, other pathways of programmed cell death exist in disease conditions. For instance, pyroptosis has been recently uncovered to control the death of immune cells such as macrophages (Broz and Dixit, 2016; Kovacs and Miao, 2017; Shi et al., 2017). In response to various immune stimuli, for example, intracellular pathogenic infection, activating caspase-1, caspase-11, or other caspases leads to the cleavage of gasdermin proteins. The cleaved gasdermins, for example, gasdermin D

(GSDMD), then oligomerize and insert into the plasma membrane to form the pore structure. Like the MLKL-mediated necroptosis described above, gasdermin-triggered membrane permeabilization causes rapid leakage of proteins and ions, leading to pyroptotic cell death. Although the GSDMD cleavage and pyroptosis of retinal neurons or enteric neurons were reported under specific disease conditions in mice (Huang et al., 2021; Ye et al., 2020), whether the pyroptotic pathway might directly participate in pathological axonal degeneration has been untested. Also, certain types of neuronal cells, for example, cortical neurons, exhibit the minor expression of gasdermins (Tsuchiya et al., 2019), likely precluding the involvement of the pyroptotic pathway in the pathological loss of their axons.

Besides pyroptosis, several additional types of programmed cell death, for example, ferroptosis, parthanatos, and NETosis, have garnered attention for their potential roles in disease scenarios. Ferroptosis is an iron-dependent death pathway characterized by significant oxidative stress and excessive oxidation of lipids within cells (Lei et al., 2019; Xie et al., 2016). Accordingly, ferroptotic cell death can be alleviated by antioxidant molecules. Parthanatos is induced when cells suffer extensive DNA damage resulting in the overactivation of poly(ADP-ribose) polymerases (PARPs) proteins (David et al., 2009; Fatokun et al., 2014). The overactive PARPs produce a significant amount of poly(ADP-ribose) in cells. This poly(ADP-ribose) accumulation induces the release of apoptosis-inducing factor (AIF) and endonuclease G proteins from mitochondria, which then causes nuclear condensation and cell death. NETosis is a unique type of cell death occurring in neutrophils (Remijsen et al., 2011; Thiam et al., 2020). Neutrophils shed their genomic DNA to entrap invading pathogens through the NETosis process. Although these different pathways have been indicated in various pathological conditions, their potential roles in neurodegenerative diseases remain mostly uncharted. Moreover, it is worth noting that novel pathways of programmed cell death are still being discovered and might act in specific contexts of pathological axonal degeneration.

6.5 NAD⁺-dependent Pathway

Significant research advances have revealed that pathological axonal degeneration can intrinsically link to energy metabolism, particularly NAD^+, within axons. This research direction is traced back to 1850 when the British physiologist Augustus Waller reported that the traumatic injury of peripheral nerves in frogs could lead to the stereotyped dismantling of axonal structures in the following days or weeks (Waller, 1850). In recognition of this historical discovery, pathological axonal degeneration is also known as Wallerian degeneration. As stated in his original publication, "...*it is particularly with reference to nervous diseases that it will be most desirable to extend these researches....*" Augustus Waller predicted the potential significance of pathological axonal degeneration in human diseases. However, the relevance of Wallerian degeneration to neurodegenerative conditions had been long overlooked. In particular, it has been a common belief, even till now, that an axon cannot maintain its own survival independently of the neuronal cell body. Indeed, as described above, neuronal cell bodies provide many essential cellular components via axonal transport, for example, mRNAs, ribosomes, proteins, vesicles, and mitochondria. Therefore, a traumatic injury to axons disconnects such axonal transport and, as a result, deprives the critical trophic support of neuronal cell bodies. In light of such a view, Wallerian degeneration occurring in the context of traumatic neural injuries had been regarded as merely a passive, necrotic process of axonal destruction, denying any involvement of molecular mechanisms.

6.5.1 WLDˢ Mutant Protein

Modern research into Wallerian degeneration was re-ignited in the 1980s when British neuroscientists challenged the long-held view of Wallerian degeneration as a passive death event. They serendipitously identified a mutant mouse line, now called *Wallerian degeneration slow* (*Wld*ˢ), in which the breakdown of traumatically injured axons in sciatic nerves was delayed for weeks (Lunn et al., 1989). Moreover, such axons completely disconnected from neuronal cell bodies in the *Wld*ˢ mice could still sustain the ability to transduce action potentials after injury. This observation indicated for the first time that Wallerian degeneration would be an active process of axonal death instructed by some unknown signaling mechanisms. With this discovery of the *Wld*ˢ mutant mouse, the research field has embarked on the endeavor to unravel the signaling pathway of Wallerian degeneration in the following decades.

Studies then showed that the *Wld*ˢ mutant gene functions in a neuron-intrinsic manner (Perry et al., 1990a) and is autosomal dominant (Perry et al., 1990b). The decade-long research of map-based cloning eventually identified *Wld*ˢ as the triplication mutation of an 85-kb region on chromosome 4 of the mouse genome (Coleman et al., 1998; Conforti et al., 2000). This 85-kb region originally contains the entire coding sequences of nicotinamide mononucleotide adenylyltransferase 1 (NMNAT1) and retinol binding protein 7 and also the partial 5'-coding sequence of ubiquitin conjugation factor E4B (UBE4b).

Notably, a new mutant protein is generated on the boundary between every two triplicated regions by the in-frame fusion of the N-terminal 70 amino acids of UBE4b with the full-length protein of NMNAT1. This UBE4b/NMNAT1 fusion protein has been proven as the causative factor conferring axonal protection against neurodegenerative insults, thereby named the WLD[s] mutant protein (Mack et al., 2001). However, studies have later demonstrated that the axonal protection afforded by the WLD[s] protein does not directly involve the ubiquitin system as implicated by UBE4b. On the other hand, NMNAT1 is one of the enzymes catalyzing the last step of NAD[+] synthesis from nicotinamide mononucleotide (NMN) in mammalian cells, including neurons. Notably, this enzymatic activity of NMNAT1 is indispensable for the axonal protective effect of WLD[s] (Araki et al., 2004). Moreover, the overexpression of an NMNAT protein derived from the archaebacterium *Methanococcus jannaschii*, which exhibits almost no sequence homology to mammalian NMNATs, could still be sufficient to delay the pathological axonal degeneration upon traumatic neural injuries (Sasaki et al., 2009). This observation is in accordance with the view that the enzymatic activity is solely responsible for the axonal protection by the WLD[s] mutant protein. Further, it has been unequivocally proven that the WLD[s] protein exerts its action explicitly in axons but not in neuronal cell bodies (Sasaki and Milbrandt, 2010). These results have suggested that Wallerian degeneration is linked to the NAD[+]-related signaling mechanism.

With such insight into the potential link between Wallerian degeneration and NAD[+] metabolism, it was then noted that the intracellular NAD[+] levels in axons decrease significantly upon traumatic neural injuries (Wang et al., 2005). Such NAD[+] depletion further triggers the blockage of energy production, particularly by glycolysis and the tricarboxylic acid cycle, resulting in the consequential decrease of axonal ATP levels. Conversely, manipulations that sustained the axonal NAD[+] or ATP levels in traumatically injured axons effectively delay Wallerian degeneration (Wang et al., 2005; Yang et al., 2015). This evidence has demonstrated that the metabolic energy deficit underlies pathological axonal degeneration.

Understandably, the research field has been prompted to examine the axonal protective effect of WLD[s] in the context of various neurodegenerative diseases in addition to traumatic neural injuries. Indeed, the axonal structures of dopaminergic neurons were protected by WLD[s] in the mouse models of Parkinson's disease (Cheng and Burke, 2010; Sajadi et al., 2004). Also, the WLD[s] protein inhibited the axonal damage in the mouse model of experimental autoimmune encephalomyelitis (Kaneko et al., 2006). Moreover, WLD[s] can prevent axonal pathology in other rodent models of pathological axonal degeneration, for example, gracile axonal dystrophy (Mi et al., 2005), Charcot–Marie–Tooth disease (Meyer zu Horste et al., 2011), chemotherapy-induced periphery neuropathy (Wang et al., 2002), progressive motor neuronopathy (Ferri et al., 2003), and glaucoma (Beirowski et al., 2008; Howell et al., 2007). Till now, only a few exceptions have been reported in which the WLD^s mutant protein fails to confer axonal protection, for example, the mouse model of amyotrophic lateral sclerosis induced by the mutant human SOD1 protein (Fischer et al., 2005; Vande Velde et al., 2004) or the mouse model of spinal muscular atrophy (Kariya et al., 2009). These accumulating research efforts have given rise to a consensus that pathological axonal losses under most disease scenarios share a common signaling pathway regulated by the WLD^s protein.

6.5.2 NMNAT2 Protein

Given that the WLD^s mutant protein functions exclusively in axons, it was suggested that WLD^s might act to substitute an endogenous NMNAT protein. There are three isoforms of NMNATs in mammalian cells, that is, NMNAT1, NMNAT2, and NMNAT3. These three isoforms have distinct subcellular localizations (Belenky et al., 2007; Cambronne and Kraus, 2020). NMNAT1 is primarily concentrated in the nucleus. NMNAT2 is present in the cytosol and may be associated with membrane-bound vesicles via protein palmitoylation (Lau et al., 2010). NMNAT3 was reported to reside in mitochondria, though its precise localization has been debated. It was then found that while NMNAT2 and NMNAT3 are both detectable in axons, the protein level of NMNAT2 rapidly decreased upon traumatic injuries (Gilley and Coleman, 2010). This phenomenon is due to proteosome-mediated degradation as the specific proteasomal inhibitors suppress the loss of NMNAT2 protein in traumatically injured axons. Significantly, such inhibition of the proteasomal activity also delayed pathological axonal degeneration (Gilley and Coleman, 2010; Zhai et al., 2003), supporting its functional relevance in this process. Furthermore, at least in the in vitro cultured neurons, the NMNAT2 protein is initially synthesized in cell bodies and then continuously transported into distal axons (Gilley and Coleman, 2010). Once arriving in axons, NMNAT2 exhibits a short half-life time of several hours because of the proteasomal degradation primed by the PHR1-SKP1-FBXO45 ubiquitin E3 ligase complex. Therefore, traumatic injuries cut off NMNAT2 transported from neuronal cell bodies, leading to its depletion within axons. Accordingly, the genetic deletion of PHR1, SKP1, or FBXO45 could all delay the degeneration of traumatically injured axons (Babetto et al., 2013; Yamagishi and

Tessier-Lavigne, 2016). The protein stability of NMNAT2 within axons may also be modulated by the mitogen-activated protein kinase (MAPK) signal (Walker et al., 2017).

As additional evidence substantiating the essential role of NMNAT2 in axonal survival, recent studies have identified the rare loss-of-function mutations of NMNAT2 associated with severe neural defects resulting in embryonic lethality or childhood polyneuropathy in humans (Huppke et al., 2019; Lukacs et al., 2019). Similarly, the genetic deficiency of NMNAT2 in mice causes widespread defects of axonal projections within the central and peripheral nervous systems at the embryonic stage (Gilley et al., 2013). Of particular importance, the WLD^s mutant protein rescues most of the neural defects associated with the NMNAT2 deficiency (Gilley et al., 2013), confirming that WLD^s can functionally replace the endogenous NMNAT2 protein in maintaining axonal survival. These research findings have highlighted that NAD$^+$ metabolism is crucial for designating pathological axonal degeneration.

6.5.3 SARM1 Protein

Several research groups conducted genetic screenings in the 2010s in the hope of revealing new molecular components in pathological axonal degeneration. Mutagenesis screening in flies revealed that the genetic deletion of *Drosophila* sterile alpha and Armadillo motif (dSARM) or its mouse ortholog sterile alpha and Toll/interleukin-1 receptor motif-containing protein 1 (SARM1) could significantly prolong the survival of traumatically injured axons (Osterloh et al., 2012). In parallel, gene knockdown screening in cultured mouse neurons identified SARM1 as a central regulator of pathological axonal degeneration induced by traumatic injuries (Gerdts et al., 2013). SARM1 or dSARM has an ortholog in Caenorhabditis *elegans*, that is, *tir-1*, originally identified as an essential gene controlling asymmetric neuronal differentiation (Chuang and Bargmann, 2005). The mammalian SARM1 protein belongs to the Toll/interleukin-1 receptor (TIR) domain-containing adaptor family (O'Neill and Bowie, 2007). This protein family also contains MYD88, TRIF, TRAM, and TIRAP. These other four family members have been extensively studied in the context of various immune responses. For instance, MYD88 and TRIF are central for transducing the innate immune response mediated by Toll-like receptors (TLRs) upon pathogenic infections. Although SARM1 or its ortholog *tir-1* was reported to modulate innate immune signals (Carty et al., 2006; Couillault et al., 2004), the precise function of SARM1 in immunity has remained controversial.

Studies have demonstrated that the SARM1 expression is highly enriched in all types of neurons but limited in immune cells (Kim et al., 2007). SARM1 is present in the cytosol of neurons and axons and may be associated with mitochondria through its N-terminal mitochondria-targeting sequence, though its precise subcellular localization remains to be unequivocally determined. Importantly, the genetic deletion of SARM1 delays the pathological axonal degeneration in traumatically injured mouse nerves, and the protective effect is comparable to, if not more robust than, that observed in the *Wld^s* mutant mice (Gerdts et al., 2013; Osterloh et al., 2012). Also, the SARM1 deletion can effectively mitigate chemotherapy-induced peripheral neuropathy triggered by vincristine or paclitaxel (Geisler et al., 2016; Wang et al., 2019). Similarly, the axonal structures of dopaminergic neurons in the mouse model of Parkinson's disease induced by 6-hydroxydopamine are protected by the SARM1 deletion (Peters et al., 2021). In addition, the SARM1 deletion suppresses the pathological axonal degeneration in several other common models of neurodegenerative diseases, for example, amyotrophic lateral sclerosis induced by the mutant human TAR DNA-binding protein 43 kDa (TDP-43) protein (White et al., 2019), experimental autoimmune encephalomyelitis (Viar et al., 2020), and diabetic peripheral neuropathy (Turkiew et al., 2017). Moreover, recent studies have reported that SARM1 participates in some previously-unrecognized events of pathological axonal degeneration, for example, the sympathetic neuropathy in the liver under metabolic stress (Liu et al., 2021) or the loss of catecholaminergic axons in the enteric nervous system in acute inflammation (Sun et al., 2021). The disease spectrum of axonal protective effects by the SARM1 deletion factually mirrors that observed with the WLD^s mutant protein, suggesting that SARM1 and WLD^s may act with the related molecular mechanism. Till now, among all the examined models of neurodegeneration, there are two exceptions in which the SARM1 deletion cannot confer axonal protection, that is, amyotrophic lateral sclerosis induced by the mutant human SOD1 (Peters et al., 2018) and Parkinson's disease caused by the overexpression of human alpha-Synuclein protein (Peters et al., 2021). SARM1 appears dispensable for normal neurodevelopment in mice, particularly for developmental axonal degeneration (Kim et al., 2007; Osterloh et al., 2012). Similarly, the neuron-specific deletion of dSARM in *Drosophila* does not affect the developmental loss of neurons or axons (Osterloh et al., 2012). At the same time, the WLD^s mutant protein also does not affect developmental axonal degeneration (Hoopfer et al., 2006). This functional similarity shared by SARM1 and WLD^s further supports their convergence into the same signaling pathway dedicated to pathological axonal degeneration.

Surprisingly, the SARM1 deletion reverts the aforementioned severe neural defects observed with the NMNAT2 deficiency in mice (Gilley et al., 2015). This finding implicated for the first time the involvement of SARM1 in NAD^+ metabolism. Studies then revealed that the recombinant TIR domain of SARM1 from different species, including fruit flies, fish, mice, and humans, can catalyze the in vitro degradation of NAD^+ (Essuman et al., 2017). Such NAD^+ breakdown produces nicotinamide and adenosine diphosphate ribose (ADPR) or cyclic ADPR. In contrast, the recombinant TIR domain derived from other TIR domain-containing proteins in mammals, such as MYD88 and TLR4, does not possess such NAD^+-degrading ability. On the other hand, many TIR domain-containing proteins from bacteria, archaebacteria, and plants exhibit a similar NADase activity (Essuman et al., 2018; Wan et al., 2019), which may represent a conserved, ancient family of NAD^+-consuming enzymes. Of importance, the NADase activity of mammalian SARM1 proteins critically depends on a glutamate residue of the TIR domain, that is, E642 residue in the mouse or human SARM1. The E642A mutation abolishes the NADase activity of SARM1 and its ability to prime the degeneration of traumatically injured axons (Essuman et al., 2017). This research breakthrough has identified the critical mechanistic link of SARM1 to the NAD^+ metabolism during pathological axonal degeneration.

The SARM1 protein is consistently present inside axons, but the NAD^+ depletion only occurs in response to neurodegenerative insults. This fact clearly implies that SARM1 must be relatively inactive under healthy, undamaged conditions. Several recent studies have achieved the high-resolution protein structure of SARM1 (Bratkowski et al., 2020; Figley et al., 2021; Horsefield et al., 2019; Jiang et al., 2020; Shen et al., 2021; Sporny et al., 2020), showing that it is organized as an octamer (i.e., eight protein molecules) via the interaction of its sterile alpha motif (SAM) domain (Figure 6.2). Moreover, the NADase activity of the TIR domain is inhibited through its binding to the N-terminal Armadillo motif (ARM) domain within the octamer complex. In particular, the TIR domain resides on a hydrophobic interface with the ARM domain. Such interactions result in the physical blockage of the enzymatic pocket of the TIR domain, thus precluding the NAD^+ access to the catalytic site. The mutations of several hydrophobic residues within this interface could disrupt the interaction between TIR and ARM domains and cause the enhanced NADase activity of SARM1 that is sufficient to trigger the spontaneous axonal degeneration in the absence of any neurodegenerative insult (Jiang et al., 2020). It has been implicated that the TIR domain needs to dimerize or oligomerize to become activated, though research efforts are ongoing to pursue the high-resolution SARM1 structure in an active status (Shi et al., 2022).

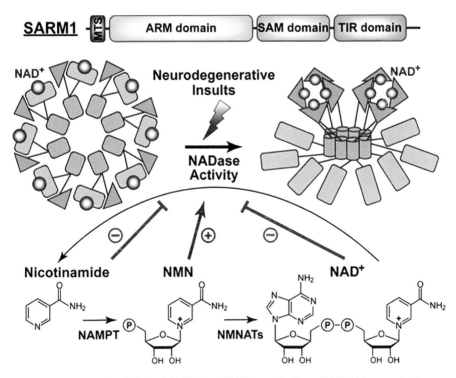

Figure 6.2 Functional link of SARM1 to NAD⁺ metabolism. SARM1 is organized as an octamer and maintained inactive through the NAD⁺ binding to the ARM domain. Upon neurodegenerative insults, the NADase activity of the TIR domain is triggered to convert NAD⁺ back into its metabolic precursor, nicotinamide. Notably, nicotinamide inhibits, but the NAD⁺ synthesis intermediate nicotinamide mononucleotide (NMN) stimulates, the NADase activity of SARM1. MTS, mitochondria-targeting sequence; NAMPT, nicotinamide phosphoribosyltransferase; NMNATs, nicotinamide mononucleotide adenylyltransferases.

Complexity has been realized in the functional link between SARM1 and axonal NAD⁺ metabolism. In the structural analyses of the SARM1 protein, it was observed unexpectedly that the ARM domain contains a new site of NAD⁺ binding (Jiang et al., 2020; Sporny et al., 2020). The mutations of critical residues involved in such NAD⁺ binding significantly boost the NADase activity of SARM1 and initiate the degeneration of uninjured axons. This surprising discovery has revealed that NAD⁺ is not only an enzymatic substrate of SARM1 but also acts as an inhibitor of the protein via allosteric regulation. In support of this view, the detailed biochemical tests showed that the NADase activity of SARM1 was suppressed by high concentrations of NAD⁺ (e.g., over 0.5 mM) but would increase when the NAD⁺ concentration dropped (e.g., below 0.1 mM). Notably, intracellular NAD⁺ levels are reported to be approximately 0.5 mM (Yang et al., 2007; Yang et al., 2019). Therefore, it becomes conceivable that such high levels of NAD$^+$ within healthy axons suffice to maintain the SARM1 protein in the inactive status. On the other hand, following traumatic axonal injuries or other neurodegenerative insults, an initial decrease of local NAD$^+$ levels due to the membrane breakage or the NMNAT2 depletion interferes with this NAD$^+$-mediated inhibition of SARM1. The active SARM1 then degrades more NAD$^+$ molecules, establishing a positive feedforward cascade along the entire length of damaged axons. Conversely, the WLD^s mutant protein or other NMNATs can effectively replenish axonal NAD$^+$ levels and prevent such a cascade. This delicate NAD$^+$-mediated regulation of SARM1 has formed the central mechanism controlling pathological axonal degeneration.

Moreover, the link between SARM1 and axonal NAD$^+$ metabolism extends beyond the NAD$^+$ molecule itself. Accumulating evidence has demonstrated that the NADase activity of SARM1 is also influenced by the NAD$^+$ metabolic precursors, that is, nicotinamide and NMN. Nicotinamide can inhibit the NADase activity of the TIR domain, though such inhibition requires high concentrations of nicotinamide (Essuman et al., 2017). At the same time, the administration of high dosages of nicotinamide decreased neural damage in the mouse model of traumatic brain injury (Goffus et al., 2010). Also, it preserved the axonal structures inflicted in the mouse model of experimental autoimmune encephalomyelitis (Kaneko et al., 2006). Notably, nicotinamide is catalyzed into NMN by the enzyme nicotinamide phosphoribosyltransferase (NAMPT) in mammalian cells, including neurons. Under normal conditions, NMN is further synthesized into NAD$^+$ by the NMNAT proteins. However, the NMNAT2 depletion occurring in damaged axons abolishes the conversion of NMN to NAD$^+$. Indeed, at least in the in vitro cultured neurons, axonal NMN levels increase significantly after traumatic injuries (Di Stefano et al., 2015). Intriguingly, recent studies have shown that NMN is an activator of the NADase activity of SARM1 (Angeletti et al., 2022; Loreto et al., 2015; Zhao et al., 2019). As a result, the NMN accumulation in damaged axons likely contributes to the SARM1 activation triggered by NAD$^+$ depletion. In addition, certain neurotoxins such as Vacor (a rodenticide) or 3-acetylpyridine can be metabolized into the NMN mimetics capable of activating SARM1 to cause pathological axonal degeneration (Loreto et al., 2021; Wu et al., 2021). Although the detailed mechanism underlying this NMN-mediated SARM1 activation remains to be determined, a paradigm has emerged that the NAD$^+$ metabolic pathway regulates SARM1 and the onset of pathological axonal degeneration.

6.5.4 Ca²⁺ and Calpains

NAD^+ has a central role in energy-producing metabolic processes, particularly in the catalytic steps by glyceraldehyde-3-phosphate dehydrogenase in glycolysis, or pyruvate dehydrogenase, isocitrate dehydrogenase, alpha-ketoglutarate dehydrogenase, and malate dehydrogenase in the tricarboxylic acid cycle. Therefore, the NAD^+ depletion in damaged axons inevitably causes the blockage of such essential processes, resulting in the continuous decrease of axonal ATP levels. As expected, this axonal energy deficit is prevented by maintaining NAD^+ levels via the WLD^s mutant protein or the SARM1 deletion (Wang et al., 2005; Yang et al., 2015). Otherwise, the lasting energy deficit severely interferes with many cellular events, for example, axonal transport, protein synthesis or degradation, and ion gradients across the plasma membrane. Among them, the significant accumulation of Ca^{2+} within axons has been documented as a common hallmark under neurodegenerative conditions, often occurring immediately before the final dismantling of axonal structures. As discussed above, such Ca^{2+} overload can be attributed to the failure of Ca^{2+}-ATPases and Na^+/Ca^{2+} exchangers to clear out Ca^{2+} influx into axons through various channels.

It has already been discovered in the 1970s that high levels (e.g., tens of micromolar concentrations) of intracellular Ca^{2+} are sufficient to induce the destruction of axonal structures (Schlaepfer, 1971; Schlaepfer, 1974). This process is executed by a group of Ca^{2+}-activated proteases known as calpains (Goll et al., 2003; Liu et al., 2004). Calpains are broadly expressed in mammalian cells, and the predominant forms in the cytosol of neurons and axons include calpain-1 and calpain-2. Under low Ca^{2+} concentrations (i.e., submicromolar concentrations), calpain-1 and calpain-2 remain mostly inactive. When Ca^{2+} levels increase, the two calpains are triggered into action. Accordingly, removing extracellular Ca^{2+} or chelating intracellular Ca^{2+} effectively prevents the calpain activation and preserves the structural integrity of traumatically injured axons (George et al., 1995; Schlaepfer, 1974). However, such manipulations could not rescue the depletion of ATP levels in damaged axons (Yang et al., 2015), consistent with the metabolic energy deficit being the upstream causative event.

Because of their promiscuous specificity for protein substrates, the active calpains cleave many essential proteins in axons, such as neurofilaments, microtubules, and motor proteins. Calpain-mediated proteolysis is the final stage of pathological axonal degeneration, reminiscent of apoptotic cell death executed by active effector caspases. Conversely, the specific small-molecule inhibitors of calpains preserve the structural integrity of damaged axons while not reverting the metabolic energy defect (Yang et al., 2015). Notably, the neurofilament proteins proteolyzed by calpains may be released from degenerating neurons or axons into the cerebrospinal fluid or the blood circulation. Such neuron-derived protein fragments, for example, serum neurofilament light chain (sNf-L), have been exploited as biomarkers to diagnose certain neurodegenerative diseases (Kapoor et al., 2020; Khalil et al., 2020; Rohrer et al., 2016).

Importantly, due to this irreversible calpain activation, the safety mechanism exists in axons. Calpastatin is an endogenous specific protein inhibitor of calpains and is abundantly distributed within neurons and axons (Goll et al., 2003). By directly binding to calpains, calpastatin prevents the inadvertent activation of the proteases by physiological fluctuations of intracellular Ca^{2+} levels, for example, that occurring in action potentials. Interestingly, calpastatin is a calpain substrate and can be degraded by prolonged calpain activity. As a result, the Ca^{2+} overload caused by the metabolic energy deficits in damaged axons continuously activates calpains and thus overrides this safety mechanism enforced by calpastatin. Conversely, calpastatin overexpression suppresses the calpain activity and the structural destruction of axons under neurodegenerative insults (Yang et al., 2013).

In retrospect, the original discovery of the WLD^s mutant protein has served as the prelude to the characterization of the NAD$^+$-dependent pathway, composed of several sequential events, that is, NMNAT2 depletion, SARM1 activation, metabolic energy deficit, Ca^{2+} overload, and calpain activation. This central mechanism, distinct from all the known types of programmed cell death, represents a common signal instructing pathological axonal degeneration in many neurodegenerative conditions.

6.6 Future Perspectives

We have summarized the current knowledge of the molecular mechanisms underlying pathological axonal degeneration. However, it is essential to emphasize that this unique axonal pathology represents the stereotyped self-destruction of axons under different neurodegenerative insults. Importantly, it can occur independently of or even preceding neuronal cell death in many circumstances. Therefore, in-depth investigations into pathological axonal degeneration are crucial for effectively treating neurodegenerative diseases. Indeed, we have witnessed some of the tremendous advances built upon the decades of accumulating efforts in the field. Meanwhile, we would like to highlight several critical questions that still await to be addressed in future research:

1. Whether unknown signaling pathways may exist to control pathological axonal degeneration demands more examinations. For instance, at least in the mouse model of amyotrophic lateral sclerosis induced by the mutant human SOD1, the genetic deletion of the central apoptotic component BAX did not prevent the death of motor axons (Gould et al., 2006). At the same time, the WLD^s mutant protein (Vande Velde et al., 2004) or the SARM1 deletion (Peters et al., 2018) failed to delay this SOD1-induced axonal pathology. In addition, the RIPK3 deletion only modestly preserved the motor axons in this disease model (Ito et al., 2016). Therefore, unknown mechanisms other than the apoptotic, necroptotic, and NAD$^+$-dependent pathways may be involved in this particular type of pathological axonal degeneration. Detailed studies need to focus on molecular or biochemical alterations beyond those known signaling pathways in the motor axons inflicted by amyotrophic lateral sclerosis, which could pave the way to the mechanistic dissection of this axonal degeneration process.

2. It remains an open question whether some common neurodegenerative diseases, particularly Alzheimer's disease, may involve the currently known pathways. The challenge related to this question is that most of the available rodent disease models are based on the genetic overexpression or knock-in of the mutant forms of human amyloid precursor protein (APP) or gamma-secretase. However, although such disease models recapitulate several neuropathological features in vivo, for example, amyloid plaques, neurofibrillary tangles of TAU proteins, and synaptic defects, they cannot reproduce the massive loss of neurons and axons in the cortex or the hippocampus as that occurring in patients. As a result, the genetic evidence either proving or precluding the involvement of apoptosis, necroptosis, or the NAD$^+$-dependent pathway in the axonal degeneration of Alzheimer's disease is still lacking. Developing more efficient animal models in other species, such as nonhuman primates, will be instructive in answering this vital question (Capitanio and Emborg, 2008; Verdier et al., 2015).

3. Although it has been demonstrated that the NAD$^+$-dependent pathway is essential for pathological axonal degeneration in many disease scenarios, how this mechanism is triggered remains incompletely understood. For instance, SARM1-dependent axonal degeneration occurs upon exposure to neurotoxins such as 6-hydroxydopamine or rotenone (Peters et al., 2021; Sur et al., 2018). However, how such neurotoxins would alter the NAD$^+$ metabolism and activate SARM1 is unclear. Those neurotoxins

disrupt the electron transport chain, leading to mitochondrial damage. Meanwhile, the SARM1 protein may be anchored to mitochondria via its N-terminal mitochondria-targeting sequence. Whether this unique subcellular localization of SARM1 would be linked to mitochondrial damage becomes an attractive question. Also, though SARM1 has an essential role in chemotherapy-induced peripheral neuropathy (Geisler et al., 2016; Wang et al., 2019), how axonal NAD^+ metabolism is affected by chemotherapeutic agents such as vincristine or paclitaxel is unknown. The interference of microtubules by those chemotherapeutic agents may cause the reduced transport of NMNAT2 protein from neuronal cell bodies, resulting in the disrupted NAD^+ metabolism in axons. More in-depth research on the engagement of the NAD^+-dependent pathway under specific disease conditions is warranted.

4. It has been intriguing whether different signaling pathways may be synergetically involved in a particular neurodegenerative condition. For example, the apoptotic pathway partially controls the degeneration of axonal projections of dopaminergic neurons in mouse models of Parkinson's disease (Kim et al., 2011; Vila et al., 2001). The WLD^s mutant protein (Cheng and Burke, 2010; Sajadi et al., 2004) or the SARM1 deletion (Peters et al., 2021) could also mitigate the pathological axonal degeneration in such disease models. Therefore, how the apoptotic pathway and the NAD^+-dependent pathway crosstalk with each other need to be explored. Similarly, recent studies have reported that the TNF-alpha-induced pathological degeneration of mouse optic, sensory, or sympathetic axons depends on the SARM1 signal (Ko et al., 2020; Liu et al., 2021). Meanwhile, the pharmacological induction of MLKL oligomerization, which is the core step of necroptosis, is sufficient to trigger the SARM1 activation (Ko et al., 2020). Such results have implicated the potential intertwining between necroptosis and the NAD^+-dependent pathway. If the crosstalk of signaling pathways exists in the context of specific diseases, it will emphasize the necessity of simultaneously targeting individual pathways for more efficient therapeutic strategies.

5. While the current focus has been mainly on the intrinsic molecular mechanisms of pathological axonal degeneration, extensive evidence has demonstrated that non-neuronal cells, especially glial cells, and immune cells, also exert critical roles in neurodegenerative diseases. For instance, myelinating oligodendrocytes and Schwann cells shuttle essential metabolic intermediates to axons (Boucanova and Chrast,

2020; Simons and Nave, 2015). As a result, the myelin destruction by aberrant autoimmunity occurring in multiple sclerosis or Guillain–Barré syndrome leads to the death of demyelinated axons. Accordingly, targeting such autoimmune responses has been proven effective in mitigating the progression of those diseases (Dobson and Giovannoni, 2019; van den Berg et al., 2014). How the functions of non-neuronal cells, for example, metabolic shuttling, inflammation, and phagocytosis, may modulate pathological axonal degeneration is still incompletely understood and is becoming a new frontier in the research field.

6. Although the specific mechanisms of pathological axonal degeneration have been extensively explored for decades, it remains daunting that most neurodegenerative diseases are still incurable. This reality could indicate our incomplete understanding of such signaling pathways and reflect the challenge of translating basic research into therapeutic applications. However, with recent research advances, especially the breakthrough revelation of the NAD$^+$-dependent pathway, novel entry points for combatting pathological axonal degeneration have emerged. In particular, different approaches such as small-molecule inhibitors, macromolecules, or genetic manipulations to target axonal NAD$^+$ metabolism could hold promise and have been pursued.

In our great hope, the combination of enduring basic research and pioneering translational endeavor could eventually conquer those dreadful, debilitating neurodegenerative diseases in years to come.

Acknowledgements

We wish to apologize to colleagues for the omission of many important references due to space limitations. Research in Jing Yang's lab has been funded by the National Natural Science Foundation of China (#31970974, #32061143007, #32125017, and #32150008) and the National Key Research and Development Program of China (2019YFA0802003). Ying Cao has been supported by the China Postdoctoral Science Foundation (#2022M710219) and the Postdoctoral Fellowship of the Center for Life Sciences at Peking University.

References

Albrecht, S., Bogdanovic, N., Ghetti, B., Winblad, B., and LeBlanc, A.C. (2009) Caspase-6 activation in familial alzheimer disease brains carrying amyloid precursor protein or presenilin i or presenilin II mutations. *J Neuropathol Exp Neurol.* **68**, 1282–1293. DOI: 10.1097/ NEN.0b013e3181c1da10.

Angeletti, C., Amici, A., Gilley, J., Loreto, A., Trapanotto, A.G., Antoniou, C., Merlini, E., Coleman, M.P., and Orsomando, G. (2022) SARM1 is a multi-functional NAD(P)ase with prominent base exchange activity, all regulated bymultiple physiologically relevant NAD metabolites. *iScience.* **25**, 103812. DOI: 10.1016/j.isci.2022.103812.

Araki, T., Sasaki, Y., and Milbrandt, J. (2004) Increased nuclear NAD biosynthesis and SIRT1 activation prevent axonal degeneration. *Science.* **305**, 1010–1013. DOI: 10.1126/science.1098014.

Babetto, E., Beirowski, B., Russler, E.V., Milbrandt, J., and DiAntonio, A. (2013) The Phr1 ubiquitin ligase promotes injury-induced axon self-destruction. *Cell Rep.* **3**, 1422–1429. DOI: 10.1016/j.celrep.2013.04.013.

Beirowski, B., Babetto, E., Coleman, M.P., and Martin, K.R. (2008) The WldS gene delays axonal but not somatic degeneration in a rat glaucoma model. *Eur J Neurosci.* **28**, 1166–1179. DOI: 10.1111/j.1460-9568.2008.06426.x.

Belenky, P., Bogan, K.L., and Brenner, C. (2007) NAD+ metabolism in health and disease. *Trends Biochem Sci.* **32**, 12–19. DOI: 10.1016/j. tibs.2006.11.006.

Boucanova, F., and Chrast, R. (2020) Metabolic Interaction Between Schwann Cells and Axons Under Physiological and Disease Conditions. *Front Cell Neurosci.* **14**, 148. DOI: 10.3389/fncel.2020.00148.

Bratkowski, M., Xie, T., Thayer, D.A., Lad, S., Mathur, P., Yang, Y.S., Danko, G., Burdett, T.C., Danao, J., Cantor, A., Kozak, J.A., Brown, S.P., Bai, X., and Sambashivan, S. (2020) Structural and Mechanistic Regulation of the Pro-degenerative NAD Hydrolase SARM1. *Cell Rep.* **32**, 107999. DOI: 10.1016/j.celrep.2020.107999.

Broz, P., and Dixit, V.M. (2016) Inflammasomes: mechanism of assembly, regulation and signalling. *Nat Rev Immunol.* **16**, 407–420. DOI: 10.1038/nri.2016.58.

Budihardjo, I., Oliver, H., Lutter, M., Luo, X., and Wang, X. (1999) Biochemical pathways of caspase activation during apoptosis. *Annu Rev Cell Dev Biol.* **15**, 269–290. DOI: 10.1146/annurev.cellbio.15.1.269.

Cambronne, X.A., and Kraus, W.L. (2020) Location, Location, Location: Compartmentalization of NAD(+) Synthesis and Functions in Mammalian Cells. *Trends Biochem Sci.* **45**, 858–873. DOI: 10.1016/j. tibs.2020.05.010.

Capitanio, J.P., and Emborg, M.E. (2008) Contributions of non-human primates to neuroscience research. *Lancet.* **371**, 1126–1135. DOI: 10.1016/ S0140-6736(08)60489-4.

Carty, M., Goodbody, R., Schroder, M., Stack, J., Moynagh, P.N., and Bowie, A.G. (2006) The human adaptor SARM negatively regulates adaptor protein TRIF-dependent Toll-like receptor signaling. *Nat Immunol.* **7**, 1074–1081. DOI: 10.1038/ni1382.

Cheng, H.C., and Burke, R.E. (2010) The Wld(S) mutation delays antero-grade, but not retrograde, axonal degeneration of the dopaminergic nigro-striatal pathway *in vivo. J Neurochem.* **113**, 683–691. DOI: 10.1111/j.1471-4159.2010.06632.x.

Chiesa, R., Piccardo, P., Dossena, S., Nowoslawski, L., Roth, K.A., Ghetti, B., and Harris, D.A. (2005) Bax deletion prevents neuronal loss but not neurological symptoms in a transgenic model of inherited prion disease. *Proc Natl Acad Sci U S A.* **102**, 238–243. DOI: 10.1073/pnas.0406173102.

Christofferson, D.E., and Yuan, J. (2010) Necroptosis as an alternative form of programmed cell death. *Curr Opin Cell Biol.* **22**, 263–268. DOI: 10.1016/j.ceb.2009.12.003.

Chuang, C.F., and Bargmann, C.I. (2005) A Toll-interleukin 1 repeat protein at the synapse specifies asymmetric odorant receptor expression via ASK1 MAPKKK signaling. *Genes Dev.* **19**, 270–281. DOI: 10.1101/gad.1276505.

Clark, R.S., Kochanek, P.M., Chen, M., Watkins, S.C., Marion, D.W., Chen, J., Hamilton, R.L., Loeffert, J.E., and Graham, S.H. (1999) Increases in Bcl-2 and cleavage of caspase-1 and caspase-3 in human brain after head injury. *FASEB J.* **13**, 813–821. DOI: 10.1096/fasebj.13.8.813.

Coleman, M. (2005) Axon degeneration mechanisms: commonality amid diversity. *Nat Rev Neurosci.* **6**, 889–898. DOI: 10.1038/nrn1788.

Coleman, M.P., Conforti, L., Buckmaster, E.A., Tarlton, A., Ewing, R.M., Brown, M.C., Lyon, M.F., and Perry, V.H. (1998) An 85-kb tandem trip-lication in the slow Wallerian degeneration (Wlds) mouse. *Proc Natl Acad Sci U S A.* **95**, 9985–9990. DOI: 10.1073/pnas.95.17.9985.

Coleman, M.P., and Hoke, A. (2020) Programmed axon degeneration: from mouse to mechanism to medicine. *Nat Rev Neurosci.* **21**, 183–196. DOI: 10.1038/s41583-020-0269-3.

Conforti, L., Tarlton, A., Mack, T.G., Mi, W., Buckmaster, E.A., Wagner, D., Perry, V.H., and Coleman, M.P. (2000) A Ufd2/D4Cole1e chimeric protein and overexpression of Rbp7 in the slow Wallerian degenera-tion (WldS) mouse. *Proc Natl Acad Sci U S A.* **97**, 11377–11382. DOI: 10.1073/pnas.97.21.11377.

Couillault, C., Pujol, N., Reboul, J., Sabatier, L., Guichou, J.F., Kohara, Y., and Ewbank, J.J. (2004) TLR-independent control of innate immunity in Caenorhabditis elegans by the TIR domain adaptor protein TIR-1, an ortholog of human SARM. *Nat Immunol.* **5**, 488–494. DOI: 10.1038/ni1060.

David, K.K., Andrabi, S.A., Dawson, T.M., and Dawson, V.L. (2009) Parthanatos, a messenger of death. *Front Biosci (Landmark Ed).* **14**, 1116–1128. DOI: 10.2741/3297.

De Vos, K.J., Grierson, A.J., Ackerley, S., and Miller, C.C. (2008) Role of axonal transport in neurodegenerative diseases. *Annu Rev Neurosci.* **31**, 151–173. DOI: 10.1146/annurev.neuro.31.061307.090711.

Di Stefano, M., Nascimento-Ferreira, I., Orsomando, G., Mori, V., Gilley, J., Brown, R., Janeckova, L., Vargas, M.E., Worrell, L.A., Loreto, A., Tickle, J., Patrick, J., Webster, J.R., Marangoni, M., Carpi, F.M., Pucciarelli, S., Rossi, F., Meng, W., Sagasti, A., Ribchester, R.R., Magni, G., Coleman, M.P., and Conforti, L. (2015) A rise in NAD precursor nicotinamide mononucleotide (NMN) after injury promotes axon degeneration. *Cell Death Differ.* **22**, 731–742. DOI: 10.1038/cdd.2014.164.

DiAntonio, A. (2019) Axon degeneration: mechanistic insights lead to therapeutic opportunities for the prevention and treatment of peripheral neuropathy. *Pain.* **160** Suppl 1, S17–S22. DOI: 10.1097/j.pain.0000000000001528.

Dobson, R., and Giovannoni, G. (2019) Multiple sclerosis - a review. *Eur J Neurol.* **26**, 27–40. DOI: 10.1111/ene.13819.

Elmore, S. (2007) Apoptosis: a review of programmed cell death. *Toxicol Pathol.* **35**, 495–516. DOI: 10.1080/01926230701320337.

Essuman, K., Summers, D.W., Sasaki, Y., Mao, X., DiAntonio, A., and Milbrandt, J. (2017) The SARM1 Toll/Interleukin-1 Receptor Domain Possesses Intrinsic NAD(+) Cleavage Activity that Promotes Pathological Axonal Degeneration. *Neuron.* **93**, 1334–1343 e1335. DOI: 10.1016/j.neuron.2017.02.022.

Essuman, K., Summers, D.W., Sasaki, Y., Mao, X., Yim, A.K.Y., DiAntonio, A., and Milbrandt, J. (2018) TIR Domain Proteins Are an Ancient Family of NAD(+)-Consuming Enzymes. *Curr Biol.* **28**, 421–430 e424. DOI: 10.1016/j.cub.2017.12.024.

Fan, H., Zhang, K., Shan, L., Kuang, F., Chen, K., Zhu, K., Ma, H., Ju, G., and Wang, Y.Z. (2016) Reactive astrocytes undergo M1 microglia/macrohpages-induced necroptosis in spinal cord injury. *Mol Neurodegener.* **11**, 14. DOI: 10.1186/s13024-016-0081-8.

Fatokun, A.A., Dawson, V.L., and Dawson, T.M. (2014) Parthanatos: mitochondrial-linked mechanisms and therapeutic opportunities. *Br J Pharmacol.* **171**, 2000–2016. DOI: 10.1111/bph.12416.

Ferri, A., Sanes, J.R., Coleman, M.P., Cunningham, J.M., and Kato, A.C. (2003) Inhibiting axon degeneration and synapse loss attenuates apoptosis and disease progression in a mouse model of motoneuron disease. *Curr Biol.* **13**, 669–673. DOI: 10.1016/s0960-9822(03)00206-9.

Figley, M.D., Gu, W., Nanson, J.D., Shi, Y., Sasaki, Y., Cunnea, K., Malde, A.K., Jia, X., Luo, Z., Saikot, F.K., Mosaiab, T., Masic, V., Holt, S., Hartley-Tassell, L., McGuinness, H.Y., Manik, M.K., Bosanac, T., Landsberg, M.J., Kerry, P.S., Mobli, M., Hughes, R.O., Milbrandt, J., Kobe, B., DiAntonio, A., and Ve, T. (2021) SARM1 is a metabolic sensor activated by an increased NMN/NAD(+) ratio to trigger axon degeneration. *Neuron.* **109**, 1118–1136 e1111. DOI: 10.1016/j. neuron.2021.02.009.

Fischer, L.R., Culver, D.G., Davis, A.A., Tennant, P., Wang, M., Coleman, M., Asress, S., Adalbert, R., Alexander, G.M., and Glass, J.D. (2005) The WldS gene modestly prolongs survival in the SOD1G93A fALS mouse. *Neurobiol Dis.* **19**, 293–300. DOI: 10.1016/j.nbd.2005.01.008.

Geden, M.J., and Deshmukh, M. (2016) Axon degeneration: context defines distinct pathways. *Curr Opin Neurobiol.* **39**, 108–115. DOI: 10.1016/j. conb.2016.05.002.

Geisler, S., Doan, R.A., Strickland, A., Huang, X., Milbrandt, J., and DiAntonio, A. (2016) Prevention of vincristine-induced peripheral neuropathy by genetic deletion of SARM1 in mice. *Brain.* **139**, 3092–3108. DOI: 10.1093/brain/aww251.

George, E.B., Glass, J.D., and Griffin, J.W. (1995) Axotomy-induced axonal degeneration is mediated by calcium influx through ion-specific channels. *J Neurosci.* **15**, 6445–6452. DOI.

Gerdts, J., Summers, D.W., Sasaki, Y., DiAntonio, A., and Milbrandt, J. (2013) Sarm1-mediated axon degeneration requires both SAM and TIR interactions. *J Neurosci.* **33**, 13569–13580. DOI: 10.1523/ JNEUROSCI.1197-13.2013.

Gilley, J., Adalbert, R., Yu, G., and Coleman, M.P. (2013) Rescue of peripheral and CNS axon defects in mice lacking NMNAT2. *J Neurosci.* **33**, 13410–13424. DOI: 10.1523/JNEUROSCI.1534-13.2013.

Gilley, J., and Coleman, M.P. (2010) Endogenous Nmnat2 is an essential survival factor for maintenance of healthy axons. *PLoS Biol.* **8**, e1000300. DOI: 10.1371/journal.pbio.1000300.

Gilley, J., Orsomando, G., Nascimento-Ferreira, I., and Coleman, M.P. (2015) Absence of SARM1 rescues development and survival of NMNAT2-deficient axons. *Cell Rep.* **10**, 1974–1981. DOI: 10.1016/j. celrep.2015.02.060.

Goffus, A.M., Anderson, G.D., and Hoane, M. (2010) Sustained delivery of nicotinamide limits cortical injury and improves functional recovery following traumatic brain injury. *Oxid Med Cell Longev.* **3**, 145–152. DOI: 10.4161/oxim.3.2.11315.

Goldstein, L.S., and Yang, Z. (2000) Microtubule-based transport systems in neurons: the roles of kinesins and dyneins. *Annu Rev Neurosci.* **23**, 39–71. DOI: 10.1146/annurev.neuro.23.1.39.

Goll, D.E., Thompson, V.F., Li, H., Wei, W., and Cong, J. (2003) The calpain system. *Physiol Rev.* **83**, 731–801. DOI: 10.1152/physrev.00029.2002.

Gould, T.W., Buss, R.R., Vinsant, S., Prevette, D., Sun, W., Knudson, C.M., Milligan, C.E., and Oppenheim, R.W. (2006) Complete dissociation of motor neuron death from motor dysfunction by Bax deletion in a mouse model of ALS. *J Neurosci.* **26**, 8774–8786. DOI: 10.1523/JNEUROSCI.2315-06.2006.

Hartmann, A., Hunot, S., Michel, P.P., Muriel, M.P., Vyas, S., Faucheux, B.A., Mouatt-Prigent, A., Turmel, H., Srinivasan, A., Ruberg, M., Evan, G.I., Agid, Y., and Hirsch, E.C. (2000) Caspase-3: A vulnerability factor and final effector in apoptotic death of dopaminergic neurons in Parkinson's disease. *Proc Natl Acad Sci U S A.* **97**, 2875–2880. DOI: 10.1073/pnas.040556597.

Hoopfer, E.D., McLaughlin, T., Watts, R.J., Schuldiner, O., O'Leary, D.D., and Luo, L. (2006) Wlds protection distinguishes axon degeneration following injury from naturally occurring developmental pruning. *Neuron.* **50**, 883–895. DOI: 10.1016/j.neuron.2006.05.013.

Horsefield, S., Burdett, H., Zhang, X., Manik, M.K., Shi, Y., Chen, J., Qi, T., Gilley, J., Lai, J.S., Rank, M.X., Casey, L.W., Gu, W., Ericsson, D.J., Foley, G., Hughes, R.O., Bosanac, T., von Itzstein, M., Rathjen, J.P., Nanson, J.D., Boden, M., Dry, I.B., Williams, S.J., Staskawicz, B.J., Coleman, M.P., Ve, T., Dodds, P.N., and Kobe, B. (2019) NAD(+) cleavage activity by animal and plant TIR domains in cell death pathways. *Science.* **365**, 793–799. DOI: 10.1126/science.aax1911.

Howell, G.R., Libby, R.T., Jakobs, T.C., Smith, R.S., Phalan, F.C., Barter, J.W., Barbay, J.M., Marchant, J.K., Mahesh, N., Porciatti, V., Whitmore, A.V., Masland, R.H., and John, S.W. (2007) Axons of retinal ganglion cells are insulted in the optic nerve early in DBA/2J glaucoma. *J Cell Biol.* **179**, 1523–1537. DOI: 10.1083/jcb.200706181.

Huang, Y., Wang, S., Huang, F., Zhang, Q., Qin, B., Liao, L., Wang, M., Wan, H., Yan, W., Chen, D., Liu, F., Jiang, B., Ji, D., Xia, X., Huang, J., and Xiong, K. (2021) c-FLIP regulates pyroptosis in retinal neurons following oxygen-glucose deprivation/recovery via a GSDMD-mediated pathway. *Ann Anat.* **235**, 151672. DOI: 10.1016/j.aanat.2020.151672.

Huppke, P., Wegener, E., Gilley, J., Angeletti, C., Kurth, I., Drenth, J.P.H., Stadelmann, C., Barrantes-Freer, A., Bruck, W., Thiele, H., Nurnberg, P., Gartner, J., Orsomando, G., and Coleman, M.P. (2019) Homozygous NMNAT2 mutation in sisters with polyneuropathy and erythromelalgia. *Exp Neurol.* **320**, 112958. DOI: 10.1016/j.expneurol.2019.112958.

Inoue, H., Tsukita, K., Iwasato, T., Suzuki, Y., Tomioka, M., Tateno, M., Nagao, M., Kawata, A., Saido, T.C., Miura, M., Misawa, H., Itohara, S., and Takahashi, R. (2003) The crucial role of caspase-9 in the disease progression of a transgenic ALS mouse model. *EMBO J.* **22**, 6665–6674. DOI: 10.1093/emboj/cdg634.

Ito, Y., Ofengeim, D., Najafov, A., Das, S., Saberi, S., Li, Y., Hitomi, J., Zhu, H., Chen, H., Mayo, L., Geng, J., Amin, P., DeWitt, J.P., Mookhtiar, A.K., Florez, M., Ouchida, A.T., Fan, J.B., Pasparakis, M., Kelliher, M.A., Ravits, J., and Yuan, J. (2016) RIPK1 mediates axonal degeneration by promoting inflammation and necroptosis in ALS. *Science.* **353**, 603–608. DOI: 10.1126/science.aaf6803.

Jiang, Y., Liu, T., Lee, C.H., Chang, Q., Yang, J., and Zhang, Z. (2020) The NAD(+)-mediated self-inhibition mechanism of pro-neurodegenerative SARM1. *Nature.* **588**, 658–663. DOI: 10.1038/s41586-020-2862-z.

Kaneko, S., Wang, J., Kaneko, M., Yiu, G., Hurrell, J.M., Chitnis, T., Khoury, S.J., and He, Z. (2006) Protecting axonal degeneration by increasing nicotinamide adenine dinucleotide levels in experimental autoimmune encephalomyelitis models. *J Neurosci.* **26**, 9794–9804. DOI: 10.1523/JNEUROSCI.2116-06.2006.

Kapoor, R., Smith, K.E., Allegretta, M., Arnold, D.L., Carroll, W., Comabella, M., Furlan, R., Harp, C., Kuhle, J., Leppert, D., Plavina, T., Sellebjerg, F., Sincock, C., Teunissen, C.E., Topalli, I., von Raison, F., Walker, E., and Fox, R.J. (2020) Serum neurofilament light as a biomarker in progressive multiple sclerosis. *Neurology.* **95**, 436–444. DOI: 10.1212/WNL.0000000000010346.

Kariya, S., Mauricio, R., Dai, Y., and Monani, U.R. (2009) The neuroprotective factor Wld(s) fails to mitigate distal axonal and neuromuscular junction (NMJ) defects in mouse models of spinal muscular atrophy. *Neurosci Lett.* **449**, 246–251. DOI: 10.1016/j.neulet.2008.10.107.

Khalil, M., Pirpamer, L., Hofer, E., Voortman, M.M., Barro, C., Leppert, D., Benkert, P., Ropele, S., Enzinger, C., Fazekas, F., Schmidt, R., and Kuhle, J. (2020) Serum neurofilament light levels in normal aging and their association with morphologic brain changes. *Nat Commun.* **11**, 812. DOI: 10.1038/s41467-020-14612-6.

Kim, T.W., Moon, Y., Kim, K., Lee, J.E., Koh, H.C., Rhyu, I.J., Kim, H., and Sun, W. (2011) Dissociation of progressive dopaminergic neuronal death and behavioral impairments by Bax deletion in a mouse model of Parkinson's diseases. *PLoS One.* **6**, e25346. DOI: 10.1371/journal. pone.0025346.

Kim, Y., Zhou, P., Qian, L., Chuang, J.Z., Lee, J., Li, C., Iadecola, C., Nathan, C., and Ding, A. (2007) MyD88-5 links mitochondria, microtubules, and JNK3 in neurons and regulates neuronal survival. *J Exp Med.* **204**, 2063–2074. DOI: 10.1084/jem.20070868.

Ko, K.W., Milbrandt, J., and DiAntonio, A. (2020) SARM1 acts downstream of neuroinflammatory and necroptotic signaling to induce axon degeneration. *J Cell Biol.* **219**. DOI: 10.1083/jcb.201912047.

Kovacs, S.B., and Miao, E.A. (2017) Gasdermins: Effectors of Pyroptosis. *Trends Cell Biol.* **27**, 673–684. DOI: 10.1016/j.tcb.2017.05.005.

Krajewska, M., You, Z., Rong, J., Kress, C., Huang, X., Yang, J., Kyoda, T., Leyva, R., Banares, S., Hu, Y., Sze, C.H., Whalen, M.J., Salmena, L., Hakem, R., Head, B.P., Reed, J.C., and Krajewski, S. (2011) Neuronal deletion of caspase 8 protects against brain injury in mouse models of controlled cortical impact and kainic acid-induced excitotoxicity. *PLoS One.* **6**, e24341. DOI: 10.1371/journal.pone.0024341.

Lau, C., Dolle, C., Gossmann, T.I., Agledal, L., Niere, M., and Ziegler, M. (2010) Isoform-specific targeting and interaction domains in human nicotinamide mononucleotide adenylyltransferases. *J Biol Chem.* **285**, 18868–18876. DOI: 10.1074/jbc.M110.107631.

Lei, P., Bai, T., and Sun, Y. (2019) Mechanisms of Ferroptosis and Relations With Regulated Cell Death: A Review. *Front Physiol.* 10, **139**. DOI: 10.3389/fphys.2019.00139.

Libby, R.T., Li, Y., Savinova, O.V., Barter, J., Smith, R.S., Nickells, R.W., and John, S.W. (2005) Susceptibility to neurodegeneration in a glaucoma is modified by Bax gene dosage. *PLoS Genet.* **1**, 17–26. DOI: 10.1371/journal.pgen.0010004.

Liu, K., Yang, L., Wang, G., Liu, J., Zhao, X., Wang, Y., Li, J., and Yang, J. (2021) Metabolic stress drives sympathetic neuropathy within the liver. *Cell Metab.* **33**, 666–675 e664. DOI: 10.1016/j.cmet.2021.01.012.

Liu, X., Van Vleet, T., and Schnellmann, R.G. (2004) The role of calpain in oncotic cell death. *Annu Rev Pharmacol Toxicol.* **44**, 349–370. DOI: 10.1146/annurev.pharmtox.44.101802.121804.

Liu, Z.M., Chen, Q.X., Chen, Z.B., Tian, D.F., Li, M.C., Wang, J.M., Wang, L., Liu, B.H., Zhang, S.Q., Li, F., Ye, H., and Zhou, L. (2018) RIP3 deficiency protects against traumatic brain injury (TBI) through suppressing oxidative stress, inflammation and apoptosis: Dependent on AMPK pathway. *Biochem Biophys Res Commun.* **499**, 112–119. DOI: 10.1016/j.bbrc.2018.02.150.

Loreto, A., Angeletti, C., Gu, W., Osborne, A., Nieuwenhuis, B., Gilley, J., Merlini, E., Arthur-Farraj, P., Amici, A., Luo, Z., Hartley-Tassell, L., Ve, T., Desrochers, L.M., Wang, Q., Kobe, B., Orsomando, G., and Coleman, M.P. (2021) Neurotoxin-mediated potent activation of the axon degeneration regulator SARM1. *Elife.* **10**. DOI: 10.7554/eLife.72823.

Loreto, A., Di Stefano, M., Gering, M., and Conforti, L. (2015) Wallerian Degeneration Is Executed by an NMN-SARM1-Dependent Late Ca(2+) Influx but Only Modestly Influenced by Mitochondria. *Cell Rep.* **13**, 2539–2552. DOI: 10.1016/j.celrep.2015.11.032.

Lukacs, M., Gilley, J., Zhu, Y., Orsomando, G., Angeletti, C., Liu, J., Yang, X., Park, J., Hopkin, R.J., Coleman, M.P., Zhai, R.G., and Stottmann, R.W. (2019) Severe biallelic loss-of-function mutations in nicotinamide mononucleotide adenylyltransferase 2 (NMNAT2) in two fetuses with fetal akinesia deformation sequence. *Exp Neurol.* **320**, 112961. DOI: 10.1016/j.expneurol.2019.112961.

Lunn, E.R., Perry, V.H., Brown, M.C., Rosen, H., and Gordon, S. (1989) Absence of Wallerian Degeneration does not Hinder Regeneration in Peripheral Nerve. *Eur J Neurosci.* **1**, 27–33. DOI: 10.1111/j.1460-9568.1989.tb00771.x.

Mack, T.G., Reincr, M., Beirowski, B., Mi, W., Emanuelli, M., Wagner, D., Thomson, D., Gillingwater, T., Court, F., Conforti, L., Fernando, F.S., Tarlton, A., Andressen, C., Addicks, K., Magni, G., Ribchester, R.R., Perry, V.H., and Coleman, M.P. (2001) Wallerian degeneration of injured axons and synapses is delayed by a Ube4b/Nmnat chimeric gene. *Nat Neurosci.* **4**, 1199–1206. DOI: 10.1038/nn770.

Maday, S., Twelvetrees, A.E., Moughamian, A.J., and Holzbaur, E.L. (2014) Axonal transport: cargo-specific mechanisms of motility and regulation. *Neuron.* **84**, 292–309. DOI: 10.1016/j.neuron.2014.10.019.

Meyer zu Horste, G., Miesbach, T.A., Muller, J.I., Fledrich, R., Stassart, R.M., Kieseier, B.C., Coleman, M.P., and Sereda, M.W. (2011) The Wlds transgene reduces axon loss in a Charcot-Marie-Tooth disease 1A rat model and nicotinamide delays post-traumatic axonal degeneration. *Neurobiol Dis.* **42**, 1–8. DOI: 10.1016/j.nbd.2010.12.006.

Mi, W., Beirowski, B., Gillingwater, T.H., Adalbert, R., Wagner, D., Grumme, D., Osaka, H., Conforti, L., Arnhold, S., Addicks, K., Wada, K., Ribchester, R.R., and Coleman, M.P. (2005) The slow

Wallerian degeneration gene, WldS, inhibits axonal spheroid pathology in gracile axonal dystrophy mice. *Brain.* **128**, 405–416. DOI: 10.1093/brain/awh368.

Mifflin, L., Ofengeim, D., and Yuan, J. (2020) Receptor-interacting protein kinase 1 (RIPK1) as a therapeutic target. *Nat Rev Drug Discov.* **19**, 553–571. DOI: 10.1038/s41573-020-0071-y.

Millecamps, S., and Julien, J.P. (2013) Axonal transport deficits and neurodegenerative diseases. *Nat Rev Neurosci.* **14**, 161–176. DOI: 10.1038/nrn3380.

Neukomm, L.J., and Freeman, M.R. (2014) Diverse cellular and molecular modes of axon degeneration. *Trends Cell Biol.* **24**, 515–523. DOI: 10.1016/j.tcb.2014.04.003.

O'Neill, L.A., and Bowie, A.G. (2007) The family of five: TIR-domain-containing adaptors in Toll-like receptor signalling. *Nat Rev Immunol.* **7**, 353–364. DOI: 10.1038/nri2079.

Ofengeim, D., Ito, Y., Najafov, A., Zhang, Y., Shan, B., DeWitt, J.P., Ye, J., Zhang, X., Chang, A., Vakifahmetoglu-Norberg, H., Geng, J., Py, B., Zhou, W., Amin, P., Berlink Lima, J., Qi, C., Yu, Q., Trapp, B., and Yuan, J. (2015) Activation of necroptosis in multiple sclerosis. *Cell Rep.* **10**, 1836–1849. DOI: 10.1016/j.celrep.2015.02.051.

Osterloh, J.M., Yang, J., Rooney, T.M., Fox, A.N., Adalbert, R., Powell, E.H., Sheehan, A.E., Avery, M.A., Hackett, R., Logan, M.A., MacDonald, J.M., Ziegenfuss, J.S., Milde, S., Hou, Y.J., Nathan, C., Ding, A., Brown, R.H., Jr., Conforti, L., Coleman, M., Tessier-Lavigne, M., Zuchner, S., and Freeman, M.R. (2012) dSarm/Sarm1 is required for activation of an injury-induced axon death pathway. *Science.* **337**, 481–484. DOI: 10.1126/science.1223899.

Perry, V.H., Brown, M.C., Lunn, E.R., Tree, P., and Gordon, S. (1990a) Evidence that Very Slow Wallerian Degeneration in C57BL/Ola Mice is an Intrinsic Property of the Peripheral Nerve. *Eur J Neurosci.* **2**, 802–808. DOI: 10.1111/j.1460-9568.1990.tb00472.x.

Perry, V.H., Lunn, E.R., Brown, M.C., Cahusac, S., and Gordon, S. (1990b) Evidence that the Rate of Wallerian Degeneration is Controlled by a Single Autosomal Dominant Gene. *Eur J Neurosci.* **2**, 408–413. DOI: 10.1111/j.1460-9568.1990.tb00433.x.

Peters, O.M., Lewis, E.A., Osterloh, J.M., Weiss, A., Salameh, J.S., Metterville, J., Brown, R.H., and Freeman, M.R. (2018) Loss of Sarm1 does not suppress motor neuron degeneration in the SOD1G93A mouse model of amyotrophic lateral sclerosis. *Hum Mol Genet.* **27**, 3761–3771. DOI: 10.1093/hmg/ddy260.

Peters, O.M., Weiss, A., Metterville, J., Song, L., Logan, R., Smith, G.A., Schwarzschild, M.A., Mueller, C., Brown, R.H., and Freeman, M. (2021) Genetic diversity of axon degenerative mechanisms in models of Parkinson's disease. *Neurobiol Dis.* **155**, 105368. DOI: 10.1016/j.nbd.2021.105368.

Remijsen, Q., Kuijpers, T.W., Wirawan, E., Lippens, S., Vandenabeele, P., and Vanden Berghe, T. (2011) Dying for a cause: NETosis, mechanisms behind an antimicrobial cell death modality. *Cell Death Differ.* **18**, 581–588. DOI: 10.1038/cdd.2011.1.

Rohn, T.T., Vyas, V., Hernandez-Estrada, T., Nichol, K.E., Christie, L.A., and Head, E. (2008) Lack of pathology in a triple transgenic mouse model of Alzheimer's disease after overexpression of the anti-apoptotic protein Bcl-2. *J Neurosci.* **28**, 3051–3059. DOI: 10.1523/JNEUROSCI.5620-07.2008.

Rohrer, J.D., Woollacott, I.O., Dick, K.M., Brotherhood, E., Gordon, E., Fellows, A., Toombs, J., Druyeh, R., Cardoso, M.J., Ourselin, S., Nicholas, J.M., Norgren, N., Mead, S., Andreasson, U., Blennow, K., Schott, J.M., Fox, N.C., Warren, J.D., and Zetterberg, H. (2016) Serum neurofilament light chain protein is a measure of disease intensity in frontotemporal dementia. *Neurology.* **87**, 1329–1336. DOI: 10.1212/WNL.0000000000003154.

Sajadi, A., Schneider, B.L., and Aebischer, P. (2004) Wlds-mediated protection of dopaminergic fibers in an animal model of Parkinson disease. *Curr Biol.* **14**, 326–330. DOI: 10.1016/j.cub.2004.01.053.

Sasaki, Y., and Milbrandt, J. (2010) Axonal degeneration is blocked by nicotinamide mononucleotide adenylyltransferase (Nmnat) protein transduction into transected axons. *J Biol Chem.* **285**, 41211-41215. DOI: 10.1074/jbc.C110.193904.

Sasaki, Y., Vohra, B.P., Lund, F.E., and Milbrandt, J. (2009) Nicotinamide mononucleotide adenylyl transferase-mediated axonal protection requires enzymatic activity but not increased levels of neuronal nicotinamide adenine dinucleotide. *J Neurosci.* **29**, 5525–5535. DOI: 10.1523/JNEUROSCI.5469-08.2009.

Schlaepfer, W.W. (1971) Experimental alterations of neurofilaments and neurotubules by calcium and other ions. *Exp Cell Res.* **67**, 73–80. DOI: 10.1016/0014-4827(71)90622-7.

Schlaepfer, W.W. (1974) Calcium-induced degeneration of axoplasm in isolated segments of rat peripheral nerve. *Brain Res.* **69**, 203–215. DOI: 10.1016/0006-8993(74)90002-x.

Schroer, T.A. (2004) Dynactin. *Annu Rev Cell Dev Biol.* **20**, 759–779. DOI: 10.1146/annurev.cellbio.20.012103.094623.

Schuldiner, O., and Yaron, A. (2015) Mechanisms of developmental neurite pruning. *Cell Mol Life Sci.* **72**, 101–119. DOI: 10.1007/s00018-014-1729-6.

Selznick, L.A., Holtzman, D.M., Han, B.H., Gokden, M., Srinivasan, A.N., Johnson, E.M., Jr., and Roth, K.A. (1999) In situ immunodetection of neuronal caspase-3 activation in Alzheimer disease. *J Neuropathol Exp Neurol.* **58**, 1020–1026. DOI: 10.1097/00005072-199909000-00012.

Shen, C., Vohra, M., Zhang, P., Mao, X., Figley, M.D., Zhu, J., Sasaki, Y., Wu, H., DiAntonio, A., and Milbrandt, J. (2021) Multiple domain interfaces mediate SARM1 autoinhibition. *Proc Natl Acad Sci U S A.* **118**. DOI: 10.1073/pnas.2023151118.

Shi, J., Gao, W., and Shao, F. (2017) Pyroptosis: Gasdermin-Mediated Programmed Necrotic Cell Death. *Trends Biochem Sci.* **42**, 245–254. DOI: 10.1016/j.tibs.2016.10.004.

Shi, Y., Kerry, P.S., Nanson, J.D., Bosanac, T., Sasaki, Y., Krauss, R., Saikot, F.K., Adams, S.E., Mosaiab, T., Masic, V., Mao, X., Rose, F., Vasquez, E., Furrer, M., Cunnea, K., Brearley, A., Gu, W., Luo, Z., Brillault, L., Landsberg, M.J., DiAntonio, A., Kobe, B., Milbrandt, J., Hughes, R.O., and Ve, T. (2022) Structural basis of SARM1 activation, substrate recognition, and inhibition by small molecules. *Mol Cell.* **82**, 1643–1659 e1610. DOI: 10.1016/j.molcel.2022.03.007.

Simon, D.J., Weimer, R.M., McLaughlin, T., Kallop, D., Stanger, K., Yang, J., O'Leary, D.D., Hannoush, R.N., and Tessier-Lavigne, M. (2012) A caspase cascade regulating developmental axon degeneration. *J Neurosci.* **32**, 17540–17553. DOI: 10.1523/JNEUROSCI.3012-12.2012.

Simons, M., and Nave, K.A. (2015) Oligodendrocytes: Myelination and Axonal Support. *Cold Spring Harb Perspect Biol.* **8**, a020479. DOI: 10.1101/cshperspect.a020479.

Sporny, M., Guez-Haddad, J., Khazma, T., Yaron, A., Dessau, M., Shkolnisky, Y., Mim, C., Isupov, M.N., Zalk, R., Hons, M., and Opatowsky, Y. (2020) Structural basis for SARM1 inhibition and activation under energetic stress. *Elife.* **9**. DOI: 10.7554/eLife.62021.

Sun, L., and Wang, X. (2014) A new kind of cell suicide: mechanisms and functions of programmed necrosis. *Trends Biochem Sci.* **39**, 587–593. DOI: 10.1016/j.tibs.2014.10.003.

Sun, Y., Wang, Q., Wang, Y., Ren, W., Cao, Y., Li, J., Zhou, X., Fu, W., and Yang, J. (2021) Sarm1-mediated neurodegeneration within the enteric nervous system protects against local inflammation of the colon. *Protein Cell.* **12**, 621–638. DOI: 10.1007/s13238-021-00835-w.

Sur, M., Dey, P., Sarkar, A., Bar, S., Banerjee, D., Bhat, S., and Mukherjee, P. (2018) Sarm1 induction and accompanying inflammatory response mediates age-dependent susceptibility to rotenone-induced neurotoxic-ity. *Cell Death Discov.* **4**, 114. DOI: 10.1038/s41420-018-0119-5.

Thiam, H.R., Wong, S.L., Wagner, D.D., and Waterman, C.M. (2020) Cellular Mechanisms of NETosis. *Annu Rev Cell Dev Biol.* **36**, 191–218. DOI: 10.1146/annurev-cellbio-020520-111016.

Tsuchiya, K., Nakajima, S., Hosojima, S., Thi Nguyen, D., Hattori, T., Manh Le, T., Hori, O., Mahib, M.R., Yamaguchi, Y., Miura, M., Kinoshita, T., Kushiyama, H., Sakurai, M., Shiroishi, T., and Suda, T. (2019) Caspase-1 initiates apoptosis in the absence of gasdermin D. *Nat Commun.* **10**, 2091. DOI: 10.1038/s41467-019-09753-2.

Turkiew, E., Falconer, D., Reed, N., and Hoke, A. (2017) Deletion of Sarm1 gene is neuroprotective in two models of peripheral neuropathy. *J Peripher Nerv Syst.* **22**, 162–171. DOI: 10.1111/jns.12219.

van den Berg, B., Walgaard, C., Drenthen, J., Fokke, C., Jacobs, B.C., and van Doorn, P.A. (2014) Guillain-Barre syndrome: pathogenesis, diagnosis, treatment and prognosis. *Nat Rev Neurol.* **10**, 469–482. DOI: 10.1038/nrneurol.2014.121.

Vande Velde, C., Garcia, M.L., Yin, X., Trapp, B.D., and Cleveland, D.W. (2004) The neuroprotective factor Wlds does not attenuate mutant SOD1-mediated motor neuron disease. *Neuromolecular Med.* **5**, 193–203. DOI: 10.1385/NMM:5:3:193.

Verdier, J.M., Acquatella, I., Lautier, C., Devau, G., Trouche, S., Lasbleiz, C., and Mestre-Frances, N. (2015) Lessons from the analysis of nonhuman primates for understanding human aging and neurodegenerative diseases. *Front Neurosci.* **9**, 64. DOI: 10.3389/fnins.2015.00064.

Viar, K., Njoku, D., Secor McVoy, J., and Oh, U. (2020) Sarm1 knockout protects against early but not late axonal degeneration in experimental allergic encephalomyelitis. *PLoS One.* **15**, e0235110. DOI: 10.1371/journal.pone.0235110.

Vila, M., Jackson-Lewis, V., Vukosavic, S., Djaldetti, R., Liberatore, G., Offen, D., Korsmeyer, S.J., and Przedborski, S. (2001) Bax ablation prevents dopaminergic neurodegeneration in the 1-methyl- 4-phenyl-1,2,3,6-tetrahydropyridine mouse model of Parkinson's disease. *Proc Natl Acad Sci U S A.* **98**, 2837–2842. DOI: 10.1073/pnas.051633998.

Walker, L.J., Summers, D.W., Sasaki, Y., Brace, E.J., Milbrandt, J., and DiAntonio, A. (2017) MAPK signaling promotes axonal degeneration by speeding the turnover of the axonal maintenance factor NMNAT2. *Elife.* **6**. DOI: 10.7554/eLife.22540.

Waller, A. (1850) Experiments on the section of the glossopharyngeal and hypoglossal nerves of the frog, and observations of the alterations produced thereby in the structure of their primitive fibres. *Philos Trans R Soc Lond.* **140**, 423–429. DOI.

Wan, L., Essuman, K., Anderson, R.G., Sasaki, Y., Monteiro, F., Chung, E.H., Osborne Nishimura, E., DiAntonio, A., Milbrandt, J., Dangl, J.L., and Nishimura, M.T. (2019) TIR domains of plant immune receptors are NAD(+)-cleaving enzymes that promote cell death. *Science.* **365**, 799–803. DOI: 10.1126/science.aax1771.

Wang, J., Zhai, Q., Chen, Y., Lin, E., Gu, W., McBurney, M.W., and He, Z. (2005) A local mechanism mediates NAD-dependent protection of axon degeneration. *J Cell Biol.* **170**, 349–355. DOI: 10.1083/jcb.200504028.

Wang, J.T., Medress, Z.A., and Barres, B.A. (2012) Axon degeneration: molecular mechanisms of a self-destruction pathway. *J Cell Biol.* **196**, 7–18. DOI: 10.1083/jcb.201108111.

Wang, M.S., Davis, A.A., Culver, D.G., and Glass, J.D. (2002) WldS mice are resistant to paclitaxel (taxol) neuropathy. *Ann Neurol.* **52**, 442–447. DOI: 10.1002/ana.10300.

Wang, Q., Liu, K., Yang, L., Wang, H., and Yang, J. (2019) BoneClear: whole-tissue immunolabeling of the intact mouse bones for 3D imaging of neural anatomy and pathology. *Cell Res.* **29**, 870–872. DOI: 10.1038/s41422-019-0217-9.

Wang, T., Perera, N.D., Chiam, M.D.F., Cuic, B., Wanniarachchillage, N., Tomas, D., Samson, A.L., Cawthorne, W., Valor, E.N., Murphy, J.M., and Turner, B.J. (2020) Necroptosis is dispensable for motor neuron degeneration in a mouse model of ALS. *Cell Death Differ.* **27**, 1728–1739. DOI: 10.1038/s41418-019-0457-8.

White, M.A., Lin, Z., Kim, E., Henstridge, C.M., Pena Altamira, E., Hunt, C.K., Burchill, E., Callaghan, I., Loreto, A., Brown-Wright, H., Mead, R., Simmons, C., Cash, D., Coleman, M.P., and Sreedharan, J. (2019) Sarm1 deletion suppresses TDP-43-linked motor neuron degeneration and cortical spine loss. *Acta Neuropathol Commun.* **7**, 166. DOI: 10.1186/s40478-019-0800-9.

Whitmore, A.V., Lindsten, T., Raff, M.C., and Thompson, C.B. (2003) The proapoptotic proteins Bax and Bak are not involved in Wallerian degeneration. *Cell Death Differ.* **10**, 260–261. DOI: 10.1038/sj.cdd.4401147.

Wu, T., Zhu, J., Strickland, A., Ko, K.W., Sasaki, Y., Dingwall, C.B., Yamada, Y., Figley, M.D., Mao, X., Neiner, A., Bloom, A.J., DiAntonio, A., and Milbrandt, J. (2021) Neurotoxins subvert the allosteric activation mechanism of SARM1 to induce neuronal loss. *Cell Rep.* **37**, 109872. DOI: 10.1016/j.celrep.2021.109872.

Xie, Y., Hou, W., Song, X., Yu, Y., Huang, J., Sun, X., Kang, R., and Tang, D. (2016) Ferroptosis: process and function. *Cell Death Differ.* **23**, 369–379. DOI: 10.1038/cdd.2015.158.

Xu, D., Zou, C., and Yuan, J. (2021) Genetic Regulation of RIPK1 and Necroptosis. *Annu Rev Genet.* **55**, 235–263. DOI: 10.1146/annurev-genet-071719-022748.

Yamagishi, Y., and Tessier-Lavigne, M. (2016) An Atypical SCF-like Ubiquitin Ligase Complex Promotes Wallerian Degeneration through Regulation of Axonal Nmnat2. *Cell Rep.* **17**, 774–782. DOI: 10.1016/j.celrep.2016.09.043.

Yang, H., Yang, T., Baur, J.A., Perez, E., Matsui, T., Carmona, J.J., Lamming, D.W., Souza-Pinto, N.C., Bohr, V.A., Rosenzweig, A., de Cabo, R., Sauve, A.A., and Sinclair, D.A. (2007) Nutrient-sensitive mitochondrial NAD+ levels dictate cell survival. *Cell.* **130**, 1095–1107. DOI: 10.1016/j.cell.2007.07.035.

Yang, J., Weimer, R.M., Kallop, D., Olsen, O., Wu, Z., Renier, N., Uryu, K., and Tessier-Lavigne, M. (2013) Regulation of axon degeneration after injury and in development by the endogenous calpain inhibitor calpastatin. *Neuron.* **80**, 1175–1189. DOI: 10.1016/j.neuron.2013.08.034.

Yang, J., Wu, Z., Renier, N., Simon, D.J., Uryu, K., Park, D.S., Greer, P.A., Tournier, C., Davis, R.J., and Tessier-Lavigne, M. (2015) Pathological axonal death through a MAPK cascade that triggers a local energy deficit. *Cell.* **160**, 161–176. DOI: 10.1016/j.cell.2014.11.053.

Yang, Y., Mohammed, F.S., Zhang, N., and Sauve, A.A. (2019) Dihydronicotinamide riboside is a potent NAD(+) concentration enhancer in vitro and in vivo. *J Biol Chem.* **294**, 9295–9307. DOI: 10.1074/jbc.RA118.005772.

Ye, L., Li, G., Goebel, A., Raju, A.V., Kong, F., Lv, Y., Li, K., Zhu, Y., Raja, S., He, P., Li, F., Mwangi, S.M., Hu, W., and Srinivasan, S. (2020) Caspase-11-mediated enteric neuronal pyroptosis underlies Western diet-induced colonic dysmotility. *J Clin Invest.* **130**, 3621–3636. DOI: 10.1172/JCI130176.

Yuan, J., Amin, P., and Ofengeim, D. (2019) Necroptosis and RIPK1-mediated neuroinflammation in CNS diseases. *Nat Rev Neurosci.* **20**, 19–33. DOI: 10.1038/s41583-018-0093-1.

Zhai, Q., Wang, J., Kim, A., Liu, Q., Watts, R., Hoopfer, E., Mitchison, T., Luo, L., and He, Z. (2003) Involvement of the ubiquitin-proteasome system in the early stages of wallerian degeneration. *Neuron.* **39**, 217–225. DOI: 10.1016/s0896-6273(03)00429-x.

Zhang, S., Su, Y., Ying, Z., Guo, D., Pan, C., Guo, J., Zou, Z., Wang, L., Zhang, Z., Jiang, Z., Zhang, Z., and Wang, X. (2019) RIP1 kinase inhibitor halts the progression of an immune-induced demyelination disease at the stage of monocyte elevation. *Proc Natl Acad Sci U S A.* **116**, 5675–5680. DOI: 10.1073/pnas.1819917116.

Zhang, X., Graham, S.H., Kochanek, P.M., Marion, D.W., Nathaniel, P.D., Watkins, S.C., and Clark, R.S. (2003) Caspase-8 expression and proteolysis in human brain after severe head injury. *FASEB J.* **17**, 1367–1369. DOI: 10.1096/fj.02-1067fje.

Zhao, Z.Y., Xie, X.J., Li, W.H., Liu, J., Chen, Z., Zhang, B., Li, T., Li, S.L., Lu, J.G., Zhang, L., Zhang, L.H., Xu, Z., Lee, H.C., and Zhao, Y.J. (2019) A Cell-Permeant Mimetic of NMN Activates SARM1 to Produce Cyclic ADP-Ribose and Induce Non-apoptotic Cell Death. *iScience.* **15**, 452–466. DOI: 10.1016/j.isci.2019.05.001.

7

Roles of mRNA Axonal Localization and Translation in Neurodegenerative Diseases

Madeleine Le Coz[#], Sarah Zakhia[#], and Marco Terenzio

Molecular Neuroscience Unit, Okinawa Institute of Science and Technology
Graduate University, Japan
Corresponding Email: marco.terenzio@oist.jp
[#]These authors contributed equally to the work.

Abstract

Neurons are highly polarized cells with processes that extend over a meter in humans, thus requiring careful management of the structural and metabolic needs of their network. Indeed, neurons need to tightly regulate the flux of information from the periphery to the center, and transport defects of a variety of peripheral signaling complexes, including endosomes, mitochondria, and mRNP granules, have been shown to result in neuronal degeneration. Axonal local translation has emerged as a way of maintaining axonal homeostasis and achieving signaling compartmentalization in neurons. Though an established hallmark of neuronal development and injury, axonal local translation has also been implicated in neurodegeneration and may be an important regulatory mechanism. Alteration in the local synthesis of key proteins involved in the establishment of neurodegenerative diseases and axonal survival could be central to the dying back phenomenon observed in neurodegenerative disorders, whereby axons degenerate before toxicity is manifested in the corresponding cell bodies. In this book chapter, we will briefly review the history and the mechanisms behind axonal translation and its involvement in neurodegenerative diseases.

7.1 Introduction

Neurons are a highly diverse group of polarized cells with a complex morphology linked to their various functions in the nervous system (Zeng &

Sanes, 2017). Indeed, nerve cells are characterized by long cytoplasmic extensions, axons, and dendrites, with lengths ranging from millimeters to meters in large vertebrates, while still retaining the ability to appropriately and timely respond to both internal and external stimuli. Human motor neurons might be over one meter long, while basal brain cholinergic neurons might reach a combined length of a hundred meters, due to their complex arborization (Wu et al., 2014). Thus, functional compartmentalization coupled with a certain degree of subcellular autonomy is critical for neurons (Jung et al., 2014, 2012; Turner-Bridger et al., 2020; Sahoo et al., 2018).

To overcome the hurdles posed by their extreme morphology, neurons transport, localize, and translate mRNAs within specific subcellular domains at different stages of axonal development, from initial growth to maintenance and regeneration (Glock et al., 2017; Rangaraju et al., 2017). In addition, axonal biology is supported by a constant flow of organelles, such as mitochondria, lysosomes, and endosomes. These organelles require a cohort of proteins for their movement and function, which need to be constantly replenished (Vargas et al., 2022). Thus, the presence of an axonal pool of mRNAs is critical to the support of organelle maintenance and transport, with recent evidence showing a direct linkage of mRNAs to axonal organelles, allowing for fast and localized translation (Vargas et al., 2022). Indeed, the use of "on-demand" stored mRNA for axonal protein synthesis enables spatial and temporal regulation of the protein content of subcellular compartments (Jung et al., 2014), allowing for a rapid response to external and/ or internal stimuli.

Several attempts have been made to define the pool of axonal mRNAs and its size has been expanding as a function of the technological progress in the sensitivity of sequencing and the development of new tools for specific labeling and retrieval of RNA, ribosomes, and newly translated proteins (Koppel & Fainzilber, 2018; Holt et al., 2019). While an in-depth discussion about these technologies is outside the scope of this chapter, a comprehensive review of the tools developed to study RNA localization and local synthesis, including fluorescence-based techniques (e.g., FISH and FRAP), modern genomic approaches (e.g., RNAseq), metabolic bio-orthogonal labeling (e.g. Puromycin), and combination of the aforementioned tools (e.g., FUNCAT, Puro-PLA, MERFISH, ExSeq), can be found in (Holt et al., 2019; Taliaferro, 2022). To date, more than 2500 mRNAs, albeit some at low levels, have been shown to localize to neuronal distal compartments (Glock et al., 2017; Vargas et al., 2022). Given the extent of the phenomena, axonal protein synthesis is involved in an increasing amount of physiological and pathological processes (Costa & Willis, 2018; Batista & Hengst, 2016; Spaulding &

Burgess, 2017). In this book chapter, we will briefly address axonal translation and its implications in neuronal pathologies

7.2 Axonal Polyribosomes as a Pre-requisite for Local Translation

Neuronal subcellular compartments need to spatially and temporally control their protein content to respond to local intercellular and extracellular cues. For proteins to be synthesized locally, mRNA needs to be transcribed in the nucleus and transported to the site of synthesis. mRNA transport and localization of the translational machinery are evolutionarily conserved mechanisms critical to the spatial regulation of protein synthesis (Martin & Ephrussi, 2009; Andreassi & Riccio, 2009). Indeed, early electron microscopy (EM) studies in the 1980s identified synapse-associated polyribosomes as well as the post-translational machinery in dendrites of the rat dentate gyrus and hippocampus (Steward & Levy, 1982; Steward & Reeves, 1988). These findings suggested a supportive role for local translation in the maintenance of synapses and their activity, possibly modulating the strength of synapses, a mechanism known to play a role in learning and memory (Steward & Levy, 1982; Steward & Reeves, 1988; Steward & Schuman, 2001). Pulse labeling of de novo proteins with 3H-leucine was performed to prove that the local protein synthesis machinery was active. The use of a compartmentalized culture system in which neurites were allowed to pass through a porous membrane, while the soma remained on either side, revealed extensive dendritic labeling after minutes of exposure to 3H-leucine (Torre & Steward, 1992). A similar study by Sherry Fieg and Peter Lipton in 1993, measured the rate of 3H-leucine incorporation into dendrites in hippocampal slices that had been afferently stimulated using electrical stimulation and exposure to the cholinergic agonist, carbachol (Feig & Lipton, 1993). The presence of the cholinergic agonist coupled with a level of stimulation similar to that of CA1 and CA3 neuronal activity was able to initiate protein synthesis in target dendrites (Feig & Lipton, 1993). Further studies provided evidence for the localization of a specific mRNA subset to synaptic sites in dendrites using RNA fluorescence in situ hybridization (RNA-FISH) (Berry & Brown, 1996; Cox & Racca, 2013; Glock et al., 2017; Steward & Reeves, 1988). For instance, calmodulin I (CaM I) mRNA (Berry & Brown, 1996) and Ca2+/calmodulin-dependent protein kinase type II (CaM-KII) mRNA (Burgin et al., 1990) were found to be localized in the dendrites of cortical neurons in postnatal and developing rat brains respectively.

In contrast to dendrites, axonal mRNA localization, and local translation has been historically subject of debate. As early as 1965, biochemical evidence hinted at the possibility of axonal protein synthesis (Koenig, 1965a, 1965b, 1967a, 1967b). These studies suggested local synthesis of acetylcholinesterase (AChE) in axotomized hypoglossal nerve and the presence of RNA in unmyelinated motor axons of the accessory nerve of adult cats. A series of contrasting observations over the next couple of decades, however, casted doubts on the presence of the translational machinery in axons. For instance, while EM studies from the 1970s provided evidence of ribosomes and smooth endoplasmic reticulum in the growth cone of dorsal root ganglion axons undergoing elongation (Yamada et al., 1971, Bunge 1973, Tennyson 1970, Koenig 1967 a and b), other studies failed to detect polysomes in mature axons of hippocampal neurons (Steward & Levy, 1982). In addition, while mRNA was found in axons of olfactory and hypothalamic neurons, neither ribosomes nor golgi apparatus could be detected in the same system (Mohr & Richter, 1992; Denis-Donini et al., 1998). Critical studies of the 80s and 90s performed in the squid giant axon showed clear evidence of intra-axonal proteins synthesis in invertebrate neurons (Giuditta et al., 1980, 1986, 1991; Sotelo et al., 1999; Crispino et al., 1997). This notion was later expanded to vertebrates, where mature axons of adult neurons were shown to contain mRNA associated with ribosomes and be capable of de novo protein synthesis even during adult life (Twiss & Minnen, 2006; Sotelo-Silveira et al., 2008; Perry & Fainzilber, 2014; Kalinski et al., 2015; Taliaferro et al., 2016; Kun et al., 2007; Bassell et al., 1998). Interestingly, a recent study showed evidence supporting local protein synthesis at axon branches by revealing the presence of microtubules, ER, compact mitochondria, and locally clustered ribosomes using in situ cellular cryo-electron tomography (Nedozralova et al., 2022).

The origin of axonal ribosomes has also been the topic of debate (Sotelo et al., 2014; Twiss & Fainzilber, 2009), with different sets of evidence pointing to a somatic or an extra-neuronal source. As early as 1970, ribosomal transfer from glia was proposed (Lasek et al., 1977; Gainer et al., 1977). Successive studies further documented the presence of glial-derived ribosomes in axons (Court et al., 2008, 2011; Sotelo et al., 2013; Shakhbazau et al., 2016). Recent studies based on genetically tagged ribosomes have shown both the neuronal origin of axonal ribosomes *in vivo* (Shigeoka et al., 2016, 2019, 2018) and in compartmental cultures, where isolated axons are devoid of glia (Perry et al., 2016), and glial origin (Müller et al., 2018). More careful investigation is required to resolve this ongoing debate.

Following technical and experimental improvements in the detection of mRNAs and newly synthetized proteins (Terenzio et al., 2018; Holt et al.,

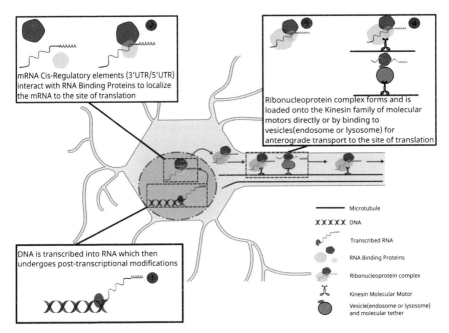

mRNA Cis-Regulatory elements (3'UTR/5'UTR) interact with RNA Binding Proteins to localize the mRNA to the site of translation

Ribonucleoprotein complex forms and is loaded onto the Kinesin family of molecular motors directly or by binding to vesicles(endosome or lysosome) for anterograde transport to the site of translation

DNA is transcribed into RNA which then undergoes post-transcriptional modifications

Microtubule
XXXXX DNA
Transcribed RNA
RNA Binding Proteins
Ribonucleoprotein complex
Kinesin Molecular Motor
Vesicle(endosome or lysosome) and molecular tether

Figure 7.1 mRNA localization and trafficking. Following transcription, RNA undergoes several post-transcriptional modifications after which trans-acting factors, namely RNA binding proteins and miRNAs, interact with the Cis-regulatory elements found in the 3'UTR and/ or 5'UTR to regulate mRNA stability, determine its subcellular localization and regulate its translation. mRNA targeted to the axons along with the bound RBPs will then be exported from the nucleus and form a ribonucleoprotein complex (RNP), which is subsequently transported anterogradely by the kinesin family of molecular motors to the site of local translation. Recent evidence has also shown the association of mRNA, mRNA granules and component of the translational machinery with vesicular organelles such as endosomes, lysosomes, and mitochondria.

2019), the repertoire of axonally localized mRNAs has exponentially grown and axonal local translation has been correlated to a variety of critical neuronal functions, which we will explore in the sections below.

7.3 Mechanisms of mRNA Transport and Peripheral Localization

In addition to localizing the translational machinery in axons and dendrites, mRNA needs to be transported to these subcellular compartments (Figure 7.1).

mRNAs carry information in their sequence and structure related to translational regulation, cellular localization, and splicing as well as their own stability and turnover (Batey, 2006). Indeed, the mRNA 3'-untranslated regions (UTRs) are known to house cis-regulatory elements (CREs), that regulate mRNA stability, cellular localization, and efficiency of translation (Andreassi & Riccio, 2009; Moore, 2005; Moore & Proudfoot, 2009; Gomes et al., 2014) by interacting with one or more trans-acting factors, such as RNA-binding proteins (RBPs) and microRNAs (Martin & Ephrussi, 2009; Andreassi & Riccio, 2009; Sahoo et al., 2018). 5'UTRs have also been implicated in axonal localization of mRNAs such as Neuritin (Merianda et al., 2013). One of the most known dynamics leading to mRNA axonal transport and localization is perhaps the interaction between β-actin mRNA and the zip code binding protein 1 (ZBP1) (Sotelo-Silveira et al., 2008; Zhang et al., 1999) and 2 (ZBP2) (Pan et al., 2009). Interestingly, longer 3'UTRs are overrepresented in axonal transcripts compared to their somatodendritic counterparts, suggesting the presence of specific CREs in axonal mRNAs and the possibility of their involvement in modulating mRNA axonal localization (Tushev et al., 2018).

The interaction between RBPs and axonal localization motifs in either the 5' or 3' UTR results in the formation of ribonucleoprotein complexes (RNPs), which are actively transported into the axon by molecular motors (Andreassi & Riccio, 2009; Gomes et al., 2014; Sahoo et al., 2018). A differential sedimentation approach was used to isolate and characterize RNA granule composition (Krichevsky & Kosik, 2001), while in a study published in 2004, researchers isolated RNPs associated with the anterograde molecular motor Kif5 and were able to identify 42 proteins and the mRNA for CaMKIIα and Arc (Kanai et al., 2004). Importantly, these studies were looking at a mixture of RNA granules, thus the identified proteins could belong to different granules. Nucleolin is another known axonal RBP associated with axonally localized mRNAs, including importin β1 mRNA. 3' UTR deletion of importin β1, small interfering RNA (siRNA) mediated knockdown of Kif5A and Kif5B, and treatment with AS1411, an aptamer that binds nucleolin thereby inhibiting its binding to kinesin molecular motors, reduced the levels of importin β1 mRNA from the axons of sensory neurons (Perry et al., 2016). Several other RBPs have been linked to the regulation of translation and mRNA localization in both dendrites and axons. Mutations in these RBPs or their aggregation and mislocalization have also been implicated in neurodegenerative diseases (Lagier-Tourenne et al., 2010; Sahoo et al., 2018) (Table 7.1.).

Recent evidence has also shown the association of some axonal mRNAs with organelles such as endosomes, multivesicular bodies, lysosomes, and proteins involved in the endoplasmic reticulum (ER)–golgi complex trafficking (Dalla Costa et al., 2021). Indeed, endosomes, lysosomes, and

Table 7.1 Summary of mutations and risk factors associated with neurodegenerative diseases.

Disease(s)	Gene	Protein	Function(s)	Reference(s)
ALS	SOD1	Superoxide dismutase [Cu-Zn]	An oxidoreductase that catalyzes the conversion of toxic superoxide species	(Rosen, Siddique et al., 1993)
ALS/FTD	UBQLN2	Ubiquilin 2	A shuttle protein involved in the ubiquitin-proteasome system (UPS) and implicated in macroautophagy and the degradation of protein aggregates	(Deng, Chen et al., 2011, Renaud, Picher-Martel et al., 2019)
ALS/FTD-ALS	OPTN	Optineurin	An autophagy adaptor reported to be involved in parkin-mediated mitophagy targeting damaged mitochondria for degradation	(Maruyama, Morino et al., 2010, Wong Yvette and Holzbaur Erika 2014)
ALS/FTD	SQSTM1	Sequestosome 1	A ubiquitin-binding protein that plays a role in protein degradation via the proteasome pathway and autophagy	(Fecto, Yan et al., 2011)
ALS/FTD, HD	VCP	Transitional endoplasmic reticulum ATPase (also known as valosin-containing protein or p97)	Involved in UPS-mediated protein degradation	(Johnson, Mandrioli et al., 2010)
ALS/FTD	TBK1	TANK-binding kinase 1 (Serine/threonine-protein kinase TBK1)	A Serine/threonine-protein kinase involved in the degradation of ubiquitinated cargo by the autophagosome	(Freischmidt, Wieland et al., 2015)
ALS	DCTN1	Dynactin-1	Part of the dynein-dynactin molecular motor complex	(Puls, Jonnakuty et al., 2003)

(continued)

Table 7.1 *Continued.*

Disease(s)	Gene	Protein	Function(s)	Reference(s)
ALS	*TUBA4A*	Tubulin α-4A chain	A microtubule subunit	(Smith, Ticozzi et al., 2014)
ALS	*PFN1*	Profilin 1	Binds to monomeric G-actin and regulates the growth of filamentous F-actin	(Wu, Fallini et al., 2012)
ALS/FTD	*TARDPB*	TAR DNA binding protein 43	RNA and DNA binding protein involves in multiple RNA processes including splicing, trafficking, stability, and translation	(Sreedharan, Blair Ian et al., 2008, Kapeli, Martinez et al., 2017)
ALS	*FUS/TLS*	Fused in Sarcoma/Translocated in Liposarcoma	Associated with several RNA processing events including splicing, trafficking, and transcription	(Kwiatkowski, Bosco et al., 2009, Vance, Rogelj et al., 2009, Kapeli, Martinez et al., 2017)
ALS/FTD	*C9orf72*	Human chromosome 9 open reading frame 72	Linked to RNA processes and autophagy	(Farg, Sundaramoorthy et al., 2014, Kapeli, Martinez et al., 2017, Shi, Lin et al. 2018)
ALS	*hnRNP A1*	heterogeneous nuclear ribonucleoproteins A1	RNA processing and stability including splicing and nuclear export	(Kapeli, Martinez et al. 2017)
ALS	*hnRNPA2/B1*	heterogeneous nuclear ribonucleoproteins A2/B1	RNA splicing, trafficking, and translational regulation	(Kapeli, Martinez et al., 2017)
ALS	*EWSR1*	EWS RNA-binding protein 1	Essential to various cellular processes including meiosis, mitosis, and homologous recombination during the DNA damage response. It has been also found to interact with RNA and RNA-binding proteins such as FUS and TAF15	(Kapeli, Martinez et al., 2017)

ALS	ANG	Angiogenin	A ribonuclease and an inducer of angiogenesis	(Taylor, Brown et al., 2016)
ALS/FTD	MATR3	Matrin	A nuclear matrix RNA and DNA binding protein that has been found to interact with TDP-43	(Taylor, Brown et al., 2016)
ALS/ FTD-ALS	ATXN2	Ataxin-2	RNA-binding protein with multiple roles in RNA metabolism	(Renton, Chiò et al., 2014, Taylor, Brown et al., 2016)
ALS	TAF15	TATA-box binding protein associated factor 15	An RNA-binding protein that plays a role in transcription and RNA splicing	(Kapeli, Martinez et al., 2017)
PD	SNCA	α-synuclein	Involved in the regulation of neurotransmitter release and synaptic vesicle trafficking	(Stefanis 2012)
PD	LRRK2	Leucine-rich repeat kinase 2	A multidomain protein kinase	(Imai, Gehrke et al., 2008)
PD	PINK1/ PARK6	Pten-induced kinase 1	A mitochondrial serine/threonine-protein kinase associated with the local translation of nuclear-encoded respiratory chain complexes (nRCC) mRNAs	(Singleton, Farrer et al., 2013, Gehrke, Wu et al., 2015)
PD	PARK2	Parkin	An E3 ubiquitin ligase involved in mitochondrial homeostasis, protein degradation, and implicated in the local translation of nuclear-encoded respiratory chain complexes (nRCC) mRNAs along with PINK1	(Singleton, Farrer et al., 2013, Gehrke, Wu et al., 2015)

(continued)

Table 7.1 *Continued.*

Disease(s)	Gene	Protein	Function(s)	Reference(s)
AD	APP	Amyloid precursor protein	A transmembrane protein involved in synaptic plasticity and synaptogenesis. It is a precursor of Aβ as a result of cleavage by β- and γ-secretases	(Thinakaran and Koo 2008, Gamarra, de la Cruz et al., 2021, Knopman, Amieva et al., 2021)
AD	PSEN1	Presenilin 1	Involved in γ-secretase activity responsible for proteolytic cleavage of APP	(Knopman, Amieva et al., 2021)
AD	PSEN2	Presenilin 2	Involved in γ-secretase activity responsible for proteolytic cleavage of APP	(Knopman, Amieva et al., 2021)
AD	APOE 4	Apolipoprotein E	Involved in lipid metabolism	(Knopman, Amieva et al., 2021)
AD	TREM2	Triggering Receptor Expressed on Myeloid Cells 2	Microglial transmembrane receptor protein	(Bellenguez, Charbonnier et al., 2017, Knopman, Amieva et al., 2021)
AD	SORL1	Sortilin-Related Receptor 1	Receptors involved in the endosomal sorting of proteins	(Rogaeva, Meng et al., 2007, Bellenguez, Charbonnier et al., 2017, Knopman, Amieva et al., 2021)
AD	ABCA7	ATP-Binding Cassette Subfamily A Member 7	Involved in lipid metabolism and phagocytosis of apoptotic cells	(Bellenguez, Charbonnier et al., 2017, Knopman, Amieva et al., 2021)
AD	BIN1	Bridging Integrator 1	An adaptor protein that functions in clathrin-mediated endocytosis and endocytic recycling and has been shown to interact with Tau	(Knopman, Amieva et al., 2021)

AD	CD2AP	CD2 Associated Protein	An adaptor protein involved in regulating signal transduction and cytoskeletal molecules	(Knopman, Amieva et al., 2021)
AD	FERMT2	Kindlin-2	A protein that localizes to focal adhesions and is associated with integrin activation	(Eysert, Coulon et al. 2021, Knopman, Amieva et al., 2021)
AD	CASS4	Cas scaffold protein family member 4	A scaffolding protein involved in tyrosine-kinase signaling and associated with focal adhesions	(Knopman, Amieva et al., 2021)
AD	PTK2B	Protein tyrosine-kinase 2 beta	A Ca^{2+}-activated non-receptor tyrosine kinase	(Knopman, Amieva et al., 2021)
HD	HTT	Huntingtin	Proposed to have a flexible structure that alters its activity. It contains HEAT (Huntingtin, Elongator factor3, PR65/A regulatory subunit of PP2A, and Tor1) repeats which are through to mediate protein-protein interactions possible through scaffolding and is involved in mRNA transport	(Gauthier, Charrin et al. 2004, Schulte and Littleton 2011)
SMA	SMN1	Survival motor neuron protein	Associated with the assembly of the pre-mRNA splicing complex and plays a role in mRNA localization and regulation of RNP granules	(Fallini, Donlin-Asp et al. 2016, Khalil, Morderer et al., 2018)
FXS	FMR1	Fragile X mental retardation protein (FMRP)	An RNA-binding protein that is essential for local translation and synaptic plasticity	(Akins, Berk-Rauch et al., 2017)

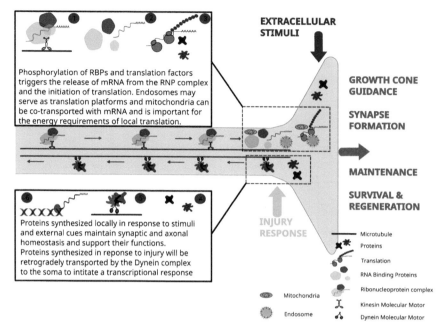

Figure 7.2   Local translation and the role of locally synthesized proteins. Upon reaching the site of local translation, RBPs will undergo modifications, such as phosphorylation, triggered by external or internal stimuli, which will then determine the release of the mRNA, the assembly of the translation complex and the initiation of translation by the phosphorylation of translation initiation factors. Locally translated proteins perform important functions in axonal maintenance, synaptogenesis, growth cone guidance and neuronal survival. In addition, local translation can be triggered by injury, upon which locally translated proteins are then retrogradely transported by the dynein-dynactin molecular motor complex to the soma, where a transcriptional cellular response is initiated.

mitochondria were shown to mediate axonal RNA transport and/or translational regulation. RNA granules were found to tether to lysosomes through Annexin 11 (ANXA11), with mutations in ANXA11 impairing their transport by disrupting their interactions with lysosomes (Liao et al., 2019). Late endosomes were also described to interact with RNA granules, translation machinery, and mitochondria (Cioni et al., 2019). Recently, the involvement of mitochondria in the axonal localization and transport of the RNAi machinery has also been described (Gershoni-Emek et al., 2018). Pink1 mRNA was shown to be co-transported with mitochondria via an RNA-binding domain in synaptojanin 2 (SYNJ2) and synaptojanin 2 binding protein (SYNJ2BP) (Harbauer, Hees et al., 2022) (Figure 7.2).

7.4 Regulation of Axonal Local Translation

Regulation of localized mRNA translation, including extracellular and chemical triggers, ribosomal heterogeneity, RBP/mRNA interaction, RNA post-transcriptional modifications, mitochondrial contribution, and non-coding RNAs, adds another layer of complexity to mRNA spatiotemporal dynamics. The coupling of receptors to ribosomes has been proposed to link extrinsic signals to the local intracellular translation machinery (Koppers et al., 2022). Receptor-ribosome coupling seems to be common to several receptors, including the Deleted in Colorectal Carcinoma (DCC) transmembrane receptor that interacts with translation components and is regulated by the extracellular cue Netrin-1 (Tcherkezian et al., 2010). Several receptors were also found to associate with distinct pools of RBPs and mRNAs (Koppers et al., 2022), which could help fine-tune the regulation of local protein synthesis in response to extracellular cues. Specific extracellular stimuli can also directly modify local mRNA levels independently of new transcription (Willis et al., 2005, 2007). Differential localization of mRNAs to specific locations in axons is yet another way to regulate the identity of the proteins synthetized locally. Furthermore, specific cues can lead to protein synthesis of subsets of mRNAs by the activation of kinases, which triggers site-specific phosphorylation of RBPs and translation factors, resulting in the local release of associated mRNAs, which are then available for translation (Hörnberg & Holt, 2013; Jung et al., 2012). Netrin-1, for instance, induces hyperphosphorylation of growth factor receptor-bound protein 7 (Grb7), decreasing its RNA-binding and translation repressive activity, and resulting in increased translation of KOR mRNA (Tsai et al., 2007). Further, BDNF signaling was shown to lead to Src-mediated phosphorylation of ZBP1, which in turn initiates axonal translation of β-actin (Sasaki et al., 2010). The mechanistic target of rapamycin (mTOR) is a kinase involved in a plethora of cellular mechanisms including axonal local translation (Laplante & Sabatini, 2012; Hörnberg & Holt, 2013). Indeed, activation of the mTOR pathway by extracellular signals can increase cap-dependent translation initiation of axonal mRNAs through the phosphorylation of eIF4E binding proteins, which leads to their dissociation from eIF4E (Sonenberg & Hinnebusch, 2009). For instance, NGF can activate mTOR, resulting in local protein synthesis of TC10 and Par3, which are involved in membrane expansion and cytoskeletal dynamics, thus triggering dorsal root ganglion (DRG) axonal outgrowth (Hengst et al., 2009; Gracias et al., 2014). Another level of spatiotemporal regulation of mTOR activity was shown to be the localization of its own mRNA, which is transported in axons by the RBP nucleolin (Terenzio et al., 2018).

Following sciatic nerve injury, resident mTOR protein was shown to amplify its signaling by triggering local protein synthesis of its own mRNA, leading to the translation of critical retrograde injury signals such as importin-β1 and STAT3 (Terenzio et al., 2018). Deletion of mTOR 3′UTR, which contains its axonal localization motif, negatively impacted axonal translation after injury, resulting in decreased survival of injured DRG neurons (Terenzio et al., 2018). In addition, axonal mTOR is required for the sequential axonal translation of several mRNAs in response to nerve injury, including axonal Casein Kinase 2α (CK2α) (Sahoo et al., 2020), and mTOR mRNA miss-localization negatively impacted the speed of axonal regeneration (Sahoo et al., 2020).

Another important mechanism of translational regulation hinges on mRNA post-transcriptional modifications. Indeed, it was shown that n6-methyladenosine (m6A) mRNA modification participates in axonal translation (Yu et al., 2018, 2021). Whether or not additional post-transcriptional modifications of mRNAs can modulate local translation is yet to be found.

Different RBPs can compete for the same mRNA, resulting in fine regulation of its local translation. For instance, HuD and KHSRP share the same target mRNAs, including GAP43 mRNA, and either stabilize or destabilize it (Yoo et al., 2013; Gardiner et al., 2015; Smith et al., 2004; Bird et al., 2013; Anderson et al., 2000). Multiple mRNAs can also compete for the binding to the same RBP. Indeed, β-actin and GAP43 mRNAs were shown to compete for ZBP1 (Donnelly et al., 2011).

Ribosomes are another key component of the translational machinery that might be subjected to regulation. Indeed, localization and translation of mRNA coding for ribosomal proteins were shown in dendrites and axons (Zivraj et al., 2010; Cajigas et al., 2012; Shigeoka et al., 2016; Hodas et al., 2012). Inhibition of axonal translation of ribosomal proteins also decreased local translation activity and negatively impacted axon branching *in vivo* (Shigeoka et al., 2019). Finally, the observation of variability in the half-life of neuronal ribosomes (Dörrbaum et al., 2022) compared to canonical stable "lifelong" assembly of nuclear ribosomes could suggest that, in specialized neuronal ribosomes, ribosomal proteins may be exchanged to repair or replace components in these complexes (Pulk et al., 2010; Xue & Barna, 2012; Jung et al., 2014; Fusco et al., 2021), possibly constituting a further level for regulation of spatiotemporal protein synthesis in axons.

Axonal non-coding RNAs, including microRNAs (miRNAs), were also found to inhibit or activate translation and/or promote mRNA degradation. As mentioned above, axonal mRNAs are generally defined by longer 3′UTRs, which contain miRNA binding sites (Bae & Miura, 2020). Indeed, miRNAs are localized to DRG and mature peripheral axons, together with a functional miRNA silencing machinery (Hengst et al., 2006; Murashov et al., 2007). There is also evidence of modulation of gene expression by the microRNA-mediated silencing machinery in neurons (Kosik, 2006). For instance, miR-21 and miR-199a-3p modulation of expression post-injury can regulate the axonal regeneration associated with the mTOR pathway (Kar et al., 2021), while miR-338, a brain-specific miRNA, indirectly regulates mitochondrial activity through the modulation of nuclear-encoded mitochondrial transcripts COXIV and ATP5G1, and consequently affects axon growth (Aschrafi et al., 2008, 2012). More recently, a long intergenic non-coding RNA (lincRNA) called ALAE was found enriched in axons, leading to the local translation of the GAP43 transcript (Wei et al., 2021).

Finally, mitochondria have been shown to participate in driving translation in dendrites (Rangaraju et al., 2019), while synthesis of the mitochondrial proteins ATP5G1 and COXIV was found to be regulated locally (Aschrafi et al., 2008, 2012). Mitochondria are known to be recruited not only to dendrites but also to axon branching sites to provide energy supply for local protein synthesis (Spillane et al., 2013). Interestingly, local translation of the short-lived PINK1 protein in axon has been recently described to provide distal mitochondria with the required supply of PINK1 for the activation of mitophagy (Harbauer et al., 2022), suggesting a possible role for translation in mitochondrial homeostasis.

7.5 Functions of Axonally Synthetized Proteins

Excluding their role in pathology, axonally synthesized proteins have been implicated in a variety of critical biological axonal functions, including axon growth, guidance, branching, and maintenance, synapse formation and regulation, retrograde signaling, and neuronal survival and regeneration (Figure 7.2). Here we will briefly explore some of these roles.

Growth and guidance of axons are sensed by the growth cone and mediated by extracellular stimuli. Interestingly, attractant cues have been shown to increase axonal β-actin mRNA levels in growing axons (Bassell et al., 1998; Zhang et al., 1999), and activate local translation (Campbell & Holt, 2001; Pratt et al., 2012). Moreover, external attractant or repellant stimuli can modify the localization of mRNA and translational machinery within a growth cone (Leung et al., 2006; Yao et al., 2006; Piper et al., 2006; Walker et al., 2012; Wu et al., 2005). Once axons navigate to their targets, they extend branches harboring synapses (Kalil & Dent, 2014). The enrichment of the translational machinery and mitochondria at incipient branch points was shown to result in local translation, inducing axon branching (Spillane et al., 2013; Spillane et al., 2012). Indeed, axonal β-actin mRNA and its translation drive axonal branching (Donnelly et al., 2013), while β-actin mRNA and subsequent protein localization to axonal branches were shown to predict longer-lived branching events in developing axons (Wong et al., 2017). These results suggest an essential role for local protein synthesis in axonal development.

Local translation was initially believed to be a minor contribution to synaptic protein production, activated in particular circumstances during synaptic plasticity (Kosik, 2016). The discovery of a large number of mRNAs in neurites, however, challenged this assumption (Zappulo et al., 2017; Taliaferro et al., 2016). Polyribosomes were also shown to be at the site of synapses in response to synaptic activity (Ostroff et al., 2017, 2018). Formation of the presynaptic terminal was found to require the recruitment of the SNAP25 transcript and its local translation (Batista et al., 2017). mRNAs coding for proteins involved in both presynaptic and postsynaptic zones were also shown to be present at synapses, suggesting a role for local protein production in the development, maintenance, and modulation of this structure (Shigeoka et al., 2016; Hafner et al., 2019).

Local axonal protein synthesis has also been heavily implicated in neuronal homeostasis and survival. Dynein regulators, such as Lis1 and p150glued, were shown to be axonally translated in response to survival signals, mediating the transport of vesicles presumed to contribute to axonal survival (Villarin et al., 2016). Furthermore, pro-survival transcription factors are also translated locally and delivered to the soma, resulting in retrograde signaling triggering the activation of an anti-apoptotic transcriptional response in neurons (Harrington & Ginty, 2013; Cox et al., 2008). Local synthesis of mitochondrial-related proteins might also be critical for axon viability and maintenance, given the role of axonal mitochondrial activity in regulating metabolism and energy production and the activation of apoptotic pathways (Hillefors et al., 2007). Indeed, nuclear-encoded mitochondrial mRNAs are enriched and translated in axons (Zivraj et al., 2010; Gumy et al., 2011; Shigeoka et al., 2016; Aschrafi et al., 2016).

7.6 Axonal Local Translation in Nerve Injury and Regeneration

Nerve injury triggers a catastrophic chain of molecular events in damaged axons, which leads to Wallerian degeneration and ultimately can cause loss of the neuronal cell body in absence of a robust regenerative response (Li et al., 2013; Hetz & Saxena, 2017). After an injury, neurons must be able to convert a mature damaged axon into a new growth cone that allows for its regeneration (Sahly et al., 2006; Chierzi et al., 2005; Verma et al., 2005). An interesting feature of the nervous system is the existence of a differential capacity for responses to injury in the central nervous system (CNS) as compared to the peripheral nervous system (PNS). Regeneration and functional recovery are typically much more successful in the PNS than in the CNS (Verma & Fawcett, 2005). Since regeneration after axotomy heavily depends on the capacity to locally synthetize new proteins in injured axons, providing both the components for axonal regrowth as well as cytoskeletal elements and retrograde signals that activate the regenerative response (Ben-Yaakov et al., 2012; Cox et al., 2008; Donnelly et al., 2011; Hanz et al., 2003; Michaelevski et al., 2010; Verma et al., 2005; Willis et al., 2007; Yudin et al., 2008; Perlson et al., 2005), axonal injury in the PNS has historically been used as a model to dissect the mechanisms underpinning axonal translation and its effect on neuronal survival and regeneration.

Initial studies described the presence of over 200 mRNAs in adult sensory axons of injury-conditioned DRG (Willis et al., 2007), where mRNAs related to the ribosomal/translational machinery and mitochondrial/oxidative phosphorylation were highly represented (Gumy et al., 2010). Subsequent studies reported the presence of ribosomal proteins, translation promoters, and ribosomal RNA in axons of adult sensory neurons after injury (Gumy et al., 2011; Minis et al., 2014). An early wave of Ca^{2+} from the site of injury can trigger the translation of a variety of axonal mRNAs, including Importin-β1 and STAT3, which then form an injury signaling complex that is retrogradely transported to the soma (Hanz et al., 2003; Perry et al., 2012; Ben-Yaakov et al., 2012; Rishal & Fainzilber, 2014). The Dual Leucine-zipper 1 (DLK1) is involved in retrograde injury-response signaling by phosphorylating the Mitogen-activated Protein Kinases (MAPK) (Tedeschi & Bradke, 2013; Mahar & Cavalli, 2018) and was shown to promote mRNA stability and local translation after axon injury (Yan et al., 2009). Kinases such as ERK1/2, members of the MAPK family, are also phosphorylated upon injury, bound to a locally translated proteolytic fragment of Vimentin, and retrogradely transported (Perlson et al., 2005). mTOR, a serine-threonine-protein kinase, has also been shown to be translated and phosphorylated in axons after nerve injury (Terenzio et al., 2018). Finally another major player involved in axonal regeneration are mitochondria, which normally accumulate at the site of injury, while their absence was shown to harm the regenerative capacity of injured axons, suggesting that mitochondria might provide the energy for local translation after injury (Han et al., 2016). All results taken together, it has become clear in recent years that axonal protein synthesis is crucial for retrograde injury signaling and axonal regeneration in sensory neurons (Rishal & Fainzilber, 2014; Terenzio et al., 2017; Sahoo , 2018; Koley et al, 2019).

7.7 Axonal mRNA Localization and Translation in Neurodegenerative Diseases

Due to lifespan increase and consequent population aging, neurodegenerative diseases are becoming a major public health concern worldwide (Heemels, 2016). Patients affected by neurodegenerative pathologies display an array of different clinical manifestations but share common features such as the progressive course of the disease and irreversible neuronal loss in different anatomical regions of the brain (Soto & Pritzkow, 2018). Current clinical approaches for these diseases are aimed at managing symptoms, which can help to slow down the progression of neurodegeneration but do not necessarily treat the cause of the disease. One of the hallmarks of amyotrophic lateral sclerosis (ALS), frontotemporal dementia (FTD), Parkinson's disease (PD), Alzheimer's disease (AD), and Huntington's disease (HD), is an aggregation of abnormal (misfolded/insoluble) proteins in neurons (Davis et al., 2018). Genes encoding for RBPs are also often affected, like in spinal muscular atrophy (SMA) or fragile X syndrome (FXS), and a cohort of published results suggest that impaired axonal transport, localization, and translation in axon might be involved in neurodegenerative diseases. We will explore these studies in the following sections, focusing on the contribution of mRNA localization and translation to the pathophysiology of these neurodegenerative diseases. Understanding the mechanisms of neurodegeneration and the involvement of mRNA axonal transport and local protein synthesis could be useful to propose new therapeutic approaches.

7.7.1 Amyotrophic lateral sclerosis (ALS)/frontotemporal dementia (FTD)

Amyotrophic lateral sclerosis (ALS) is a fatal disease characterized by progressive degeneration of motor neurons in the motor cortex, brainstem, and spinal cord (Taylor et al., 2016; Taylor, Brown et al., 2016). ALS symptoms vary from skeletal muscular atrophy and asymmetric weakness in the limbs (Swinnen & Robberecht, 2014), weakened muscles in the neck, jaw, and tongue (Rowland & Shneider, 2001; Swinnen & Robberecht, 2014; Taylor et al., 2016), to a respiratory onset of the disease with extremely poor prognosis (Swinnen & Robberecht, 2014). Frontotemporal dementia (FTD) is a form of dementia characterized by progressive neurodegeneration in the frontal and temporal lobes of the brain (Bang et al., 2015). Affected patients display personality and behavioral changes, and progressive impairment in language skills and executive function (Van Langenhove et al., 2012; Bang et al., 2015). Around 15–20% of patients with ALS meet the clinical criteria of FTD, the two diseases sharing some pathological and clinical features and underlying genetic mutations (Ringholz et al., 2005; Ling et al., 2013; Taylor et al., 2016). Common causes for both diseases include mutations in RBPs, disruption of proteostasis, and protein aggregation and inclusion bodies (Ling et al., 2013; Taylor et al., 2016). In the following section, we will discuss the underlying causes of both diseases with a focus on ALS to avoid redundancy.

ALS is classified into two categories, familial ALS, which accounts for about 10% of ALS cases, and sporadic ALS, accounting for 90% of cases (Renton et al., 2014; Swinnen & Robberecht, 2014; Taylor et al., 2016). In contrast, around 50% of FTD cases are familial (Ling et al., 2013; Taylor et al., 2016). Several genetic mutations have been linked to ALS, which can be roughly classified into three categories: 1) genes involved in protein homeostasis and autophagy, 2) genes related to cytoskeletal dynamics and motor protein complexes, and 3) genes associated with RNA metabolism, stability, and transport. In 1993, a study by Daniel R Rosen et al. identified the first genetic mutation associated with ALS in a gene encoding the enzyme superoxide dismutase (SOD1), an oxidoreductase that catalyzes the conversion of toxic superoxide species (Rosen et al., 1993), causing the protein to aggregate in association with mitochondria (Renton et al., 2014; Yasuda & Mili, 2016). Mutations of genes involved in the lysosomal degradation pathway were also linked to ALS, such as UBQLN2 encoding Ubiquilin 2, a shuttle protein that plays a role in the ubiquitin-proteasome system (UPS) (Rosen et al., 1993; Renaud et al., 2019), Optineurin (OPTN), an autophagy adaptor (Maruyama et al., 2010), involved in parkin-mediated mitophagy (Wong & Holzbaur, 2014), Sequestosome 1 (SQST1) (Fecto, Yan et al., 2011), the Transitional endoplasmic reticulum ATPase (VCP) (Johnson et al., 2010) and the Serine/threonine-protein kinase TBK1 (Freischmidt et al., 2015). Genes involved in cytoskeletal dynamics and motor protein complexes responsible for cargo trafficking were also found mutated in ALS, such as Dynactin-1 (DCTN1), which is part of the retrograde dynein-dynactin molecular motor complex (Puls et al., 2003); Tubulin α-4A (TUBA4A), a microtubule subunit that affects microtubule polymerization and results in the formation of ubiquitinated aggregates (Smith et al., 2014); and Profilin-1 (PFN1), which binds to monomeric G-actin and regulates the growth of filamentous F-actin

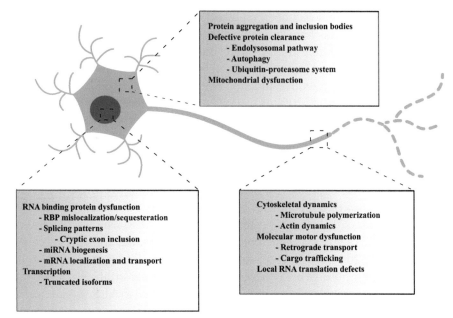

Figure 7.3   Summary of ALS pathology. ALS pathology has been linked to dysfunction in RNA binding proteins resulting in RBP sequestration, mislocalization and aggregation, which also leads to disruption of RNA processes such as transcription, splicing patterns and mRNA localization and transport. Additionally, ALS has also been linked to defects in the protein degradation pathways such as the ubiquitin-proteasome system, endo-lysosomal pathway, autophagy and mitophagy, leading to increased protein aggregation and the formation of inclusion bodies as well as mitochondrial dysfunction. Defects in the cytoskeletal dynamics such as microtubule and actin polymerization, molecular motor dysfunction and disruption of local translation have also been found to be associated with ALS pathology.

(Wu et al., 2012). Finally, genes associated with RNA metabolism, stability, and transport have also been implicated in ASL, including TARDPB (TAR DNA binding protein 43), FUS/TLS (Fused in Sarcoma/Translocated in Liposarcoma), C9orf72 (human chromosome 9 open reading frame 72), hnRNP A1 (heterogeneous nuclear ribonucleoproteins A1), hnRNPA2/B1, EWSR1 (EWS RNA-binding protein 1), ANG (Angiogenin), SETX (Senataxin), MATR3 (Matrin), ATXN2 (Ataxin-2), and TAF15 (TATA-box binding protein associated factor 15) (Kapeli et al., 2017). Indeed, a growing set of evidence suggests that defects in mRNA transport, processing, and translation caused by mutations in RBP coding genes or the impairment of RBP functions are a key factor underlying ALS and FTD pathologies (Figure 7.3).

TDP-43, a highly conserved RNA/DNA binding protein involved in multiple RNA processes, was first linked to ALS in 2008 (Sreedharan et al.,

2008). TDP-43 cytoplasmic aggregates and nuclear depletion have been reported in more than 96% of ALS and FTD cases, including both familial and sporadic ALS, except for SOD1-associated ALS, and are recognized as hallmarks of the disease (Arai et al., 2006; Neumann et al., 2006; Lagier-Tourenne et al., 2010). TDP-43 depletion in the mouse brain results in altered mRNA levels and mRNA splicing patterns in 601 and 965 mRNAs respectively (Polymenidou et al., 2011). Additionally, TDP-43 binds to the 3'UTR of Fus/Tls and Grn mRNAs, which are known to correlate with ALS (Polymenidou et al., 2011). A Drosophila study revealed an impairment in the anterograde trafficking of ALS-associated mutant TDP-43 containing RNP granules and their depletion at the neuromuscular junction (Alami et al., 2014). Additionally, two recent studies revealed how mislocalization of TDP-43 and its depletion from the nucleus result in a cryptic exon (CE) inclusion in the transcripts for UNC13A, encoding an essential neuronal protein involved in synaptic function, and STMN2, which encodes the regulator of microtubule stability stathmin-2 (Brown et al., 2022; Ma et al., 2022). The CE inclusion in STMN2 transcript results in a truncated isoform, significantly reducing stathmin-2 protein levels, a characteristic feature of ALS and FTD (Ma et al., 2022). Mutated forms of TDP-43 have been shown to reduce the movement of their associated RNP granules in the dendritic arbor of rat hippocampal neurons, likely resulting in a disruption of the transport and local translation of mRNA essential for synaptic function (Liu-Yesucevitz et al., 2014). Axonal accumulation of mutated TDP-43 RNP aggregates was also found to inhibit nuclear-encoded mitochondrial protein translation in neuromuscular junctions and distal axons (Altman et al., 2021).

Mutations of FUS/TLS, an RBP involved in several RNA processes essential for neuronal function and survival have also been linked to ALS/FTD. Like TDP-43, mutant variants of FUS were reported to mislocalize to the cytoplasm and form aggregates (Kwiatkowski et al., 2009; Vance et al., 2009). For instance, a study conducted in ALS-associated FUS-mutant motor neurons, identified increased levels of Fos-B mRNA, one of the mRNAs targeted by FUS, in correlation with irregular axonal branching (Akiyama et al., 2019). Additionally, both *in vivo*, in the mouse sciatic nerve, and *in vitro*, in primary cultured mouse hippocampal neurons, ALS/FTD-linked mutations in FUS have been reported to disrupt local axonal protein synthesis (López-Erauskin et al., 2018). Finally, the most common genetic mutation linked to both ALS and FTD is the C9orf72 hexanucleotide repeat expansion (HRE), which can lead to a decreased level of C9orf72, affecting vesicle trafficking and autophagy (Farg et al., 2014; Shi et al., 2018). C9orf72 HRE has also been linked to altered RNA processing, resulting in the formation of RNA foci due to expanding RNA repeats, which localize in the nucleus and sequester RBPs, inhibiting their function (Barker et al., 2017). The aforementioned examples highlight how defects in mRNA localization and local translation are linked to the ALS/FTD pathology either directly through mutations in the RNA-binding proteins or indirectly, like in the case of C9orf72 expanded repeats.

Recently, a previously not described interaction between RNA, RNA granules, and components of the translational machinery with vesicular organelles such as endosomes, late endosomes, lysosomes, and mitochondria has been found (Dalla Costa et al., 2021). Interestingly, ANXA11, an RNA granule-associated phosphoinositide-binding protein was shown to tether RNA granules and lysosomes (Liao et al., 2019). Mutations of ANXA11 linked to ALS were found to disrupt RNA granules binding to lysosomes, thus impairing their transport (Liao et al., 2019). In addition, miR-124 was shown to be actively transported in axons and to be associated with mito-chondria at growth cones and axonal branching points (Gershoni-Emek et al., 2018). Mitochondrial localization of this miRNA was reduced by the expression of hSOD1G93A, a gene linked to familial ALS, in motor neurons (Gershoni-Emek et al., 2018). While these observations are relatively recent, they strengthen the potential link between defects in transport observed in neurodegenerative diseases such as ALS and local translation.

7.7.2 Parkinson's disease (PD)

Parkinson's disease (PD) is a progressive neurodegenerative disease, affect-ing about 1% of the population aged 60 or above. The presence of protein aggregates called Lewy Bodies and the loss of dopaminergic (DA) neurons are hallmarks of PD (Goedert et al., 2013) and result in the characteristic motor and cognitive dysfunction observed in patients (Alexander, 2004). Unlike ALS and FTD, PD is mostly a sporadic disease with rare familial cases (Warner & Schapira, 2003; Alexander, 2004). α-synuclein was identi-fied as the main constituent of LB in both sporadic and familial cases of PD. Indeed, the first genetic mutations to be linked to familial PD mapped in the gene encoding α-synuclein (SNCA) (Stefanis 2012). Amyloid β(Aβ) and Tau accumulations are also observed in PD, and Aβ aggregates are found to be linked to cognitive decline (Lim et al., 2019).

While the disruption of the unfolded protein response has been reported in PD, a direct link between impaired mRNA localization and local protein synthesis has not been established. Protein aggregation and misfolding trig-ger ER stress, activating the UPR signaling cascade, which controls mRNA stability and the rate of protein synthesis (Hetz & Saxena, 2017). For instance, the UPR PKR-like endoplasmic reticulum kinase (PERK) has been shown to induce an increase in local translation via phosphorylation of the translation initiation factor eIF2α (Cagnetta et al., 2019). Semaphorin-3A (Sema3A) was suggested to induce mTOR and ERK1/2 mediated protein synthesis, which activates PERK and causes the subsequent eIF2α phosphorylation, accompanied by eIF2Bε dephosphorylation via GSK-3β inhibition and activation of PP1 by ERK-1/2, which increases eIF2B activity (Cagnetta et al., 2019). Aberrant protein translation has also been linked to genetic mutations in leucine-rich repeat kinase 2 (LRRK2), which are associated with both familial and sporadic PD (Imai et al., 2008). The eIF4E-binding protein (4E-BP) was shown to be a phosphorylation target of LRRK2, resulting in its activation and subsequent promotion of protein translation (Imai et al., 2008). The increase in protein synthesis was proposed to be detrimental to post-mitotic DA neurons, leading to an increase in aberrant proteins and/or a disruption of synapse integrity and neurodegeneration (Imai et al., 2008). Lastly, mutations in Pten-induced kinase 1 (PINK1/PARK6) and Parkin (PARK2) have also been associated with PD (Singleton et al., 2013). Interestingly, PINK1 and Parkin have been implicated in the local translation of a subset of nuclear-encoded respiratory chain complexes (nRCC) mRNAs essential for mitochondrial function (Gehrke et al., 2015). PINK1 interacts with Tom20 to localize nRCCs mRNA to the mitochondrial outer membrane and subsequently promote their translation in concert with Parkin (Gehrke et al., 2015). Recently, another study showed that Pink1 mRNA is co-transported with mitochondria and that its local translation along with the mitochondrial outer membrane proteins synaptojanin 2 binding protein (SYNJ2BP) and synaptojanin 2 (SYNJ2) are needed for its recruitment to the mitochondria (Harbauer, Hees et al., 2022). The local translation of PINK1 was described to be essential for the activation of mitophagy and the clearing of damaged mitochondria (Harbauer, Hees et al., 2022). These recent studies highlight the direct contribution of impaired proteostasis and aberrant protein synthesis and indirectly suggest the possibility of dysregulation of local translation and RNA metabolism in PD.

7.7.3 Alzheimer's disease (AD)

Alzheimer's disease (AD) is a genetic and sporadic neurodegenerative disease that causes dementia and cognitive impairment (Yang et al., 2016). The presence of Amyloid β (Aβ) and hyperphosphorylated forms of the microtubule-associated protein Tau-containing neurofibrillary tangles are hallmarks of AD (Knopman et al., 2021). Genetic mutations associated with AD such as PSEN1 (encoding presenilin 1) and PSEN2 (encoding presenilin 2) as well as

APP (encoding amyloid precursor protein (APP)) are rare and account for the inherited, generally early-onset, cases (Knopman et al., 2021). However, several genes have been identified as risk factors for the development of the disease. Those are APOE ε4, TREM2 (surface receptor required for microglial functions), SORL1 (neuronal sortilin-related receptor), and ABCA7(ATP-binding cassette, subfamily A member 7), as well as mutations in Tau-binding proteins such as BIN1, CD2AP, FERMT2, CASS4, and PTK2B, but not the gene encoding Tau (MAPT) (Knopman, Amieva et al., 2021). AD has also been found to be associated with α-synuclein and TDP-43 pathologies (Karanth et al., 2020).

APP is an Aβ precursor that undergoes cleavage by β- and γ-secretases to release Aβ peptides (Thinakaran & Koo, 2008). APP mutation or incorrect cleavage results in Aβ peptides prone to aggregation, resulting in fibril formation (Thinakaran & Koo, 2008; Gamarra et al., 2021). There are several examples of modulation of mRNA axonal translation in AD, which are mostly connected with Aβ induced toxicity. Aβ peptides, for instance, have been found to play a role in modulating the axonal local translation of the transcription factor ATF4, which is a component of the PERK signaling pathway (Baleriola et al., 2014). Indeed, pathogenic exposure to Aβ peptide was shown to elicit ATF4 axonal local translation and its subsequent retrograde transport to the nucleus, where it elicited a transcriptional response, which was suggested to not directly result in neurodegeneration and cell death, but rather in pathogenic changes that lead to degeneration further on (Baleriola et al., 2014). ATF4 siRNA knockdown was sufficient to rescue the degeneration phenotype in this context (Baleriola et al., 2014). Similarly, the protein Vimentin was found to be locally translated and retrogradely transported in response to Aβ exposure, in a way that is connected to ATF4 local translation (Walker et al., 2018). Additionally, Aβ oligomers were shown to impede retrograde trafficking of Brain-derived Neurotrophic Factor (BDNF), which is known to play a role in synaptic plasticity and memory, in response to altered ubiquitin homeostasis and the downregulation of Ubiquitin C-terminal hydrolase L1 (UCH-L1) (Poon et al., 2013). A similar study also described NMDAR dysfunction induced by Aβ oligomers to impair axonal trafficking of BDNF and mitochondria by regulating signaling cascades that result in the activation of Glycogen Synthase Kinase-3 (GSK-3β) (Decker et al., 2010). Furthermore, Aβ has been linked to the mislocalization and local translation of Mapt mRNA encoding Tau (Kobayashi et al., 2017; Li & Götz, 2017), with Aβ mediating the activation of Fyn via kinase-dependent activation of ERK/S6, resulting in the mislocalized translation and hyperphosphorylation of Tau, and leading to its accumulation in the somatodendritic compartment (Li & Götz, 2017). Additionally, Tau hyperphosphorylation was also shown to be triggered by AMPA and NMDA receptor stimulation (Kobayashi et al., 2017)). Finally, Aβ was recently found to regulate the translation of several mRNAs bound to FMRP, resulting in the impaired synthesis of proteins that are important for synaptic function (Ghosh et al., 2020). Interestingly, using an optical reporter where the coding sequence of Venus was flanked by short stretches of the Calcium/calmodulin-dependent Kinase IIa (CAMKIIa) 5′- and 3′-UTRs, decreased translation of CAMK2a was reported adjacent to Alzheimer-related amyloid plaques *in vivo* (Meyer-Luehmann et al., 2009).

7.7.4 Huntington's disease (HD)

Huntington's disease (HD) is an autosomal dominant neurodegenerative disorder characterized by a pathogenic unstable trinucleotide CAG repeat expansion (over 36 repeats) in the Huntingtin (HTT) gene, which manifests as abnormal uncontrolled movements (chorea), psychiatric symptoms, and cognitive deficits that worsen over time (Landles & Bates, 2004; Li & Li, 2004). Mutant HTT (mHTT) protein differs from its wild-type counterpart by an elongated polyglutamine (polyQ) region near the amino terminus of the protein, with longer polyQ expansions associated with earlier onset and increased severity (Duyao et al., 1993). Aberrant aggregation, and subsequent inactivation, of mHTT are detected in the brains of patients with Huntington's disease (Davies et al., 1997; DiFiglia et al., 1997).

HTT is transported in axons and plays a role in dendritic RNA delivery (Ma et al., 2010). Indeed, HTT protein inactivation leads to defective BDNF mRNA localization in axons of cortical neurons (Ma et al., 2010). HTT was also shown to colocalize with specific RNPs, Ago2 and Staufen, in P bodies containing translationally repressed mRNA (Savas et al., 2008) and in dendritic RNA granules regulating transport and local translation (Savas et al., 2010). Moreover, HTT can bind the 3′UTRs of mRNAs targeted to the dendrites, such as Actb or Bdnf (Ma et al., 2010; Savas et al., 2010). Interestingly, BDNF is a known regulator of local translation (Swanger & Bassell, 2013). Recently HTT protein was found in a complex with its own mRNA, RNA-binding proteins, and translation factors (Culver et al., 2016). Thus, HTT may be involved in modulating its expression through post-transcriptional pathways. Similarly, to other neurodegenerative disorders, HD is yet another example of deregulation in the interaction with RBPs or in the direct binding to mRNA 3′UTRs leading to mRNA transport impairment. While we have data regarding dendrites, it is possible that axonal translation could also be hindered in HD.

7.7.5 Spinal muscular atrophy (SMA)

Spinal muscular atrophy (SMA) is one of the most common autosomal recessive hereditary disorders, manifesting as a gradual spinal alpha motor neuron degeneration caused mostly by bi-allelic loss-of-function mutations in the SMN1 gene (Wirth, 2000; Verhaart et al., 2017; Calucho et al., 2018). Hallmarks of the disease are progressive proximal muscle weakness and atrophy, which can lead to paralysis, with the severity of the disease being modulated by the copy number variation of SMN2, a paralog of the SMN1 gene (Crawford et al., 2012). SMA patients are classified clinically into five types, from 0 to 4, according to the highest achieved motor abilities, which loosely correlate with the age of symptoms onset (Mercuri et al., 2018; Finkel et al., 2018). Currently, no cure has been found for this pathology, and symptoms management is mostly performed via mechanical supportive care, the use of disease-modifying agents, and gene therapy aimed at restoring SMN protein expression (Nicolau et al., 2021).

The SMN protein is involved in the assembly of the pre-mRNA splicing complex small-nuclear ribonucleoproteins (snRNPs) (Khalil et al., 2018) and plays a role in the modulation of mRNA localization and RNP regulation in axons (Fallini et al., 2012, 2016). Axonal SMN-RNP complexes differ from their snRNPs counterparts, suggesting an axonal function for SMN other than splicing regulation (Fallini et al., 2011). Indeed, SMN was found to control mRNA axonal transport and axonal growth in cooperation with HuD, a neuron-specific RNA binding protein (Akten et al., 2011; Hao le et al., 2017). Thus, alteration of SMN1 expression can lead to mRNA mislocalization and impairment of axonal local translation in motor neurons. For instance, β-actin (mRNA is miss-localized), and its local protein synthesis is impaired in SMN-deficient motor neurons, causing defects in axonal growth (Rossoll et al.., 2003; Rathod et al., 2012). Interestingly, GAP43 is highly expressed during neuronal growth and axonal regeneration and its axonal mRNA mislocalization leads to motor neuron axonal growth defect, and SMN was shown to control GAP43 mRNA transport and translation (Hartl & Schneider, 2019; Fallini et al., 2016). GAP43 and β-actin mRNAs can compete for their localization and translation, and, in doing so, regulate axon elongation and branching respectively (Donnelly et al., 2013). SMN deficiency also affects Annexin A2 (Anxa2) mRNA localization (Rage et al., 2013). Anxa2 is involved in actin cytoskeleton regulation and its mRNA miss-localization and impaired axonal translation, could in part explain the observed cytoskeleton defects in SMN models (Rihan et al., 2017). Finally, Axonal localization of the transcript coding for the voltage-gated calcium channel CaV2.2 is decreased in growth cones of SMA cultured neurons, leading to a reduction of Ca^{2+} signaling (Jablonka et al., 2007). SMN also regulates local protein synthesis through miRNA expression. Indeed, miR-183, which targets mTOR, a key regulator of local translation in neurons, was shown to be increased in neurites of SMN-deficient neurons leading to decreased translation (Kye et al., 2014). Interestingly, recent evidence acquired by ultrastructural analyses of ribosomes showed a 27% decrease in axonal ribosomes in motor axons of SMA mice compared to their wild-type counterpart, suggesting an overall decreased capacity for translation in axons (Bernabò et al., 2017). Altogether, these data suggest that mRNA mislocalization and local translation impairment could be among the underlying causes of neurite growth, presynaptic functions, and cytoskeleton organization defects in SMA motor neurons.

7.7.6 Fragile X syndrome (FXS)

Fragile X syndrome (FXS) is a neurodevelopmental disorder, which has not been associated with axonal loss during adult life. The initiation of the pathology is linked to mutations in the FMR1 gene, which encodes the RNA-binding protein FMRP. The symptoms of FXS are variable on the autism spectrum and depend on gender, age, genetic background, and environmental effects (Dyer-Friedman et al., 2002; Loesch et al., 2004; Hoogeveen et al., 2002). Since the FMR1 allele is localized on the X chromosome, FMRP levels also correlate with X-inactivation in females. Consequently, the disease has a lower prevalence and is less severe in females (Hagerman et al., 2017).

Abnormal trinucleotide repeats in FMR1 5'-UTR reduce FMRP protein synthesis and manifest in behavioral features associated with the autism spectrum (Maurin et al., 2014). The triplet repeats lead to DNA methylation of FMR1, transcriptional inactivation of the gene, and finally partial or complete loss of FMRP (Pieretti et al., 1991; Verkerk et al., 1991). FMRP is enriched in the brain RNA and has an essential role in synaptic plasticity and architecture (Ashley et al., 1993; Darnell et al., 2011; Siomi et al., 1993). Several pieces of evidence point to the role of FMRP in dendrite local translation (Feuge et al., 2019; Antar et al., 2004; Banerjee et al., 2018). However, FMRP-containing granules, called Fragile X granules (FXG), have also been found in a subset of axons, mostly during synapse formation and pruning (Akins et al., 2012; Christie et al., 2009). While FMRP is not required for the axonal transport of ribosomes (Akins et al., 2017), loss of FMRP in mice is linked to the regulation of local translation. FMRP is responsible for the transport of Map1b and Calm1 mRNAs together with the local translational regulator miR-181d. Upon NGF stimulation, FMRP and miR-181d mediate axon elongation by translational regulation of their targets (Wang et al., 2015). Thus, disruption of the local translation machinery due to FMRP loss or mutation might play a role in the developmental symptoms of this pathology.

7.8 Conclusion

mRNA localization and local translation are important mechanisms by which highly polarized cells with specialized functions such as neurons can spatially and temporally control the subcellular proteome. This spatiotemporal control is important for a variety of neuronal processes including synaptic function and plasticity, growth cone guidance, axonal maintenance, neuronal survival and homeostasis, and response to injury. The disruption of mRNA trafficking and local translation either directly, such as mutations in RNA-binding proteins involved in RNA processes, or indirectly thought the disruption of the proteasome, UPS, autophagy, and in general protein homeostasis has been implicated in many neurodegenerative pathologies such as ALS, FTD, HD, AD, PD, SMA and FXS. In this chapter, we tried to give an overview of the neurodegenerative pathologies, which involve defects in mRNA local translation and localization (Table 7.1). Further research on the subject, focused on understanding the physiological and pathological functions and mechanisms underlying this alteration for the individual pathology, is needed to propose efficient treatments. For instance, finding out how to promote the localization of specific mRNAs and/or activating the local translational machinery could preserve axonal integrity and ameliorate disease prognosis. Indeed, the range of technologies allowing for direct visualization of mRNA and proteins as well as de novo discovery of axonal mRNA and RBPs has been drastically expanded in recent years (Koppel & Fainzilber, 2018; Holt et al., 2019), with an increasing number of proximity-based approaches to transcriptomics and proteomics, which allows for the investigation of axonal organelle-based mRNA transport (Liao et al., 2019; Williams et al., 2014; Qin et al., 2021). Data generated via these novel technologies is likely to uncover the critical mechanism underlying neurodegeneration and recovery from injury.

Acknowledgments

M.T. acknowledges the generous support of the Okinawa Institute of Science and Technology graduate University internal funding and JSPS/Kakenhi C Research Grant (#20K07458).

References

Akins MR, Berk-Rauch HE, Kwan KY, Mitchell ME, Shepard KA, Korsak LIT, Stackpole EE, Warner-Schmidt JL, Sestan N, Cameron HA, *et al* (2017) Axonal ribosomes and mRNAs associate with fragile X granules in adult rodent and human brains. *Human Molecular Genetics* **26**: 192–209

Akins MR, LeBlanc HF, Stackpole EE, Chyung E & Fallon JR (2012) Systematic mapping of Fragile X granules in the developing mouse brain reveals a potential role for presynaptic FMRP in sensorimotor functions. *J Comp Neurol* **520**: 3687–3706

Akiyama T, Suzuki N, Ishikawa M, Fujimori K, Sone T, Kawada J, Funayama R, Fujishima F, Mitsuzawa S, Ikeda K, *et al* (2019) Aberrant axon branching via Fos-B dysregulation in FUS-ALS motor neurons. *EBioMedicine* **45**: 362–378

Akten B, Kye MJ, Hao LT, Wertz MH, Singh S, Nie D, Huang J, Merianda TT, Twiss JL, Beattie CE, *et al* (2011) Interaction of survival of motor neuron (SMN) and HuD proteins with mRNA cpg15 rescues motor neuron axonal deficits. *Proc Natl Acad Sci U S A* **108**: 10337–10342

Alami NH, Smith RB, Carrasco MA, Williams LA, Winborn CS, Han SSW, Kiskinis E, Winborn B, Freibaum BD, Kanagaraj A, *et al* (2014) Axonal Transport of TDP-43 mRNA Granules Is Impaired by ALS-Causing Mutations. *Neuron* **81**: 536–543

Alexander GE (2004) Biology of Parkinson's disease: pathogenesis and pathophysiology of a multisystem neurodegenerative disorder. *Dialogues Clin Neurosci* **6**: 259–280

Altman T, Ionescu A, Ibraheem A, Priesmann D, Gradus-Pery T, Farberov L, Alexandra G, Shelestovich N, Dafinca R, Shomron N, *et al* (2021) Axonal TDP-43 condensates drive neuromuscular junction disruption through inhibition of local synthesis of nuclear encoded mitochondrial proteins. *Nat Commun* **12**: 6914

Anderson KD, Morin MA, Beckel-Mitchener A, Mobarak CD, Neve RL, Furneaux HM, Burry R & Perrone-Bizzozero NI (2000) Overexpression of HuD, but Not of Its Truncated Form HuD I+II, Promotes GAP-43

Gene Expression and Neurite Outgrowth in PC12 Cells in the Absence of Nerve Growth Factor. *Journal of Neurochemistry* **75**: 1103–1114

Andreassi C & Riccio A (2009) To localize or not to localize: mRNA fate is in 3'UTR ends. *Trends Cell Biol* **19**: 465–474

Antar LN, Afroz R, Dictenberg JB, Carroll RC & Bassell GJ (2004) Metabotropic Glutamate Receptor Activation Regulates Fragile X Mental Retardation Protein and Fmr1 mRNA Localization Differentially in Dendrites and at Synapses. *J Neurosci* **24**: 2648–2655

Arai T, Hasegawa M, Akiyama H, Ikeda K, Nonaka T, Mori H, Mann D, Tsuchiya K, Yoshida M, Hashizume Y, *et al* (2006) TDP-43 is a component of ubiquitin-positive tau-negative inclusions in frontotemporal lobar degeneration and amyotrophic lateral sclerosis. *Biochem Biophys Res Commun* **351**: 602–611

Aschrafi A, Kar AN, Gale J, Elkahloun AG, Vargas J-N, Sales N, Wilson G, Tompkins M, Gioio AE & Kaplan BB (2016) A Heterogeneous Population of Nuclear-Encoded Mitochondrial mRNAs Is Present in the Axons of Primary Sympathetic Neurons. *Mitochondrion* **30**: 18–23

Aschrafi A, Kar AN, Natera-Naranjo O, MacGibeny MA, Gioio AE & Kaplan BB (2012) MicroRNA-338 regulates the axonal expression of multiple nuclear-encoded mitochondrial mRNAs encoding subunits of the oxidative phosphorylation machinery. *Cell Mol Life Sci* **69**: 4017–4027

Aschrafi A, Schwechter AD, Mameza MG, Natera-Naranjo O, Gioio AE & Kaplan BB (2008) MicroRNA-338 Regulates Local Cytochrome c Oxidase IV mRNA Levels and Oxidative Phosphorylation in the Axons of Sympathetic Neurons. *J Neurosci* **28**: 12581–12590

Ashley CT, Wilkinson KD, Reines D & Warren ST (1993) FMR1 protein: conserved RNP family domains and selective RNA binding. *Science* **262**: 563–566

Bae B & Miura P (2020) Emerging Roles for 3′ UTRs in Neurons. *Int J Mol Sci* **21**: 3413

Baleriola J, Walker CA, Jean YY, Crary JF, Troy CM, Nagy PL & Hengst U (2014) Axonally Synthesized ATF4 Transmits a Neurodegenerative Signal across Brain Regions. *Cell* **158**: 1159–1172

Banerjee A, Ifrim MF, Valdez AN, Raj N & Bassell GJ (2018) Aberrant RNA translation in fragile X syndrome: From FMRP mechanisms to emerging therapeutic strategies. *Brain Res* **1693**: 24–36

Bang J, Spina S & Miller BL (2015) Frontotemporal dementia. *Lancet* **386**: 1672–1682

Barker HV, Niblock M, Lee Y-B, Shaw CE & Gallo J-M (2017) RNA Misprocessing in C9orf72-Linked Neurodegeneration. *Front Cell Neurosci* **11**: 195

Bassell GJ, Zhang H, Byrd AL, Femino AM, Singer RH, Taneja KL, Lifshitz LM, Herman IM & Kosik KS (1998) Sorting of β-Actin mRNA and Protein to Neurites and Growth Cones in Culture. *J Neurosci* **18**: 251–265

Batey RT (2006) Structures of regulatory elements in mRNAs. *Curr Opin Struct Biol* **16**: 299–306

Batista AFR & Hengst U (2016) Intra-axonal protein synthesis in development and beyond. *Int J Dev Neurosci* **55**: 140–149

Batista AFR, Martínez JC & Hengst U (2017) Intra-axonal synthesis of SNAP25 is required for the formation of presynaptic terminals. *Cell Rep* **20**: 3085–3098

Ben-Yaakov K, Dagan SY, Segal-Ruder Y, Shalem O, Vuppalanchi D, Willis DE, Yudin D, Rishal I, Rother F, Bader M, *et al* (2012) Axonal transcription factors signal retrogradely in lesioned peripheral nerve. *EMBO J* **31**: 1350–1363

Bernabò P, Tebaldi T, Groen EJN, Lane FM, Perenthaler E, Mattedi F, Newbery HJ, Zhou H, Zuccotti P, Potrich V, *et al* (2017) In Vivo Translatome Profiling in Spinal Muscular Atrophy Reveals a Role for SMN Protein in Ribosome Biology. *Cell Rep* **21**: 953–965

Berry FB & Brown IR (1996) CaM I mRNA is localized to apical dendrites during postnatal development of neurons in the rat brain. *J Neurosci Res* **43**: 565–575

Bird CW, Gardiner AS, Bolognani F, Tanner DC, Chen C-Y, Lin W-J, Yoo S, Twiss JL & Perrone- Bizzozero N (2013) KSRP Modulation of GAP-43 mRNA Stability Restricts Axonal Outgrowth in Embryonic Hippocampal Neurons. *PLoS One* **8**: e79255

Brown A-L, Wilkins OG, Keuss MJ, Hill SE, Zanovello M, Lee WC, Bampton A, Lee FCY, Masino L, Qi YA, *et al* (2022) TDP-43 loss and ALS-risk SNPs drive mis-splicing and depletion of UNC13A. *Nature* **603**: 131–137

Burgin KE, Waxham MN, Rickling S, Westgate SA, Mobley WC & Kelly PT (1990) In situ hybridization histochemistry of Ca2+/calmodulin-dependent protein kinase in developing rat brain. *J Neurosci* **10**: 1788–1798

Cagnetta R, Wong HH-W, Frese CK, Mallucci GR, Krijgsveld J & Holt CE (2019) Noncanonical Modulation of the eIF2 Pathway Controls an Increase in Local Translation during Neural Wiring. *Molecular Cell* **73**: 474-489.e5

Cajigas IJ, Tushev G, Will TJ, Dieck S tom, Fuerst N & Schuman EM (2012) The Local Transcriptome in the Synaptic Neuropil Revealed by Deep Sequencing and High-Resolution Imaging. *Neuron* **74**: 453–466

Calucho M, Bernal S, Alías L, March F, Venceslá A, Rodríguez-Álvarez FJ, Aller E, Fernández RM, Borrego S, Millán JM, *et al* (2018) Correlation between SMA type and SMN2 copy number revisited: An analysis of 625 unrelated Spanish patients and a compilation of 2834 reported cases. *Neuromuscular Disorders* **28**: 208–215

Campbell DS & Holt CE (2001) Chemotropic Responses of Retinal Growth Cones Mediated by Rapid Local Protein Synthesis and Degradation. *Neuron* **32**: 1013–1026

Chierzi S, Ratto GM, Verma P & Fawcett JW (2005) The ability of axons to regenerate their growth cones depends on axonal type and age, and is regulated by calcium, cAMP and ERK. *European Journal of Neuroscience* **21**: 2051–2062

Christie SB, Akins MR, Schwob JE & Fallon JR (2009) The FXG: A Presynaptic Fragile X Granule Expressed in a Subset of Developing Brain Circuits. *J Neurosci* **29**: 1514–1524

Cioni J-M, Lin JQ, Holtermann AV, Koppers M, Jakobs MAH, Azizi A, Turner-Bridger B, Shigeoka T, Franze K, Harris WA, *et al* (2019) Late Endosomes Act as mRNA Translation Platforms and Sustain Mitochondria in Axons. *Cell* **176**: 56-72.e15

Costa CJ & Willis DE (2018) To the End of the Line: Axonal mRNA transport and local translation in health and neurodegenerative disease. *Dev Neurobiol* **78**: 209–220

Court FA, Hendriks WTJ, MacGillavry HD, Alvarez J & Minnen J van (2008) Schwann Cell to Axon Transfer of Ribosomes: Toward a Novel Understanding of the Role of Glia in the Nervous System. *J Neurosci* **28**: 11024–11029

Court FA, Midha R, Cisterna BA, Grochmal J, Shakhbazau A, Hendriks WT & Van Minnen J (2011) Morphological evidence for a transport of ribosomes from Schwann cells to regenerating axons. *Glia* **59**: 1529–1539

Cox DJ & Racca C (2013) Differential dendritic targeting of AMPA receptor subunit mRNAs in adult rat hippocampal principal neurons and interneurons. *J Comp Neurol* **521**: 1954–2007

Cox LJ, Hengst U, Gurskaya Nadya, Lukyanov KA & Jaffrey SR (2008) Intra-axonal translation and retrograde trafficking of CREB promotes neuronal survival. *Nat Cell Biol* **10**: 149–159

Crawford TO, Paushkin SV, Kobayashi DT, Forrest SJ, Joyce CL, Finkel RS, Kaufmann P, Swoboda KJ, Tiziano D, Lomastro R, *et al* (2012) Evaluation of SMN Protein, Transcript, and Copy Number in the Biomarkers for Spinal Muscular Atrophy (BforSMA) Clinical Study. *PLoS One* **7**: e33572

Crispino M, Kaplan BB, Martin R, Alvarez J, Chun JT, Benech JC & Giuditta A (1997) Active Polysomes Are Present in the Large Presynaptic Endings of the Synaptosomal Fraction from Squid Brain. *J Neurosci* **17**: 7694–7702

Culver BP, DeClercq J, Dolgalev I, Yu MS, Ma B, Heguy A & Tanese N (2016) Huntington's Disease Protein Huntingtin Associates with its own mRNA. *Journal of Huntington's Disease* **5**: 39

Dalla Costa I, Buchanan CN, Zdradzinski MD, Sahoo PK, Smith TP, Thames E, Kar AN & Twiss JL (2021) The functional organization of axonal mRNA transport and translation. *Nat Rev Neurosci* **22**: 77–91

Darnell JC, Van Driesche SJ, Zhang C, Hung KYS, Mele A, Fraser CE, Stone EF, Chen C, Fak JJ, Chi SW, *et al* (2011) FMRP stalls ribosomal translocation on mRNAs linked to synaptic function and autism. *Cell* **146**: 247–261

Davies SW, Turmaine M, Cozens BA, DiFiglia M, Sharp AH, Ross CA, Scherzinger E, Wanker EE, Mangiarini L & Bates GP (1997) Formation of Neuronal Intranuclear Inclusions Underlies the Neurological Dysfunction in Mice Transgenic for the HD Mutation. *Cell* **90**: 537–548

Davis AA, Leyns CEG & Holtzman DM (2018) Intercellular Spread of Protein Aggregates in Neurodegenerative Disease. *Annu Rev Cell Dev Biol* **34**: 545–568

Decker H, Lo KY, Unger SM, Ferreira ST & Silverman MA (2010) Amyloid-β Peptide Oligomers Disrupt Axonal Transport through an NMDA Receptor-Dependent Mechanism That Is Mediated by Glycogen Synthase Kinase 3β in Primary Cultured Hippocampal Neurons. **30**: 9166–9171

Denis-Donini S, Branduardi P, Campiglio S & Carnevali MDC (1998) Localization of calcitonin gene-related peptide mRNA in developing olfactory axons. *Cell Tissue Res* **294**: 81–91

DiFiglia M, Sapp E, Chase KO, Davies SW, Bates GP, Vonsattel JP & Aronin N (1997) Aggregation of Huntingtin in Neuronal Intranuclear Inclusions and Dystrophic Neurites in Brain. *Science* **277**: 1990–1993

Donnelly CJ, Park M, Spillane M, Yoo S, Pacheco A, Gomes C, Vuppalanchi D, McDonald M, Kim HH, Merianda TT, *et al* (2013) Axonally Synthesized β-Actin and GAP-43 Proteins Support Distinct Modes of Axonal Growth. *J Neurosci* **33**: 3311–3322

Donnelly CJ, Willis DE, Xu M, Tep C, Jiang C, Yoo S, Schanen NC, Kirn-Safran CB, van Minnen J, English A, *et al* (2011) Limited availability of ZBP1 restricts axonal mRNA localization and nerve regeneration capacity. *EMBO J* **30**: 4665–4677

Dörrbaum AR, Kochen L, Langer JD & Schuman EM (2022) Local and global influences on protein turnover in neurons and glia. *eLife* **7**: e34202

Duyao M, Ambrose C, Myers R, Novelletto A, Persichetti F, Frontali M, Folstein S, Ross C, Franz M, Abbott M, *et al* (1993) Trinucleotide repeat length instability and age of onset in Huntington's disease. *Nat Genet* **4**: 387–392

Dyer-friedman J, Glaser B, Hessl D, Johnston C, Huffman LC, Taylor A, Wisbeck J & Reiss AL (2002) Genetic and Environmental Influences on the Cognitive Outcomes of Children With Fragile X Syndrome. *Journal of the American Academy of Child & Adolescent Psychiatry* **41**: 237–244

Fallini C, Bassell GJ & Rossoll W (2012) Spinal muscular atrophy: the role of SMN in axonal mRNA regulation. *Brain Res* **1462**: 81–92

Fallini C, Donlin-Asp PG, Rouanet JP, Bassell GJ & Rossoll W (2016) Deficiency of the Survival of Motor Neuron Protein Impairs mRNA Localization and Local Translation in the Growth Cone of Motor Neurons. *J Neurosci* **36**: 3811–3820

Fallini C, Zhang H, Su Y, Silani V, Singer RH, Rossoll W & Bassell GJ (2011) The Survival of Motor Neuron (SMN) Protein Interacts with the mRNA-Binding Protein HuD and Regulates Localization of Poly(A) mRNA in Primary Motor Neuron Axons. *J Neurosci* **31**: 3914–3925

Farg MA, Sundaramoorthy V, Sultana JM, Yang S, Atkinson RAK, Levina V, Halloran MA, Gleeson PA, Blair IP, Soo KY, *et al* (2014) C9ORF72, implicated in amytrophic lateral sclerosis and frontotemporal dementia, regulates endosomal trafficking. *Hum Mol Genet* **23**: 3579–3595

Feig S & Lipton P (1993) Pairing the cholinergic agonist carbachol with patterned Schaffer collateral stimulation initiates protein synthesis in hippocampal CA1 pyramidal cell dendrites via a muscarinic, NMDA-dependent mechanism. *J Neurosci* **13**: 1010–1021

Feuge J, Scharkowski F, Michaelsen-Preusse K & Korte M (2019) FMRP Modulates Activity-Dependent Spine Plasticity by Binding Cofilin1 mRNA and Regulating Localization and Local Translation. *Cerebral Cortex* **29**: 5204–5216

Finkel RS, Mercuri E, Meyer OH, Simonds AK, Schroth MK, Graham RJ, Kirschner J, Iannaccone ST, Crawford TO, Woods S, *et al* (2018) Diagnosis and management of spinal muscular atrophy: Part 2: Pulmonary and acute care; medications, supplements and immunizations; other organ systems; and ethics. *Neuromuscular Disorders* **28**: 197–207

Freischmidt A, Wieland T, Richter B, Ruf W, Schaeffer V, Müller K, Marroquin N, Nordin F, Hübers A, Weydt P, *et al* (2015)

Haploinsufficiency of TBK1 causes familial ALS and fronto-temporal dementia. *Nat Neurosci* **18**: 631–636

Fusco CM, Desch K, Dörrbaum AR, Wang M, Staab A, Chan ICW, Vail E, Villeri V, Langer JD & Schuman EM (2021) Neuronal ribosomes exhibit dynamic and context-dependent exchange of ribosomal proteins. *Nat Commun* **12**: 6127

Gainer H, Tasaki I & Lasek RJ (1977) Evidence for the glia-neuron protein transfer hypothesis from intracellular perfusion studies of squid giant axons. *Journal of Cell Biology* **74**: 524–530

Gamarra M, de la Cruz A, Blanco-Urrejola M & Baleriola J (2021) Local Translation in Nervous System Pathologies. **15**

Gardiner AS, Twiss JL & Perrone-Bizzozero NI (2015) Competing Interactions of RNA-Binding Proteins, MicroRNAs, and Their Targets Control Neuronal Development and Function. *Biomolecules* **5**: 2903–2918

Gehrke S, Wu Z, Klinkenberg M, Sun Y, Auburger G, Guo S & Lu B (2015) PINK1 and Parkin Control Localized Translation of Respiratory Chain Component mRNAs on Mitochondria Outer Membrane. *Cell Metabolism* **21**: 95–108

Gershoni-Emek N, Altman T, Ionescu A, Costa CJ, Gradus-Pery T, Willis DE & Perlson E (2018) Localization of RNAi Machinery to Axonal Branch Points and Growth Cones Is Facilitated by Mitochondria and Is Disrupted in ALS. *Front Mol Neurosci* **11**: 311

Ghosh A, Mizuno K, Tiwari SS, Proitsi P, Gomez Perez-Nievas B, Glennon E, Martinez-Nunez RT & Giese KP (2020) Alzheimer's disease-related dysregulation of mRNA translation causes key pathological features with ageing. *Translational Psychiatry* **10**: 192

Giuditta A, Cupellot A & Lazzarini G (1980) Ribosomal RNA in the Axoplasm of the Squid Giant Axon. *Journal of Neurochemistry* **34**: 1757–1760

Giuditta A, Hunt T & Santella L (1986) Rapid important paper: Messenger RNA in squid axoplasm. *Neurochemistry International* **8**: 435–442

Giuditta A, Menichini E, Capano CP, Langella M, Martin R, Castigli E & Kaplan BB (1991) Active polysomes in the axoplasm of the squid giant axon. *Journal of Neuroscience Research* **28**: 18–28

Glock C, Heumüller M & Schuman EM (2017) mRNA transport & local translation in neurons. *Curr Opin Neurobiol* **45**: 169–177

Goedert M, Spillantini MG, Del Tredici K & Braak H (2013) 100 years of Lewy pathology. *Nature Reviews Neurology* **9**: 13–24

Gomes C, Merianda TT, Lee SJ, Yoo S & Twiss JL (2014) Molecular determinants of the axonal mRNA transcriptome. *Developmental Neurobiology* **74**: 218–232

Gracias NG, Shirkey-Son NJ & Hengst U (2014) Local translation of TC10 is required for membrane expansion during axon outgrowth. *Nat Commun* **5**: 3506

Gumy LF, Tan CL & Fawcett JW (2010) The role of local protein synthesis and degradation in axon regeneration. *Exp Neurol* **223**: 28–37

Gumy LF, Yeo GSH, Tung Y-CL, Zivraj KH, Willis D, Coppola G, Lam BYH, Twiss JL, Holt CE & Fawcett JW (2011) Transcriptome analysis of embryonic and adult sensory axons reveals changes in mRNA repertoire localization. *RNA* **17**: 85–98

Hafner A-S, Donlin-Asp PG, Leitch B, Herzog E & Schuman EM (2019) Local protein synthesis is a ubiquitous feature of neuronal pre- and postsynaptic compartments. 13

Hagerman RJ, Berry-Kravis E, Hazlett HC, Bailey DB, Moine H, Kooy RF, Tassone F, Gantois I, Sonenberg N, Mandel JL, *et al* (2017) Fragile X syndrome. *Nat Rev Dis Primers* **3**: 17065

Han SM, Baig HS & Hammarlund M (2016) Mitochondria localize to injured axons to support regeneration. *Neuron* 92: 1308–1323

Hanz S, Perlson E, Willis D, Zheng J-Q, Massarwa R, Huerta JJ, Koltzenburg M, Kohler M, van-Minnen J, Twiss JL, *et al* (2003) Axoplasmic Importins Enable Retrograde Injury Signaling in Lesioned Nerve. *Neuron* **40**: 1095–1104

Hao le T, Duy PQ, An M, Talbot J, Iyer CC, Wolman M & Beattie CE (2017) HuD and the Survival Motor Neuron Protein Interact in Motoneurons and Are Essential for Motoneuron Development, Function, and mRNA Regulation. *J Neurosci* **37**: 11559–11571

Harbauer AB, Hees JT, Wanderoy S, Segura I, Gibbs W, Cheng Y, Ordonez M, Cai Z, Cartoni R, Ashrafi G, *et al* (2022) Neuronal mitochondria transport Pink1 mRNA via synaptojanin 2 to support local mitophagy. *Neuron* **110**: 1516-1531.e9

Harrington AW & Ginty DD (2013) Long-distance retrograde neurotrophic factor signalling in neurons. *Nat Rev Neurosci* **14**: 177–187

Hartl M & Schneider R (2019) A Unique Family of Neuronal Signaling Proteins Implicated in Oncogenesis and Tumor Suppression. *Front Oncol* **9**: 289

Heemels M-T (2016) Neurodegenerative diseases. *Nature* **539**: 179

Hengst U, Cox LJ, Macosko EZ & Jaffrey SR (2006) Functional and Selective RNA Interference in Developing Axons and Growth Cones. *J Neurosci* **26**: 5727–5732

Hengst U, Deglincerti A, Kim HJ, Jeon NL & Jaffrey SR (2009) Axonal elongation triggered by stimulus-induced local translation of a polarity complex protein. *Nat Cell Biol* **11**: 1024–1030

Hetz C & Saxena S (2017) ER stress and the unfolded protein response in neurodegeneration. *Nature Reviews Neurology* **13**: 477–491

Hillefors M, Gioio AE, Mameza MG & Kaplan BB (2007) Axon Viability and Mitochondrial Function are Dependent on Local Protein Synthesis in Sympathetic Neurons. *Cell Mol Neurobiol* **27**: 701–716

Hodas JJL, Nehring A, Höche N, Sweredoski MJ, Pielot R, Hess S, Tirrell DA, Dieterich DC & Schuman EM (2012) Dopaminergic modulation of the hippocampal neuropil proteome identified by bio-orthogonal non-canonical amino-acid tagging (BONCAT). *Proteomics* **12**: 2464–2476

Holt CE, Martin KC & Schuman EM (2019) Local translation in neurons: visualization and function. *Nat Struct Mol Biol* **26**: 557–566

Hoogeveen AT, Willemsen R & Oostra BA (2002) Fragile X syndrome, the Fragile X related proteins, and animal models. *Microscopy Research and Technique* **57**: 148–155

Hörnberg H & Holt C (2013) RNA-binding proteins and translational regulation in axons and growth cones. *Front Neurosci* **7**: 81

Imai Y, Gehrke S, Wang H-Q, Takahashi R, Hasegawa K, Oota E & Lu B (2008) Phosphorylation of 4E-BP by LRRK2 affects the maintenance of dopaminergic neurons in Drosophila. *The EMBO Journal* **27**: 2432–2443

Jablonka S, Beck M, Lechner BD, Mayer C & Sendtner M (2007) Defective Ca2+ channel clustering in axon terminals disturbs excitability in motoneurons in spinal muscular atrophy. *J Cell Biol* **179**: 139–149

Johnson JO, Mandrioli J, Benatar M, Abramzon Y, Van Deerlin VM, Trojanowski JQ, Gibbs JR, Brunetti M, Gronka S, Wuu J, *et al* (2010) Exome sequencing reveals VCP mutations as a cause of familial ALS. *Neuron* **68**: 857–864

Jung H, Gkogkas CG, Sonenberg N & Holt CE (2014) Remote control of gene function by local translation. *Cell* **157**: 26–40

Jung H, Yoon BC & Holt CE (2012) Axonal mRNA localization and local protein synthesis in nervous system assembly, maintenance and repair. *Nat Rev Neurosci* **13**: 308–324

Kalil K & Dent EW (2014) Branch management: mechanisms of axon branching in the developing vertebrate CNS. *Nat Rev Neurosci* **15**: 7–18

Kalinski AL, Sachdeva R, Gomes C, Lee SJ, Shah Z, Houle JD & Twiss JL (2015) mRNAs and Protein Synthetic Machinery Localize into Regenerating Spinal Cord Axons When They Are Provided a Substrate That Supports Growth. *J Neurosci* **35**: 10357–10370

Kanai Y, Dohmae N & Hirokawa N (2004) Kinesin transports RNA: isolation and characterization of an RNA-transporting granule. *Neuron* **43**: 513–525

Kapeli K, Martinez FJ & Yeo GW (2017) Genetic mutations in RNA-binding proteins and their roles in ALS. *Hum Genet* **136**: 1193–1214

Kar AN, Lee S-J, Sahoo PK, Thames E, Yoo S, Houle JD & Twiss JL (2021) MicroRNAs 21 and 199a-3p Regulate Axon Growth Potential through Modulation of Pten and mTor mRNAs. *eNeuro* **8**

Karanth S, Nelson PT, Katsumata Y, Kryscio RJ, Schmitt FA, Fardo DW, Cykowski MD, Jicha GA, Van Eldik LJ & Abner EL (2020) Prevalence and Clinical Phenotype of Quadruple Misfolded Proteins in Older Adults. *JAMA Neurology* **77**: 1299–1307

Khalil B, Morderer D, Price PL, Liu F & Rossoll W (2018) mRNP assembly, axonal transport, and local translation in neurodegenerative diseases. *Brain Res* **1693**: 75–91

Knopman DS, Amieva H, Petersen RC, Chételat G, Holtzman DM, Hyman BT, Nixon RA & Jones DT (2021) Alzheimer disease. *Nature Reviews Disease Primers* **7**: 33

Kobayashi S, Tanaka T, Soeda Y, Almeida OFX & Takashima A (2017) Local Somatodendritic Translation and Hyperphosphorylation of Tau Protein Triggered by AMPA and NMDA Receptor Stimulation. *EBioMedicine* **20**: 120–126

Koenig E (1965a) Synthetic Mechanisms in the Axon. I. Local Axonal Synthesis of Acetylcholinesterase. *J Neurochem* **12**: 343–355

Koenig E (1965b) Synthetic Mechanisms in the Axon. II. Rna in Myelin-Free Axons of the Cat. *J Neurochem* **12**: 357–361

Koenig E (1967a) Synthetic Mechanisms in the Axon—IV. *in vitro* Incorporation of [3h]precursors into Axonal Protein and Rna *. *Journal of Neurochemistry* **14**: 437–446

Koenig E (1967b) Synthetic Mechanisms in the Axon—III. Stimulation of Acetylcholinesterase Synthesis by Actinomycin-D in the Hypoglossal Nerve *. *Journal of Neurochemistry* **14**: 429–435

Koley S, Rozenbaum M, Fainzilber M & Terenzio M (2019) Translating regeneration: Local protein synthesis in the neuronal injury response. *Neuroscience Research* **139**: 26–36

Koppel I & Fainzilber M (2018) Omics approaches for subcellular translation studies. *Mol Omics* **14**: 380–388

Koppers M, Cagnetta R, Shigeoka T, Wunderlich LC, Vallejo-Ramirez P, Qiaojin Lin J, Zhao S, Jakobs MA, Dwivedy A, Minett MS, *et al* (2022) Receptor-specific interactome as a hub for rapid cue-induced selective translation in axons. *eLife* **8**: e48718

Kosik KS (2006) The neuronal microRNA system. *Nat Rev Neurosci* **7**: 911–920

Kosik KS (2016) Life at Low Copy Number: How Dendrites Manage with So Few mRNAs. *Neuron* **92**: 1168–1180

Krichevsky AM & Kosik KS (2001) Neuronal RNA granules: a link between RNA localization and stimulation-dependent translation. *Neuron* **32**: 683–696

Kun A, Otero L, Sotelo-Silveira JR & Sotelo JR (2007) Ribosomal distributions in axons of mammalian myelinated fibers. *J Neurosci Res* **85**: 2087–2098

Kwiatkowski TJ, Bosco DA, Leclerc AL, Tamrazian E, Vanderburg CR, Russ C, Davis A, Gilchrist J, Kasarskis EJ, Munsat T, *et al* (2009) Mutations in the FUS/TLS gene on chromosome 16 cause familial amyotrophic lateral sclerosis. *Science* **323**: 1205–1208

Kye MJ, Niederst ED, Wertz MH, Gonçalves I do CG, Akten B, Dover KZ, Peters M, Riessland M, Neveu P, Wirth B, *et al* (2014) SMN regulates axonal local translation via miR-183/mTOR pathway. *Hum Mol Genet* **23**: 6318–6331

Lagier-Tourenne C, Polymenidou M & Cleveland DW (2010) TDP-43 and FUS/TLS: emerging roles in RNA processing and neurodegeneration. *Hum Mol Genet* **19**: R46–64

Landles C & Bates GP (2004) Huntingtin and the molecular pathogenesis of Huntington's disease. *EMBO Rep* **5**: 958–963

Laplante M & Sabatini DM (2012) mTOR signaling in growth control and disease. *Cell* **149**: 274–293

Lasek R, Gainer H & Barker J (1977) Cell-to-cell transfer of glial proteins to the squid giant axon: The glia- neuron protein transfer hypothesis. *Journal of Cell Biology* **74**: 501–523

Leung K-M, van Horck FP, Lin AC, Allison R, Standart N & Holt CE (2006) Asymmetrical β-actin mRNA translation in growth cones mediates attractive turning to netrin-1. *Nat Neurosci* **9**: 1247–1256

Li C & Götz J (2017) Somatodendritic accumulation of Tau in Alzheimer's disease is promoted by Fyn-mediated local protein translation. *The EMBO Journal* **36**: 3120–3138

Li S, Yang L, Selzer ME & Hu Y (2013) Neuronal ER Stress in Axon Injury and Neurodegeneration. *Ann Neurol* **74**: 768–777

Li S-H & Li X-J (2004) Huntington and its Role in Neuronal Degeneration. *Neuroscientist* **10**: 467–475

Liao Y-C, Fernandopulle MS, Wang G, Choi H, Hao L, Drerup CM, Patel R, Qamar S, Nixon-Abell J, Shen Y, *et al* (2019) RNA Granules Hitchhike on Lysosomes for Long-Distance Transport, Using Annexin A11 as a Molecular Tether. *Cell* **179**: 147-164.e20

Lim EW, Aarsland D, Ffytche D, Taddei RN, van Wamelen DJ, Wan YM, Tan EK & Ray Chaudhuri K (2019) Amyloid-β and Parkinson's disease. *Journal of neurology* **266**: 2605–2619

Ling S-C, Polymenidou M & Cleveland DW (2013) Converging mechanisms in ALS and FTD: Disrupted RNA and protein homeostasis. *Neuron* **79**: 416–438

Liu-Yesucevitz L, Lin AY, Ebata A, Boon JY, Reid W, Xu Y-F, Kobrin K, Murphy GJ, Petrucelli L & Wolozin B (2014) ALS-Linked Mutations Enlarge TDP-43-Enriched Neuronal RNA Granules in the Dendritic Arbor. *The Journal of Neuroscience* **34**: 4167

Loesch DZ, Huggins RM & Hagerman RJ (2004) Phenotypic variation and FMRP levels in fragile X. *Ment Retard Dev Disabil Res Rev* **10**: 31–41

López-Erauskin J, Tadokoro T, Baughn MW, Myers B, McAlonis-Downes M, Chillon-Marinas C, Asiaban JN, Artates J, Bui AT, Vetto AP, *et al* (2018) ALS/FTD-Linked Mutation in FUS Suppresses Intra-axonal Protein Synthesis and Drives Disease Without Nuclear Loss-of-Function of FUS. *Neuron* **100**: 816-830.e7

Ma B, Culver BP, Baj G, Tongiorgi E, Chao MV & Tanese N (2010) Localization of BDNF mRNA with the Huntington's disease protein in rat brain. *Mol Neurodegener* **5**: 22

Ma XR, Prudencio M, Koike Y, Vatsavayai SC, Kim G, Harbinski F, Briner A, Rodriguez CM, Guo C, Akiyama T, *et al* (2022) TDP-43 represses cryptic exon inclusion in the FTD-ALS gene UNC13A. *Nature* **603**: 124–130

Mahar M & Cavalli V (2018) Intrinsic mechanisms of neuronal axon regeneration. *Nat Rev Neurosci* **19**: 323–337

Martin KC & Ephrussi A (2009) mRNA localization: gene expression in the spatial dimension. *Cell* **136**: 719–730

Maruyama H, Morino H, Ito H, Izumi Y, Kato H, Watanabe Y, Kinoshita Y, Kamada M, Nodera H, Suzuki H, *et al* (2010) Mutations of optineurin in amyotrophic lateral sclerosis. *Nature* **465**: 223–226

Maurin T, Zongaro S & Bardoni B (2014) Fragile X Syndrome: From molecular pathology to therapy. *Neuroscience & Biobehavioral Reviews* **46**: 242–255

Mercuri E, Finkel RS, Muntoni F, Wirth B, Montes J, Main M, Mazzone ES, Vitale M, Snyder B, Quijano-Roy S, *et al* (2018) Diagnosis and management of spinal muscular atrophy: Part 1: Recommendations for diagnosis, rehabilitation, orthopedic and nutritional care. *Neuromuscular Disorders* **28**: 103–115

Merianda TT, Gomes C, Yoo S, Vuppalanchi D & Twiss JL (2013) Axonal Localization of Neuritin/CPG15 mRNA in Neuronal Populations through Distinct 5′ and 3′ UTR Elements. *J Neurosci* **33**: 13735–13742

Meyer-Luehmann M, Mielke M, Spires-Jones TL, Stoothoff W, Jones P, Bacskai BJ & Hyman BT (2009) A Reporter of Local Dendritic Translocation Shows Plaque- Related Loss of Neural System Function in APP-Transgenic Mice. *J Neurosci* **29**: 12636–12640

Michaelevski I, Medzihradszky KF, Lynn A, Burlingame AL & Fainzilber M (2010) Axonal Transport Proteomics Reveals Mobilization of Translation Machinery to the Lesion Site in Injured Sciatic Nerve. *Mol Cell Proteomics* **9**: 976–987

Minis A, Dahary D, Manor O, Leshkowitz D, Pilpel Y & Yaron A (2014) Subcellular transcriptomics—Dissection of the mRNA composition in the axonal compartment of sensory neurons. *Developmental Neurobiology* **74**: 365–381

Mohr E & Richter D (1992) Diversity of mRNAs in the Axonal Compartment of Peptidergic Neurons in the Rat. *Eur J Neurosci* **4**: 870–876

Moore MJ (2005) From birth to death: the complex lives of eukaryotic mRNAs. *Science* **309**: 1514–1518

Moore MJ & Proudfoot NJ (2009) Pre-mRNA processing reaches back to transcription and ahead to translation. *Cell* **136**: 688–700

Müller K, Schnatz A, Schillner M, Woertge S, Müller C, von Graevenitz I, Waisman A, van Minnen J & Vogelaar CF (2018) A predominantly glial origin of axonal ribosomes after nerve injury. *Glia* **66**: 1591–1610

Murashov AK, Chintalgattu V, Islamov RR, Lever TE, Pak ES, Sierpinski PL, Katwa LC & Van Scott MR (2007) RNAi pathway is functional in peripheral nerve axons. *The FASEB Journal* **21**: 656–670

Nedozralova H, Basnet N, Ibiricu I, Bodakuntla S, Biertümpfel C & Mizuno N (2022) In situ cryo-electron tomography reveals local cellular machineries for axon branch development. *J Cell Biol* **221**: e202106086

Neumann M, Sampathu DM, Kwong LK, Truax AC, Micsenyi MC, Chou TT, Bruce J, Schuck T, Grossman M, Clark CM, *et al* (2006) Ubiquitinated TDP-43 in frontotemporal lobar degeneration and amyotrophic lateral sclerosis. *Science* **314**: 130–133

Nicolau S, Waldrop MA, Connolly AM & Mendell JR (2021) Spinal Muscular Atrophy. *Seminars in Pediatric Neurology* **37**: 100878

Ostroff LE, Botsford B, Gindina S, Cowansage KK, LeDoux JE, Klann E & Hoeffer C (2017) Accumulation of Polyribosomes in Dendritic Spine Heads, But Not Bases and Necks, during Memory Consolidation Depends on Cap-Dependent Translation Initiation. *J Neurosci* **37**: 1862–1872

Ostroff LE, Watson DJ, Cao G, Parker PH, Smith H & Harris KM (2018) Shifting patterns of polyribosome accumulation at synapses over the course of hippocampal long-term potentiation. *Hippocampus* **28**: 416–430

Pan F, Hüttelmaier S, Singer Robert H & Gu W (2009) ZBP2 Facilitates Binding of ZBP1 to β-Actin mRNA during Transcription. *Molecular and Cellular Biology* **29**: 2481–2481

Perlson E, Hanz S, Ben-Yaakov K, Segal-Ruder Y, Seger R & Fainzilber M (2005) Vimentin-Dependent Spatial Translocation of an Activated MAP Kinase in Injured Nerve. *Neuron* **45**: 715–726

Perry RB & Fainzilber M (2014) Local translation in neuronal processes—in vivo tests of a "heretical hypothesis". *Developmental Neurobiology* **74**: 210–217

Perry RB-T, Doron-Mandel E, Iavnilovitch E, Rishal I, Dagan SY, Tsoory M, Coppola G, McDonald MK, Gomes C, Geschwind DH, *et al* (2012) Subcellular Knockout of Importin β1 Perturbs Axonal Retrograde Signaling. *Neuron* **75**: 294–305

Perry RB-T, Rishal I, Doron-Mandel E, Kalinski AL, Medzihradszky KF, Terenzio M, Alber S, Koley S, Lin A, Rozenbaum M, *et al* (2016) Nucleolin-Mediated RNA Localization Regulates Neuron Growth and Cycling Cell Size. *Cell Rep* **16**: 1664–1676

Pieretti M, Zhang F, Fu Y-H, Warren ST, Oostra BA, Caskey CT & Nelson DL (1991) Absence of expression of the FMR-1 gene in fragile X syndrome. *Cell* **66**: 817–822

Piper M, Anderson R, Dwivedy A, Weinl C, van Horck F, Leung KM, Cogill E & Holt C (2006) Signaling Mechanisms Underlying Slit2-Induced Collapse of Xenopus Retinal Growth Cones. *Neuron* **49**: 215–228

Polymenidou M, Lagier-Tourenne C, Hutt KR, Huelga SC, Moran J, Liang TY, Ling S-C, Sun E, Wancewicz E, Mazur C, *et al* (2011) Long pre-mRNA depletion and RNA missplicing contribute to neuronal vulnerability from loss of TDP-43. *Nat Neurosci* **14**: 459–468

Poon WW, Carlos AJ, Aguilar BL, Berchtold NC, Kawano CK, Zograbyan V, Yaopruke T, Shelanski M & Cotman CW (2013) β-Amyloid (Aβ) oligomers impair brain-derived neurotrophic factor retrograde trafficking by down-regulating ubiquitin C-terminal hydrolase, UCH-L1. *J Biol Chem* **288**: 16937–16948

Pratt T, Davey JW, Nowakowski TJ, Raasumaa C, Rawlik K, McBride D, Clinton M, Mason JO & Price DJ (2012) The expression and activity of β-catenin in the thalamus and its projections to the cerebral cortex in the mouse embryo. *BMC Neurosci* **13**: 20

Pulk A, Liiv A, Peil L, Maiväli Ü, Nierhaus K & Remme J (2010) Ribosome reactivation by replacement of damaged proteins. *Molecular Microbiology* **75**: 801–814

Puls I, Jonnakuty C, LaMonte BH, Holzbaur ELF, Tokito M, Mann E, Floeter MK, Bidus K, Drayna D, Oh SJ, *et al* (2003) Mutant dynactin in motor neuron disease. *Nature Genetics* **33**: 455–456

Qin W, Myers SA, Carey DK, Carr SA & Ting AY (2021) Spatiotemporally-resolved mapping of RNA binding proteins via functional proximity labeling reveals a mitochondrial mRNA anchor promoting stress recovery. *Nat Commun* **12**: 4980

Rage F, Boulisfane N, Rihan K, Neel H, Gostan T, Bertrand E, Bordonné R & Soret J (2013) Genome-wide identification of mRNAs associated with the protein SMN whose depletion decreases their axonal localization. *RNA* **19**: 1755–1766

Rangaraju V, tom Dieck S & Schuman EM (2017) Local translation in neuronal compartments: how local is local? *EMBO Rep* **18**: 693–711

Rangaraju V, Lauterbach M & Schuman EM (2019) Spatially Stable Mitochondrial Compartments Fuel Local Translation during Plasticity. *Cell* **176**: 73-84.e15

Rathod R, Havlicek S, Frank N, Blum R & Sendtner M (2012) Laminin induced local axonal translation of β-actin mRNA is impaired in SMN-deficient motoneurons. *Histochem Cell Biol* **138**: 737–748

Renaud L, Picher-Martel V, Codron P & Julien J-P (2019) Key role of UBQLN2 in pathogenesis of amyotrophic lateral sclerosis and frontotemporal dementia. *Acta Neuropathol Commun* **7**: 103

Renton AE, Chiò A & Traynor BJ (2014) State of play in amyotrophic lateral sclerosis genetics. *Nat Neurosci* **17**: 17–23

Rihan K, Antoine E, Maurin T, Bardoni B, Bordonné R, Soret J & Rage F (2017) A new cis-acting motif is required for the axonal SMN-dependent Anxa2 mRNA localization. *RNA* **23**: 899–909

Ringholz GM, Appel SH, Bradshaw M, Cooke NA, Mosnik DM & Schulz PE (2005) Prevalence and patterns of cognitive impairment in sporadic ALS. *Neurology* **65**: 586–590

Rishal I & Fainzilber M (2014) Axon–soma communication in neuronal injury. *Nat Rev Neurosci* **15**: 32–42

Rosen DR, Siddique T, Patterson D, Figlewicz DA, Sapp P, Hentati A, Donaldson D, Goto J, O'Regan JP & Deng HX (1993) Mutations in Cu/Zn superoxide dismutase gene are associated with familial amyotrophic lateral sclerosis. *Nature* **362**: 59–62

Rossoll W, Jablonka S, Andreassi C, Kröning A-K, Karle K, Monani UR & Sendtner M (2003) Smn, the spinal muscular atrophy–determining gene product, modulates axon growth and localization of β-actin mRNA in growth cones of motoneurons. *J Cell Biol* **163**: 801–812

Rowland LP & Shneider NA (2001) Amyotrophic lateral sclerosis. *N Engl J Med* **344**: 1688–1700

Sahly I, Khoutorsky A, Erez H, Prager-Khoutorsky M & Spira ME (2006) On-line confocal imaging of the events leading to structural dedifferentiation of an axonal segment into a growth cone after axotomy. *Journal of Comparative Neurology* **494**: 705–720

Sahoo PK, Smith DS, Perrone-Bizzozero N & Twiss JL (2018) Axonal mRNA transport and translation at a glance. *J Cell Sci* **131**: jcs196808

Sasaki Y, Welshhans K, Wen Z, Yao J, Xu M, Goshima Y, Zheng JQ & Bassell GJ (2010) Phosphorylation of Zipcode Binding Protein 1 Is Required for Brain-Derived Neurotrophic Factor Signaling of Local β-Actin Synthesis and Growth Cone Turning. *J Neurosci* **30**: 9349–9358

Savas JN, Ma B, Deinhardt K, Culver BP, Restituito S, Wu L, Belasco JG, Chao MV & Tanese N (2010) A Role for Huntington Disease Protein in Dendritic RNA Granules. *J Biol Chem* **285**: 13142–13153

Savas JN, Makusky A, Ottosen S, Baillat D, Then F, Krainc D, Shiekhattar R, Markey SP & Tanese N (2008) Huntington's disease protein contributes to RNA-mediated gene silencing through association with Argonaute and P bodies. *Proc Natl Acad Sci U S A* **105**: 10820–10825

Shakhbazau A, Schenk GJ, Hay C, Kawasoe J, Klaver R, Yong VW, Geurts JJG & van Minnen J (2016) Demyelination induces transport of ribosome-containing vesicles from glia to axons: evidence from animal models and MS patient brains. *Mol Biol Rep* **43**: 495–507

Shi Y, Lin S, Staats KA, Li Y, Chang W-H, Hung S-T, Hendricks E, Linares GR, Wang Y, Son EY, *et al* (2018) Haploinsufficiency leads to neurodegeneration in C9ORF72 ALS/FTD human induced motor neurons. *Nat Med* **24**: 313–325

Shigeoka T, Jung H, Jung J, Turner-Bridger B, Ohk J, Lin JQ, Amieux PS & Holt CE (2016) Dynamic Axonal Translation in Developing and Mature Visual Circuits. *Cell* **166**: 181–192

Shigeoka T, Jung J, Holt CE & Jung H (2018) Axon-TRAP-RiboTag: Affinity Purification of Translated mRNAs from Neuronal Axons in Mouse In Vivo. *Methods Mol Biol* **1649**: 85–94

Shigeoka T, Koppers M, Wong HH-W, Lin JQ, Cagnetta R, Dwivedy A, de Freitas Nascimento J, van Tartwijk FW, Ströhl F, Cioni J-M, *et al* (2019) On-Site Ribosome Remodeling by Locally Synthesized Ribosomal Proteins in Axons. *Cell Rep* **29**: 3605-3619.e10

Singleton AB, Farrer MJ & Bonifati V (2013) The genetics of Parkinson's disease: Progress and therapeutic implications. *Movement Disorders* **28**: 14–23

Siomi H, Siomi MC, Nussbaum RL & Dreyfuss G (1993) The protein product of the fragile X gene, FMR1, has characteristics of an RNA-binding protein. *Cell* **74**: 291–298

Smith BN, Ticozzi N, Fallini C, Gkazi AS, Topp S, Kenna KP, Scotter EL, Kost J, Keagle P, Miller JW, *et al* (2014) Exome-wide rare variant analysis identifies TUBA4A mutations associated with familial ALS. *Neuron* **84**: 324–331

Smith CL, Afroz R, Bassell GJ, Furneaux HM, Perrone-Bizzozero NI & Burry RW (2004) GAP-43 mRNA in growth cones is associated with HuD and ribosomes. *J Neurobiol* **61**: 222–235

Sonenberg N & Hinnebusch AG (2009) Regulation of Translation Initiation in Eukaryotes: Mechanisms and Biological Targets. *Cell* 136: 731–745

Sotelo JR, Canclini L, Kun A, Sotelo-Silveira JR, Calliari A, Cal K, Bresque M, Dipaolo A, Farias J & Mercer JA (2014) Glia to axon RNA transfer. *Dev Neurobiol* **74**: 292–302

Sotelo JR, Canclini L, Kun A, Sotelo-Silveira JR, Xu L, Wallrabe H, Calliari A, Rosso G, Cal K & Mercer JA (2013) Myosin-Va-Dependent Cell-To-Cell Transfer of RNA from Schwann Cells to Axons. *PLOS ONE* **8**: e61905

Sotelo JR, Kun A, Benech JC, Giuditta A, Morillas J & Benech CR (1999) Ribosomes and polyribosomes are present in the squid giant axon: an immunocytochemical study. *Neuroscience* **90**: 705–715

Sotelo-Silveira J, Crispino M, Puppo A, Sotelo JR & Koenig E (2008) Myelinated axons contain β-actin mRNA and ZBP-1 in periaxoplasmic ribosomal plaques and depend on cyclic AMP and F-actin integrity for in vitro translation. *Journal of Neurochemistry* **104**: 545–557

Soto C & Pritzkow S (2018) Protein misfolding, aggregation, and conformational strains in neurodegenerative diseases. *Nat Neurosci* **21**: 1332–1340

Spaulding EL & Burgess RW (2017) Accumulating Evidence for Axonal Translation in Neuronal Homeostasis. *Front Neurosci* **11**: 312

Spillane M, Ketschek A, Donnelly CJ, Pacheco A, Twiss JL & Gallo G (2012) Nerve growth factor-induced formation of axonal filopodia and collateral branches involves the intra-axonal synthesis of regulators of the actin-nucleating Arp2/3 complex. *J Neurosci* **32**: 17671–17689

Spillane M, Ketschek A, Merianda TT, Twiss JL & Gallo G (2013) Mitochondria Coordinate Sites of Axon Branching through Localized Intra-Axonal Protein Synthesis. *Cell Rep* **5**: 1564–1575

Sreedharan J, Blair IP, Tripathi VB, Hu X, Vance C, Rogelj B, Ackerley S, Durnall JC, Williams KL, Buratti E, *et al* (2008) TDP-43 mutations in familial and sporadic amyotrophic lateral sclerosis. *Science* **319**: 1668–1672

Steward O & Levy WB (1982) Preferential localization of polyribosomes under the base of dendritic spines in granule cells of the dentate gyrus. *J Neurosci* **2**: 284–291

Steward O & Reeves TM (1988) Protein-synthetic machinery beneath post-synaptic sites on CNS neurons: association between polyribosomes and other organelles at the synaptic site. *J Neurosci* **8**: 176–184

Steward O & Schuman EM (2001) Protein synthesis at synaptic sites on dendrites. *Annu Rev Neurosci* **24**: 299–325

Swanger SA & Bassell GJ (2013) Dendritic protein synthesis in the normal and diseased brain. *Neuroscience* **232**: 106–127

Swinnen B & Robberecht W (2014) The phenotypic variability of amyotrophic lateral sclerosis. *Nat Rev Neurol* **10**: 661–670

Taliaferro JM (2022) Transcriptome-scale methods for uncovering subcellular RNA localization mechanisms. *Biochim Biophys Acta Mol Cell Res* **1869**: 119202

Taliaferro JM, Vidaki M, Oliveira R, Olson S, Zhan L, Saxena T, Wang ET, Graveley BR, Gertler FB, Swanson MS, *et al* (2016) Distal Alternative Last Exons Localize mRNAs to Neural Projections. *Mol Cell* **61**: 821–833

Taylor JP, Brown RH & Cleveland DW (2016) Decoding ALS: from genes to mechanism. *Nature* **539**: 197–206

Tcherkezian J, Brittis PA, Thomas F, Roux PP & Flanagan JG (2010) Transmembrane Receptor DCC Associates with Protein Synthesis Machinery and Regulates Translation. *Cell* **141**: 632–644

Tedeschi A & Bradke F (2013) The DLK signalling pathway—a double-edged sword in neural development and regeneration. *EMBO Rep* **14**: 605–614

Terenzio M, Koley S, Samra N, Rishal I, Zhao Q, Sahoo PK, Urisman A, Marvaldi L, Oses-Prieto JA, Forester C, *et al* (2018) Locally translated mTOR controls axonal local translation in nerve injury. *Science* **359**: 1416–1421

Terenzio M, Schiavo G & Fainzilber M (2017) Compartmentalized Signaling in Neurons: From Cell Biology to Neuroscience. *Neuron* **96**: 667–679

Thinakaran G & Koo EH (2008) Amyloid Precursor Protein Trafficking, Processing, and Function *. *Journal of Biological Chemistry* **283**: 29615–29619

Torre ER & Steward O (1992) Demonstration of local protein synthesis within dendrites using a new cell culture system that permits the isolation of living axons and dendrites from their cell bodies. *J Neurosci* **12**: 762–772

Tsai N-P, Bi J & Wei L-N (2007) The adaptor Grb7 links netrin-1 signaling to regulation of mRNA translation. *EMBO J* **26**: 1522–1531

Turner-Bridger B, Caterino C & Cioni J-M (2020) Molecular mechanisms behind mRNA localization in axons. *Open Biol* **10**: 200177

Tushev G, Glock C, Heumüller M, Biever A, Jovanovic M & Schuman EM (2018) Alternative 3′ UTRs Modify the Localization, Regulatory Potential, Stability, and Plasticity of mRNAs in Neuronal Compartments. *Neuron* **98**: 495-511.e6

Twiss JL & Fainzilber M (2009) Ribosomes in axons--scrounging from the neighbors? *Trends Cell Biol* **19**: 236–243

Twiss JL & Minnen JV (2006) New Insights into Neuronal Regeneration: The Role of Axonal Protein Synthesis in Pathfinding and Axonal Extension. *Journal of Neurotrauma* **23**: 295–308

Van Langenhove T, van der Zee J & Van Broeckhoven C (2012) The molecular basis of the frontotemporal lobar degeneration-amyotrophic lateral sclerosis spectrum. *Ann Med* **44**: 817–828

Vance C, Rogelj B, Hortobágyi T, De Vos KJ, Nishimura AL, Sreedharan J, Hu X, Smith B, Ruddy D, Wright P, *et al* (2009) Mutations in FUS, an RNA processing protein, cause familial amyotrophic lateral sclerosis type 6. *Science* **323**: 1208–1211

Vargas JNS, Sleigh JN & Schiavo G (2022) Coupling axonal mRNA transport and local translation to organelle maintenance and function. *Curr Opin Cell Biol* **74**: 97–103

Verhaart IEC, Robertson A, Wilson IJ, Aartsma-Rus A, Cameron S, Jones CC, Cook SF & Lochmüller H (2017) Prevalence, incidence and carrier frequency of 5q–linked spinal muscular atrophy – a literature review. *Orphanet J Rare Dis* **12**: 124

Verkerk AJMH, Pieretti M, Sutcliffe JS, Fu Y-H, Kuhl DPA, Pizzuti A, Reiner O, Richards S, Victoria MF, Zhang F, *et al* (1991) Identification of a gene (FMR-1) containing a CGG repeat coincident with a breakpoint cluster region exhibiting length variation in fragile X syndrome. *Cell* **65**: 905–914

Verma P, Chierzi S, Codd AM, Campbell DS, Meyer RL, Holt CE & Fawcett JW (2005) Axonal Protein Synthesis and Degradation Are Necessary for Efficient Growth Cone Regeneration. *J Neurosci* **25**: 331–342

Verma P & Fawcett J (2005) Spinal Cord Regeneration. In *Regenerative Medicine II*, Yannas IV (ed) pp 43–66. Berlin, Heidelberg: Springer Berlin Heidelberg

Villarin JM, McCurdy EP, Martínez JC & Hengst U (2016) Local synthesis of dynein cofactors matches retrograde transport to acutely changing demands. *Nat Commun* **7**: 13865

Walker BA, Ji S-J & Jaffrey SR (2012) Intra-Axonal Translation of RhoA Promotes Axon Growth Inhibition by CSPG. *J Neurosci* **32**: 14442–14447a

Walker CA, Randolph LK, Matute C, Alberdi E, Baleriola J & Hengst U (2018) Aβ1–42 triggers the generation of a retrograde signaling complex from sentinel mRNAs in axons. *EMBO reports* **19**: e45435

Wang B, Pan L, Wei M, Wang Q, Liu W-W, Wang N, Jiang X-Y, Zhang X & Bao L (2015) FMRP-Mediated Axonal Delivery of miR-181d Regulates Axon Elongation by Locally Targeting Map1b and Calm1. *Cell Reports* **13**: 2794–2807

Warner TT & Schapira AHV (2003) Genetic and environmental factors in the cause of Parkinson's disease. *Annals of Neurology* **53**: S16–S25

Wei M, Huang J, Li G-W, Jiang B, Cheng H, Liu X, Jiang X, Zhang X, Yang L, Bao L, *et al* (2021) Axon-enriched lincRNA ALAE is required for axon elongation via regulation of local mRNA translation. *Cell Reports* **35**: 109053

Williams CC, Jan CH & Weissman JS (2014) Targeting and plasticity of mitochondrial proteins revealed by proximity-specific ribosome profiling. *Science* **346**: 748–751

Willis D, Li KW, Zheng J-Q, Chang JH, Smit A, Kelly T, Merianda TT, Sylvester J, van Minnen J & Twiss JL (2005) Differential Transport and Local Translation of Cytoskeletal, Injury-Response, and Neurodegeneration Protein mRNAs in Axons. *J Neurosci* **25**: 778–791

Willis DE, van Niekerk EA, Sasaki Y, Mesngon M, Merianda TT, Williams GG, Kendall M, Smith DS, Bassell GJ & Twiss JL (2007) Extracellular stimuli specifically regulate localized levels of individual neuronal mRNAs. *J Cell Biol* **178**: 965–980

Wirth B (2000) An update of the mutation spectrum of the survival motor neuron gene (SMN1) in autosomal recessive spinal muscular atrophy (SMA). *Human Mutation* **15**: 228–237

Wong HH-W, Lin JQ, Ströhl F, Roque CG, Cioni J-M, Cagnetta R, Turner-Bridger B, Laine RF, Harris WA, Kaminski CF, *et al* (2017) RNA Docking and Local Translation Regulate Site-Specific Axon Remodeling In Vivo. *Neuron* **95**: 852-868.e8

Wong YC & Holzbaur ELF (2014) Optineurin is an autophagy receptor for damaged mitochondria in parkin-mediated mitophagy that is disrupted by an ALS-linked mutation. *Proc Natl Acad Sci U S A* **111**: E4439–4448

Wu C-H, Fallini C, Ticozzi N, Keagle PJ, Sapp PC, Piotrowska K, Lowe P, Koppers M, McKenna-Yasek D, Baron DM, *et al* (2012) Mutations in the profilin 1 gene cause familial amyotrophic lateral sclerosis. *Nature* **488**: 499–503

Wu H, Williams J & Nathans J (2014) Complete morphologies of basal forebrain cholinergic neurons in the mouse. *Elife* **3**: e02444

Wu KY, Hengst U, Cox LJ, Macosko EZ, Jeromin A, Urquhart ER & Jaffrey SR (2005) Local translation of RhoA regulates growth cone collapse. *Nature* **436**: 1020–1024

Xue S & Barna M (2012) Specialized ribosomes: a new frontier in gene regulation and organismal biology. *Nat Rev Mol Cell Biol* **13**: 355–369

Yan D, Wu Z, Chisholm AD & Jin Y (2009) The DLK-1 Kinase Promotes mRNA Stability and Local Translation in C. elegans Synapses and Axon Regeneration. *Cell* **138**: 1005–1018

Yang HD, Kim DH, Lee SB & Young LD (2016) History of Alzheimer's Disease. *Dement Neurocogn Disord* **15**: 115–121

Yao J, Sasaki Y, Wen Z, Bassell GJ & Zheng JQ (2006) An essential role for β-actin mRNA localization and translation in Ca2+-dependent growth cone guidance. *Nat Neurosci* **9**: 1265–1273

Yasuda K & Mili S (2016) Dysregulated axonal RNA translation in amyotrophic lateral sclerosis. *Wiley Interdiscip Rev RNA* **7**: 589–603

Yoo S, Kim HH, Kim P, Donnelly CJ, Kalinski AL, Vuppalanchi D, Park M, Lee SJ, Merianda TT, Perrone-Bizzozero NI, *et al* (2013) A HuD-ZBP1 ribonucleoprotein complex localizes GAP-43 mRNA into axons through its 3' untranslated region AU-rich regulatory element. *J Neurochem* **126**: 792–804

Yu J, Chen M, Huang H, Zhu J, Song H, Zhu J, Park J & Ji S-J (2018) Dynamic m6A modification regulates local translation of mRNA in axons. *Nucleic Acids Res* **46**: 1412–1423

Yu J, She Y, Yang L, Zhuang M, Han P, Liu J, Lin X, Wang N, Chen M, Jiang C, *et al* (2021) The m6A Readers YTHDF1 and YTHDF2 Synergistically Control Cerebellar Parallel Fiber Growth by Regulating Local Translation of the Key Wnt5a Signaling Components in Axons. *Adv Sci (Weinh)* **8**: 2101329

Yudin D, Hanz S, Yoo S, Iavnilovitch E, Willis D, Gradus T, Vuppalanchi D, Segal-Ruder Y, Ben-Yaakov K, Hieda M, *et al* (2008) Localized regulation of axonal RanGTPase controls retrograde injury signaling in peripheral nerve. *Neuron* **59**: 241–252

Zappulo A, van den Bruck D, Ciolli Mattioli C, Franke V, Imami K, McShane E, Moreno-Estelles M, Calviello L, Filipchyk A, Peguero-Sanchez E, *et al* (2017) RNA localization is a key determinant of neurite-enriched proteome. *Nat Commun* **8**: 583

Zeng H & Sanes JR (2017) Neuronal cell-type classification: challenges, opportunities and the path forward. *Nat Rev Neurosci* **18**: 530–546

Zhang HL, Singer RH & Bassell GJ (1999) Neurotrophin regulation of beta-actin mRNA and protein localization within growth cones. *J Cell Biol* **147**: 59–70

Zivraj KH, Tung YCL, Piper M, Gumy L, Fawcett JW, Yeo GSH & Holt CE (2010) Subcellular Profiling Reveals Distinct and Developmentally Regulated Repertoire of Growth Cone mRNAs. *J Neurosci* **30**: 15464–15478

List of Abbreviations

2pFLIM	Two-photon fluorescence lifetime imaging microscopy
AD	Alzheimer's disease
ADGRG1	Adhesion G protein-coupled receptor G1
ALS	Amyotrophic lateral sclerosis
AMPA	α-amino-3-hydroxy-5-methyl-4-isoxazolepropionic acid
AMPAR	AMPA receptor
AMPK	AMP-activated protein kinase
APF	After puparium formation
APOE	Apolipoprotein E
APP	Amyloid precursor protein
ARG	Activity regulated gene
AS	Angelman syndrome
ASD	Autism spectrum disorder
BACE	β-secretase
BAI1	Brain-specific angiogenesis inhibitor 1
BD	Binocular deprivation
BDNF	Brain-derived neurotrophic factor
BFCN	Basal forebrain cholinergic neuron
BioID	Proximity dependent biotin identification
BMP	Bone morphogenetic protein
BO	Bolwig's organ
C4da	Class IV da
Calr	Calreticulin
CaM	Calmodulin
CaMKII	Calmodulin-dependent kinase II
CBP	CREB-binding protein
ced	_cell death abnormal_
cGKI	cGMP-dependent protein kinase 1
cKO	Conditional knockout
CNS	Central nervous system
CNV	Copy number variant
COP	Coat protein complex

CR3	Complement receptor 3
CRD	Cysteine-rich domain
CREB	cAMP response element binding protein
CREST	Calcium responsive transactivator
CRMP	Collapsin-response mediator protein
CryoET	Cryo-electron tomography
CSPG	Chondroitin sulfate proteoglycans
da	Dendritic arborization
DD	Death domain
DE	Differentially expressed
dJNK	c-Jun N-terminal kinase
DLK	Dual leucine zipper kinase
dLGN	Dorsolateral geniculate nucleus
DmCaBP1	Drosophila_ Calcium-Binding Protein 1
DOS	Daughter of sevenless
DR	Death receptor
DRG	Dorsal root ganglion
DRK	Downstream of receptor kinase
Drpr	Draper
Dscam	*Drosophila* down syndrome cell adhesion molecule
E6AP	E6-associated protein
Eb1	End binding protein 1
ECM	Extra-cellular matrix
EcR	Ecdysone receptor
EcR-DN	Dominant-negative mutant of ecdysone receptor
EGF	Epidermal growth factor
EGFP	Enhanced green fluorescent protein
ER	Endoplasmic reticulum
ERK	Extracellular signal-regulated kinase
FADD	Fas-associated death domain
FL	Full length
FMR1	Fragile X messenger ribonucleoprotein 1
FMRP	Fragile X mental retardation protein
FTD	Frontotempoal dementia
FXS	Fragile X Syndrome
Gas6	Growth arrest-specific-6
GEF	Guanine nucleotide exchange factor
GPI	Glycosylphosphatidylinositol
GTP	Guanosine-5'-triphosphate
HPD	Hours post dendrotomy
hrs	Hours

ID	Intellectual disability
IEG	Immediate early gene
iGluR	Ionotropic glutamate receptor
ION	infraorbital nerve
iPSCs	Induced-pluripotent stem cells
IPT	Infrapyramidal tract
ITAM	Immunoreceptor tyrosine-based activation motif
JNK	c-Jun N-terminal kinase
KO	Knockout
LGN	Lateral geniculate nucleus
LNv	Ventral lateral neuron
LOF	Loss-of-function
LPS	Local protein synthesis
LTD	Long-term depression
LTP	Long-term potentiation
MAP	Microtubule associated protein
MAPK	Mitogen-activated protein kinase
MB	Mushroom body
Mbc	Myoblast City
MD	Monocular deprivation
Mecp2	Methyl-CpG binding protein 2
MFD	Microfluidic Device
MFG-E8	Milk fat globule-EGF factor 8
mGluR	Metabotropic glutamate receptor
MHC	Major histocompatibility complex
MLKL	Mixed lineage kinase domain like pseudokinase
MMP 9	Matrix metalloproteinase 9
mPTP	Mitochondrial permeability transition pore
MS	Multiple sclerosis
mTOR	Mammalian Target of Rapamycin
nAchR	Nicotinic acetylcholine receptor
NAD⁺	Nicotinamide adenine dinucleotide
nBAF	neuron Brg/Brm Associated Factors
NCX	Sodium-calcium exchanger
NDEL1	Nuclear distribution element-like 1
NF-κB	Nuclear factor kappa light chain enhancer of activated B-cells
NGF	Nerve growth factor
NMDA	N-methyl-D-aspartate
NMJ	Neuromuscular junction
NMNAT1	Nicotinamide mononucleotide adenylyltransferase 1

NPXY	Asn-Pro-any amino acid-Tyr
NRCAM	Neuronal cell adhesion molecule
NRE	Neuron-receptive ending
Nrgs	Neuregulins
ODP	Ocular dominance plasticity
OE	Overexpression
ORNs	Olfactory receptor neurons
P	Postnatal day
PCD	Programmed cell death
PD	Parkinson's disease
PI3K	Phosphoinositide 3-kinase
PI3K-AKT	phosphoinositide 3-kinase-AKT/protein kinase B
PIP3	Phosphatidylinositol 3,4,5-trisphosphate
PKMz	Protein kinase Mζ
PND4	Postnatal day 4
PNS	Peripheral nervous system
POS	Photoreceptor outer segments
PP1	protein phosphatase 1
PRG2	Plasticity-related gene 2
PRMT1	Protein arginine methyltransferase 1
Prtp	Pretaporter
PS	Phosphatidylserine
PSD	Postsynaptic density
pSIVA	Polarity-sensitive annexin-based biosensor
PTB	Phosphotyrosine-binding-domain protein
PTEN	Phosphatase and tensin homolog
PTM	Posttranslational modification
RAG	Regeneration-associated gene
RCS	Royal College of Surgeons
RGC	Retinal ganglion cell
RhoGAP	Rho GTPase activating protein
Rho-GDI	Rho guanine nucleotide dissociation inhibitor
RhoGEF	Rho Guanine nucleotide exchange factor
RISC	RNA induced silencing complex
RNA-seq	RNA sequencing
ROS	Reactive oxygen species
RPE	Retinal pigment epithelium
RTK	Receptor tyrosine kinase
RTT	Rett syndrome
S1	Primary Somatosensory cortex

scRNA-seq	Single-cell RNA sequencing
SCYL1	SCY1-like pseudokinase 1
SFARI	Simons Foundation Autism Research Initiative
Shh	Sonic hedgehog
SOCE	Store-operated calcium entry
SOS	Son of sevenless
SPARC	Secreted protein acidic and rich in cysteine
STIM1	Stromal interacting molecule 1
SZ	Schizophrenia
TAM	_Tyro3, Axl, and Mer_
TARA	Trio-associated repeat on actin
TBI	Traumatic brain injury
TGF	Transforming growth factor
TIM4	T-cell immunoglobulin- and mucin-domain-containing 4
TNF	Tumor necrosis factor
TNFR	Tumor necrosis factor receptor
TNFRSF	Tumor necrosis factor receptor superfamily
Tok	Tolkin
TRADD	TNFR-associated DD
TRAF4	Tissue necrosis factor receptor associated factor 4
TREM2	Triggering receptor expressed on myeloid cells 2
TRIM	TRIpartitite Motif
TRPC	Transient receptor potential canonical
TS	Timothy syndrome
TSP	Thrombospondin
Tyr	tyrosine
UBE3A	Ubiquitin protein ligase E3a
Ulk	Unc-51 Like Autophagy Activating Kinase 1
V1	Primary visual cortex
VASP	Vasodilator-stimulated phosphoprotein
VGCC	Voltage-gated calcium channel
VNC	Ventral nerve cord
VTA	Ventral tegmental area
WD	Wallerian degeneration
wl	Wabbler-lethal
Wld^{s}	Wallerian degeneration-slow
WT	Wild-type
XIAP	X-linked inhibitor of apoptosis protein
Xkr8	Xk-related protein 8

Index

About the Editors

Born in Ho Chi Minh City, Vietnam, **Dr. Tracy S. Tran** earned her B.Sc. degree (with *cum laude*) in Neuroscience, M.Sc.and Ph.D. degrees (with *summa cum laude*) in Physiological Sciences and Molecular, Cellular & Integrative Physiology, respectively, from the University of California Los Angeles (UCLA) with Dr. Patricia E. Phelps. Dr. Tran conducted her post-doctoral training in The Solomon H. Synder Department of Neuroscience, Johns Hopkins University School of Medicine with Drs. Alex Kolodkin and David Ginty. Currently, Dr. Tran is an Associate Professor in the Department of Biological Sciences at Rutgers University, NJ, USA and the Director of Undergraduate Program in Biology. Dr. Tran studies the molecular and cellular mechanisms controlling neuronal morphogenesis and wiring of the mammalian nervous system. Her research investigates the molecular signaling involved in how neurons assume their diverse morphologies, the axons and dendrites, which enables the assembly of neural circuits required for complex behavior and cognitive function. Moreover, her lab is interested to better understand and identify the molecular and genetic correlates of developmental neurological disorders, such as autism spectrum disorder.

Born in Jerusalem, Israel, **Dr. Avraham Yaron** earned a B.Sc. degree(with *cum laude*) in Biology from the Hebrew University of Jerusalem, and a Ph.D.degree (with *summa cum laude*)from Hebrew University-Hadassah Medical School's Department of Immunology with Dr. Yinon Ben-Neriah, and conducted postdoctoral training with Dr. Marc Tessier-Lavigne. Dr. Yaronis currently a faculty member and incumbent of the Jack & Simon Djanogly Professorial Chair in Biochemistry in the Weizmann Institute. Dr. Yaronstudies the mechanisms by which the wiring of the nervous system is established during development. His research concentrates on two aspects of the wiring process: the operation of chemical cues that guide axons to their targets; and, the mechanisms that govern the elimination of certain axons during fetal development, a process termed axonalpruning. Moreover, his lab explores the functional and behavioral outcomes of miswiring, and examining how genetic wiring programs are modulated by experience.